Percutaneous Mitral Leaflet Repair

Percutaneous Mitral Leaflet Repair:
MitraClip® Therapy for Mitral Regurgitation

Edited by

Ted Feldman MD FESC FACC FSCAI

*Director, Cardiac Catheterization Laboratory, Evanston Hospital,
Mr and Mrs Charles R. Walgreen, Chair in Interventional Cardiology,
NorthShore University Health System, Evanston, Illinois, USA*

Frederick St Goar MD FACC

*Director, Fogarty Institute for Innovation,
El Camino Hospital, Mountain View, California, USA*

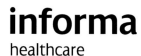

First published in 2012 by Informa Healthcare, 119 Farringdon Road, London EC1R 3DA, UK.

Simultaneously published in the USA by Informa Healthcare, 52 Vanderbilt Avenue, 7th Floor, New York, NY 10017, USA.

Informa Healthcare is a trading division of Informa UK Ltd. Registered Office: Informa House, 30–32 Mortimer Street W1W 7RE. Registered in England and Wales, number 1072954.

A CIP record for this book is available from the British Library.

ISBN-13: 978-1-84184-965-2
eISBN: 978-1-84184-966-9

Orders may be sent to: Informa Healthcare, Sheepen Place, Colchester, Essex CO3 3LP, UK
Telephone: +44 (0)20 7017 6682
Email: Books@Informa.com
Website: http://informahealthcarebooks.com

For corporate sales please contact: CorporateBooksIHC@informa.com
For foreign rights please contact: RightsIHC@informa.com
For reprint permissions please contact: PermissionsIHC@informa.com

Typeset by Exeter Premedia Services Pvt Ltd, India
Printed and bound in the United Kingdom

Contents

Contributors

John C. Alexander MD
NorthShore University Health System,
Cardiac & Thoracic Surgery Division,
Evanston, Illinois, USA

Ottavio Alfieri MD
Department of Cardiac Surgery,
San Raffaele University Hospital,
Milan, Italy

Michael Argenziano MD
Chief, Section of Adult Cardiac Surgery, Director,
Minimally Invasive Cardiac Surgery and Arrhythmia Surgery,
New York-Presbyterian Hospital/
Columbia University Medical Center,
New York, NY, USA

Ehrin J. Armstrong MD
Interventional Cardiology Fellow, UC Davis Trainee,
Mentored Clinical Research Program

Margot M. Bartelings MD PhD
Department of Anatomy and Embryology,
Leiden University Medical Center,
Leiden, The Netherlands

Peter C. Block MD
Emory University School of Medicine
Atlanta, Georgia, USA

Blase A. Carabello MD
The W.A. "Tex" and Deborah Moncrief, Jr Professor of Medicine
Vice-Chairman, Department of Medicine
Baylor College of Medicine
Medical Care Line Executive
Veterans Affairs Medical Center,
Houston, Texas, USA

Valeria Cammalleri MD
Division of Cardiology, Ferrarotto Hospital,
University of Catania,
Catania, Italy

Subhasis Chatterjee MD
NorthShore University Health System
Cardiac & Thoracic Surgery Division
Evanston, Illinois, USA

Michele De Bonis MD
Department of Cardiac Surgery
San Raffaele University Hospital
Milan, Italy

Ted Feldman MD FESC FACC FSCAI
Evanston Hospital
Cardiology Division-Walgreen Building
Evanston, Illinois, USA

Elyse Foster MD
Director of adult Echocardiography and Congenital
Heart Disease
University California San Francisco Medical Center,
San Francisco, California

Olaf Franzen MD
Rigshospitalet,
Copenhagen, Denmark

Stephan von Bardeleben MD
University Heart Center
Mainz, Germany

Susanna Price MD
Royal Brompton Hospital,
London, UK

Gretchen Gary
Director, Worldwide Sales Training
Abbott Vascular Structural Heart
Abbott Park, Illinois, USA

David A. Heimansohn MD
St Vincent Heart Center of Indiana,
Indianapolis, Indiana, USA

James B Hermiller MD FACCC FSCAI
St Vincent Heart Center of Indiana,
Indianapolis, Indiana, USA

Douglas S. Segar MD
St Vincent Heart Center of Indiana,
Indianapolis, Indiana, USA

Nauman Siddiqi MD
St Vincent Heart Center of Indiana,
Indianapolis, Indiana, USA

Howard C. Herrmann MD
Professor of Medicine
Perelman School of Medicine at the University of Pennsylvania
Director, Interventional Cardiology Program and
Cardiac Catheterization Laboratories
Hospital of the University of Pennsylvania
Philadelphia, Pennsylvania, USA

Sophie Jones MD
Department of Cardiac Surgery
New York-Presbyterian Hospital/
Columbia University Medical Center
New York, NY, USA

Saibal Kar MD FACC
Director of Interventional Cardiac Research
Cedars-Sinai Heart Institute
Los Angeles, California, USA

Elena Ladich MD
Chief, Cardiovascular Pathology
CVPath Institute, Inc.
Gaithersburg, MD, USA

Scott D. Lim MD
Associate Professor of Medicine & Pediatrics
University of Virginia
Charlottesville, Virginia, USA

Francesco Maisano MD
Department of Cardiac Surgery
San Raffaele University Hospital
Milan, Italy

Liz McDermott
Divisional Vice President, Regulatory and Clinical Affairs
Abbott Vascular Structural Heart
Menlo Park, California, USA

Jackie S. McGhie BSc
Department of Cardiology,
Thorax Center, Erasmus Medical Center,
Rotterdam, The Netherlands

Masataka Nakano MD
CVPath Institute, Inc.,
Gaithersburg and Chevy Chase,
Maryland, USA

Dr Gian Paolo Ussia
Division of Cardiology,
Ferrarotto Hospital, University of Catania,
Catania, Italy

Alice Perlowski MD
NorthShore University HealthSystem,
Evanston, Illinois, USA

Jason H. Rogers MD
Director, Interventional Cardiology,
Division of Cardiovascular Medicine,
University of California, Davis Medical Center,
Sacramento, California, USA

Allan Schwartz MD
Chief, Division of Cardiology
New York-Presbyterian Hospital/
Columbia University Medical Center
New York, NY, USA

Frank E. Silvestry MD FACC FASE
Associate Professor of Medicine
Cardiovascular Division
University of Pennsylvania School of Medicine
Philadelphia, Pennsylvania, USA

Lori K. Soni MD
Columbia University
New York, NY, USA

Frederick St Goar MD FACC
Fogarty Institute for Innovation
El Camino Hospital
Mountain View, California, USA

Corrado Tamburino MD
Chair of Cardiology, Cardiovascular Department
Ferrarotto Hospital, University of Catania
Catania, Italy

Troy Thornton
Divisional Vice President, R&D
Abbott Vascular Structural Heart
Menlo Park, California, USA

Nicolas M. Van Mieghem MD
Department of Interventional Cardiology
Thorax Center, Erasmus Medical Center
Rotterdam, The Netherlands

Renu Virmani MD
President and Medical Director,
CVPath Institute, Inc., Gaithersburg and Chevy Chase,
Maryland, USA

Patrick Whitlow MD
Cleveland Clinic
Cleveland, Ohio, USA

Willis Wu MD
Cleveland Clinic
Cleveland, Ohio, USA

Wen-Loong Yeow MBBS MRCP
Research Fellow
Cedars-Sinai Heart Institute
Los Angeles, California, USA

Foreword

Mitral regurgitation is a very serious medical condition that affects millions of patients in the United States and worldwide annually. Medical therapy is only marginally effective, but surgery for degenerative mitral regurgitation, in appropriate patients, is a tried and true therapy. However for functional mitral regurgitation, surgical intervention has its limitations and has generally been employed in conjunction with coronary artery bypass surgery or other valve operations, and less commonly as a stand-alone procedure.

Early in my career as a cardiac surgeon I took special interest in the mitral valve. I was intrigued by the elegant complexity and symphonic function of the mitral valve. After completing my cardiac surgery fellowship, I traveled the world to train with the "Masters of the Mitral Valve" including Alain Carpentier, Tirone David, Sir Madgi Yacoub, and Larry Cohen. I came away from this traveling fellowship with an even greater appreciation of the subtleties and complexities of the mitral valve apparatus. During this time I was exposed to the description of edge-to-edge mitral repair by Ottavio Alfieri and felt that it might provide an opportunity for a less invasive method for mitral repair. Given the need to open the heart for traditional annuloplasty or leaflet repair, a technique adaptable to beating heart surgery was attractive. In my animal laboratory at Columbia I created an approach for beating heart, "transapical edge-to-edge repair." We also demonstrated that the A2P2 coaptation point was the sweet spot, the "fulcrum" for the mitral valve apparatus. My team showed, using both mathematical fluid modeling and also in a sheep model, that stabilizing the A2P2 touch point reestablished effective coaptation of a dysfunctional mitral valve without compromising left ventricular function. We subsequently developed an approach for transapical edge-to-edge repair technique to facilitate off-pump mitral surgery. This pursuit of a less invasive approach led to a close association with Frederick St Goar's effort to develop an entirely percutaneous approach. I found the potential to move forward from a less invasive approach to mitral leaflet repair extremely exciting.

After more than a decade of development since these early concepts, percutaneous mitral valve repair totally has become, for selected patients, a reality. It's absolutely amazing.

This book represents the aggregation of the knowledge and experience accumulated with this approach during this exciting time of discovery. It has led to the creation of a new field and has fostered novel collaboration among cardiovascular specialties. It is especially exciting to see the accomplished path from open surgery, to beating heart surgical approaches, and finally to catheter-based therapy for a disease state that has resisted therapy for so many years and to appreciate the tremendous number of patients who will benefit from these efforts.

Mehmet Oz MD
Professor and Vice Chair of Surgery
New York Presbyterian Hospital
Columbia University Medical Center
New York, USA

My journey to develop and commercialize the MitraClip® system began more than 12 years ago. As president and CEO of Evalve, the start-up company that first developed and initially commercialized the technology, and later as general manager of the Structural Heart division of Abbott Vascular, I have had a unique vantage point to experience the challenges and opportunities involved in developing a first-in-class medical device.

Many people, including the distinguished coauthors of this book, took this journey with me. From the early bench tests and challenging preclinical studies, to first-in-human use and controlled clinical trials, this team of multidisciplinary leaders has provided wisdom, counsel, and perspective based on years of experience in cardiovascular medicine, interventional cardiology, cardiac surgery, echo-cardiology, pathology, and product development.

Mitral regurgitation is a progressive disease that continues to worsen when left untreated. Mitral regurgitation causes compensatory remodeling of the left ventricle, which results in reduced functional capacity, poor quality of life, repeat hospitalizations, and eventually in death from heart failure. Surgeons have successfully repaired the mitral valve to reduce mitral regurgitation in open, arrested heart surgery for over 50 years. However, many patients who are too sick to undergo traditional heart surgery continue to suffer from severe mitral regurgitation. The quest to help these patients through the development and application of the MitraClip® system, which has impacted more than 5000 patients and their families throughout the world, is chronicled in this book.

This collective work provides a broad and deep knowledge of the origin, history, and rapid evolution of the MitraClip® therapy. The first MitraClip® procedure was performed more than eight years ago and it took five years from that first procedure to perform 300 procedures. As of January 2012, more than 300 procedures are performed every month. Over this time, technology in the catheterization laboratory has advanced providing better methods for imaging the procedure. For example, when the early MitraClip® procedures were performed, real-time three-dimensional transesophageal echocardiography was a research tool, but today this widely available technology is routinely used to help guide MitraClip® procedures. As the therapy continues to advance at a fast pace, it is important that this text is available as a core reference on the MitraClip® system, as well a foundation for future learning on percutaneous mitral valve therapies.

All of the work described in this text also has a larger role to play in illuminating the critical junctures along the path of medical device innovation. For example, we see the importance of conducting multiple clinical studies to answer the many and evolving questions presented by a first-in-class therapy. Insight is gained into the need to compare new therapies to the gold standard of care (to clearly define the relative risks and benefits) while often in practice, adoption of a new therapy is primarily in patients for whom the standard of care is not an option.

Ultimately, the evidence presented in this book provides extensive support for the MitraClip® therapy as a therapeutic alternative for patients who currently have no good options for reduction of mitral regurgitation. I believe that the next generation of clinical and scientific advancement will expand the availability of the therapy to more patients as the clinical community works to ensure patients have options that best suit their needs.

Advancing healthcare technology is an exceptionally rewarding career. It is a privilege to witness the joy of patients and their families as they start life anew thanks to the hard work and dedication of many clinicians, scientists, and company employees. Improvement in patient care does not happen without clinical leaders who are tireless advocates for their patients. Dr Ted Feldman, without whom this book would not have been possible, is the very personification of this type of leader. For his guidance, leadership, clinical expertise, and friendship, I will always be grateful.

Ferolyn Powell
President & CEO Evalve, Inc. 1999–2009
DVP & General Manager Abbott Vascular Structural Heart,
2009–2012

Preface

When, 20 years ago, I successfully performed an edge–to-edge repair for the first time on a patient with anterior leaflet segmental flail due to primary chordal rupture, I immediately had the perception that such a procedure could have an impact of some relevance in the treatment of patients with mitral regurgitation. As a matter of fact, the functional result in that case was perfect: the newly created double-orifice mitral valve was totally competent and the global mitral area was well above 3 cm^2 even after implantation of a prosthetic ring. Besides being effective, the edge-to-edge repair was extraordinarily simple. Only few minutes were required to correct a lesion which was considered complex and well known to be historically associated with suboptimal surgical results. At that time many surgeons used to replace the mitral valve when the anterior leaflet was involved in the mechanism producing mitral regurgitation. It was clear to me after that initial experience that a double orifice repair could be easily reproducible by every surgeon and therefore be a useful addition to the armamentarium of the techniques used for mitral valve reconstructive surgery.

In the following years our surgical experience expanded and the validity of the concept was repeatedly demonstrated in a variety of clinical subsets. Rigorous follow-up data were collected including echo findings at rest and under exercise, and highly satisfactory mid-term results were reported in patients who received the edge-to-edge repair in conjunction with annuloplasty. Simultaneously the pathophysiology of the operation was extensively studied using computer modeling methods. In well-selected patients without annular dilatation, the prosthetic ring was intentionally avoided without compromising the outcome, at least at mid term.

Our enthusiasm for the procedure, however, was always somehow mitigated by the skepticism of the surgical community. The main criticism was that the edge-to-edge repair was not reproducing the configuration of a normal mitral valve and was a sort of convenient short cut for those who were unable to properly reconstruct the mitral valve. The occurrence of mitral stenosis was considered a potential problem, and the long-term durability of a double-orifice mitral valve was questioned. On the other hand, our referring cardiologists could observe excellent results even in complex cases and had a positive attitude in regard to the edge-to-edge technique. Thanks to the pragmatism of these cardiologists, we have been able to develop one of the largest practices in Europe in the field of mitral valve repair.

The simplicity and the effectiveness of this type of mitral repair were particularly attractive to innovators exploring methods to correct mitral regurgitation percutaneously via transcatheter interventions. Several grasping devices have been developed and tested in animal experiments to approximate the mitral leaflets and duplicate the Alfieri stitch. The MitraClip® system currently widely used in the clinical practice is definitely the most effective and reproducible.

The role of the percutaneous clip procedure in the clinical practice is still controversial at this point in time. Data from the EVEREST studies and from the rapidly growing clinical experience in Europe provide useful information which can be the basis for some recommendations. It has been definitely shown that the clip procedure is relatively safe and generally well tolerated even by patients in poor clinical condition, with serious comorbidities and/or severe left ventricular dysfunction. On the other hand, the clip reduces mitral regurgitation not so effectively as mitral valve surgery, and recurrence or worsening of mitral regurgitation is more likely to occur in the follow-up. It has to be recognized, however, that in sick patients with severe mitral regurgitation, some reduction of mitral regurgitation is providing meaningful clinical benefit. The applicability of the clip procedure is limited, since precise echocardiographic criteria have to be respected to make a patient eligible. A less rigorous adherence to the criteria of eligibility could allow increased applicability. Mitral valve repair after an unsuccessful clip procedure has been reported in many patients, although the preferred surgical option cannot always be maintained and valve replacement is occasionally necessary.

Considering all the above, the ideal candidate for the clip procedure could be an inoperable or high-risk symptomatic patients with severe mitral regurgitation (organic or functional), fulfilling the echocardiographic criteria of eligibility. In my opinion, for the time being, patients who can be offered mitral valve surgery with an acceptable risk should not be considered for percutaneous interventions. Along with rapid advancements in technology and progresses in imaging modalities, indications are expected to expand in the near future. Improvements in the first-generation device will take place, and some of the intrinsic limitations of the current system will be abolished. Furthermore, new sophisticated imaging modalities will be introduced and facilitate the procedure. Importantly, an effective catheter-based annuloplasty technique (not available at present) is badly needed to enhance the effectiveness and the durability of the clip procedure.

From a historical perspective, I think that the most important merit of the edge-to-edge technique was to make percutaneous mitral repair possible.

Ottavio Alfieri MD

Acknowledgments

I am grateful, especially to our first U.S. MitraClip® patient. He presented with dyspnea after being treated for 10 years, with a then new and relatively untested coronary therapy called rotational atherectomy. He sought me out because he wanted "whatever is newest" for his recurrent symptoms. Immediately upon laying a stethoscope on his chest and hearing a 4/6 murmur of new mitral regurgitation I recognized the serendipity of his presentation. It is the rare patient who seeks to be the first for a novel therapy, and this man launched all that has led to this comprehensive book on MitraClip®.

Ted Feldman MD

1   Anatomy of the mitral valvular complex
Nicolas M. Van Mieghem, Jackie S. McGhie, and Margot M. Bartelings

INTRODUCTION

> *"…mitral insufficiency begets mitral insufficiency…."*
> *Jesse E. Edwards and Howard B. Burchell, 1958* (1).

The mitral valvular apparatus is the complex anatomical and functional entity (2) that separates the left atrium from the left ventricle. The both famous and infamous Belgian anatomist and physician Andreas Vesalius described the bicuspid left atrioventricular valve as resembling a bishop's mitre, hence the term mitral valve (3). The mitral valve as such (the annulus with two leaflets) is encapsulated within surrounding structures: the left atrium, the left ventricle, the aortic valve, the papillary muscles, the tendinous cords, and the cardiac central fibrous body. In 1972, Perloff and Roberts introduced the concept of the "mitral apparatus" to underscore this essential and harmonious structural relationship (2).

One or more flaws in the machinery can impair adequate mitral valve functioning. The pathophysiology can be functional, structural, or mixed. Inadequate apposition and coaptation of the mitral leaflets during systole will result in mitral regurgitation, whereas obstruction to diastolic forward flow into the left ventricle marks mitral stenosis. In all age groups, mitral regurgitation is the most common valvular disorder with a global prevalence of 1.7%, increasing to 10% in the ≥75-year olds (4). Practical knowledge of the anatomy of the mitral valvular apparatus forms the base of understanding the pathophysiology of mitral valve disorders in general and mitral regurgitation in particular and is an evident prerequisite for successful treatment of mitral valve pathology.

The Mitral Valvular Complex

Adequate mitral valve closure requires alignment and contact of the two mitral leaflets in one single plane (apposition and coaptation). An optimal annulus size, a geometrically correct orientation of the papillary muscles with the tendinous cords attached and the closing forces generated by the left ventricle catalyze this sophisticated process. From an anatomical perspective the mitral apparatus is intimately related to surrounding structures like the electrical conduction system, the aortic valve, the coronary sinus (CS), and the left circumflex coronary artery. Evidently this integrated anatomy is relevant for surgical and catheter-bound mitral valve therapies (5).

The Mitral Annulus

The mitral annulus is D-shaped and is defined by the confluence of the fibrous cardiac skeleton and mitral valvular tissue on the one hand and left atrial and ventricular myocardium on the other (6). It has a longer intercommissural and a shorter aortic-mural (septal-to-lateral) axis. From a three-dimensional (3D) perspective it has a non-planar configuration with elevated anteroseptal and posterolateral segments toward the atrium and complementary depressed medial (septal) and anterolateral segments (at the commissures) toward the ventricle, giving the annulus its typical "saddle shape" appearance (Fig. 1.1) (7–9). The mitral valve is located posterior and inferior to the aortic valve, which can be regarded as the centrepiece of the heart. The left and non-coronary leaflets (often inappropriately called cusps) of the aortic valve and the anterior (aortic) leaflet of the mitral valve form continuity. This so-called aortic-mitral curtain is bordered by fibrous expansions, the left and right fibrous trigones (Fig. 1.2). The cardiac skeleton is formed by the fusion of both the membranous septum (interventricular and atrioventricular) and the aortic-mitral curtain and houses the bundle of His, which is the prolongation of the atrioventricular node and represents the main connection of the atrial and ventricular electrical conduction system (10).

Fibroelastic tissue extends from the fibrous trigones to mark the virtual annulus; anteriorly, it is a semicircular solid structure. From a pathological perspective this rigid structure makes the anterior annular segment resistant to dilatation but also more vulnerable to so-called skip or direct extension lesions from aortic valve endocarditis given its continuity with the aortic valve. Especially in its posterior aspects several blanks in the annular structure are filled with atrial myocardium and adipose tissue. Hutchins et al. introduced the term "disjunction" to define this absence of a complete cord-like ring of connective tissue encircling the atrioventricular junction (11). The absence of a well-formed fibrous cord in this particular position opposite the aortic-mitral curtain explains its predilection for annular dilation and calcification resulting in a disproportional increase in the aortic-mural (septal-to-lateral) diameter. The virtual annulus is not a static structure; during systole it exhibits a sphincteric contraction, which can reduce the annular surface by up to 25% and a translational excursion toward the apex, reflecting the propagation of the ventricular torsion at the base of the heart (12–15).

Mitral Leaflets

The mitral valve is bicuspid. What is classically referred to as the anterior mitral leaflet is closely related to the aortic valve and the septum, hence the alternative term "aortic leaflet" (2,3,10). As a corollary, the posterior mitral leaflet is also called the "mural leaflet." The anterior leaflet is long with a narrow base that encloses one-third of the annular circumference. It separates the inflow and outflow tracts of the left ventricle. The posterior leaflet is short but has a wide base that extends over

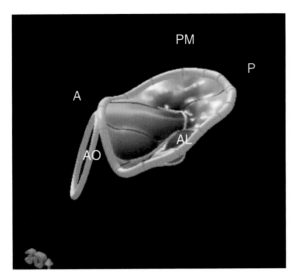

Figure 1.1 Three-dimensional echocardiographic illustration of the "mitral annulus" demonstrating the saddle shape. The anteroseptal (A) and posterolateral (P) segments toward the atrium are elevated whereas the complementary medial (septal) (PM) and anterolateral segments (AL) (at the commissures) toward the ventricle are depressed. *Abbreviations:* Ao, aorta.

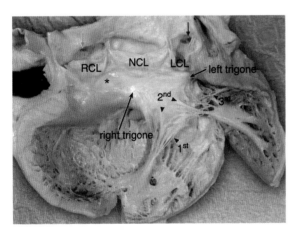

Figure 1.2 The aortic-mitral curtain. *: membranous septum. RCL: right coronary leaflet with ostium of the right coronary artery (*green arrow*). NCL: non-coronary leaflet. LCL: left coronary leaflet with ostium of left main stem (*red arrow*). Arrowheads 1st, 2nd, 3rd: primary, secondary, tertiary cords.

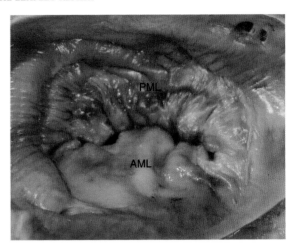

Figure 1.3 View on the closed mitral valve (systolic position) from a left atrial perspective. The anterior mitral leaflet (AML) has a longer surface with a shorter base and encloses one-third of the annular circumference. The posterior mitral leaflet (PML) is short but extending over two-thirds of the annular circumference.

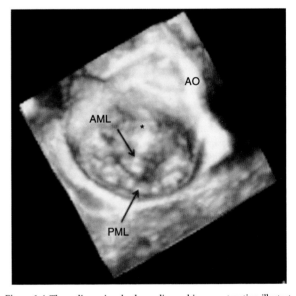

Figure 1.4 Three-dimensional echocardiographic reconstruction illustrating the "surgical view." The zone of apposition has an oblique orientation relative to the orthogonal planes of the body and is recognized as the "mitral smile." Ao: aorta. *: aortic-mitral curtain (fibrous continuity).

two-thirds of the annular circumference (Fig. 1.3). The surface area of both leaflets together is 2.5 times the area of the annular orifice. In systole, normal mitral valve leaflets coapt over a height of, on an average, 8 mm giving an "overlapping reserve" or "coaptation reserve" in case of annular dilation. The zone of apposition has an oblique orientation relative to the orthogonal planes of the body and is recognized as the "mitral smile" by short axis echocardiography (Figs. 1.3 and 1.4). It is bordered by the posteromedial and anterolateral commissures. Slits in the posterior leaflet create three scallops. Together with the

commissures these indentations are areas with less and thinner leaflet material contributing to a more flexible posterior leaflet and complying with the dynamic motions of the annulus (the so-called sphincter mechanism).

Aortic-Mitral Curtain
As mentioned earlier the aortic-mitral curtain is formed by the confluence of the left and non-coronary leaflets of the aortic

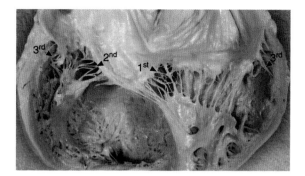

Figure 1.5 Atrial aspect of the mitral valve with three generations of cords. Arrowheads 1st, 2nd, 3rd: primary, secondary, tertiary cords.

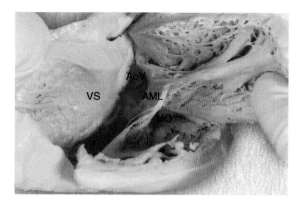

Figure 1.6 The left ventricular outflow tract is sandwiched between the ventricular septum (VS) and the anterior mitral leaflet (AML). *Abbreviations:* AoV, aortic valve; MO, mitral orifice.

valve and the anterior (aortic) leaflet of the mitral valve. It is underpinned by strut (principal) cords, which connect the papillary muscles and the anterior mitral leaflet and contribute to its virtually inert state throughout the cardiac cycle (15). As such, the aortic-mitral curtain functions as an anchor and hinge point for the aortic and mitral valve dynamics. Animal experiments and 3D transoesophageal echocardiography studies in humans elegantly demonstrated the coupled reciprocal behavior of the aortic and mitral annulus (16,17). The mitral valve annulus reaches its maximum area in early diastole when the aortic annulus area is minimal. Conversely, the aortic annulus obtains its maximal surface area in open position in systole when the mitral annulus area is the smallest area. Furthermore, during systole the angle between the aortic and mitral annulus decreases due to a flexion motion of both structures around the inert anchoring of the aortic-mitral curtain. Both principles may hypothetically optimize left ventricular contraction since the aortic annulus contraction facilitates mitral annulus expansion and vice versa and the geometric changes in systole (the "aortic-mitral flexion") may optimize ejection of blood toward the aorta. If the tension of the strut cords is released, the aortic-mitral curtain angulation (approximately 90°) is dissolved and the aortic and mitral annuli are drawn together which may impact LV geometry and performance.

Tendinous Cords and Papillary Muscles
The mitral valve leaflets are connected to the left ventricular free wall like a parachute (2,3,10). Fibro-elastic collagen-bound tendinous cords (chordae tendineae) arise from the papillary muscles, bifurcate several times, and attach to the ventricular side of both leaflets (18). The cords intermingle within the fibrous components of leaflets, annulus, and even trigones. The thinnest part is near the insertion site on the leaflets and is the predilection site for chordal rupture. There are three orders of tendinous cords (Figs. 1.2 and 1.5): the primary or marginal cords insert on the free margin of the leaflets to prevent marginal prolapse, align the coaptation zone, and maintain leaflet apposition during valve closure; secondary or intermediate cords attach onto the ventricular surface to preclude billowing and distribute tension on the leaflet tissue. Among the

secondary cords, the stay, strut, or principal cords are longer and thicker and insert on the ventricular surface of the anterior mitral leaflet ensuring direct continuity between the LV myocardium through the papillary muscles and the mitral annulus at the fibrous trigones. These struts are under continuous tension and contribute to LV geometry and angulation between the aortic and mitral annulus through the aortic-mitral curtain (see the previous section) (15). Tertiary or basal cords originate directly from the ventricular wall and attach exclusively to the posterior leaflet contributing to ventricular geometry and annular fortification (Figs. 1.2 and 1.5).

There are two papillary muscles entrenched into the apical to middle thirds of the left ventricular free wall, each with a variable number of composing subdivisional heads. The classic and somewhat simplified paradigm is that the blood supply to the anterolateral papillary muscle is provided by one or more branches of the left circumflex or diagonal branches, whereas the posteromedial papillary muscle is supplied by a single branch of the left circumflex or right coronary artery depending on coronary dominance. Due to its single vascular supply, the posteromedial papillary muscle in particular is susceptible to coronary ischemia.

Left Atrium and Left Ventricle Integration
From the previous description, it is clear that the myocardium of the left atrium and ventricle is intimately connected to the mitral valve. The term disjunction has already been proposed to mark the fact that rather than being separated by an anatomic cord-like structure, myocardium hinges directly to the valvular tissue (11). More specifically, this disjunction is apparent at the posterior segment where the left atrial posterior wall hinges directly onto the posterior leaflet. This particular continuity might render the posterior leaflet more vulnerable to being displaced in the case of left atrial enlargement hypothetically causing annular dilatation and valvular malcoaptation (2). The insertion of the left atrial myocardium follows the general contour of the annulus. This does

not hold true (3,18) for the left ventricular myocardium, which at the level of the aortic-mitral curtain doesn't hinge onto the anterior leaflet nor to the annular structure per se; so the left ventricular outflow tract gets sandwiched between the ventricular septum and the anterior mitral leaflet (Fig. 1.6). The free wall of the left ventricle on the other hand is directly connected to the posterior leaflet through the mural or tertiary cords and hinges onto the anterolateral commissure. Finally, the papillary muscles can be viewed as extensions of the apical to lateral left ventricle wall and are connected to the ventricular surface and the free edge of both mitral leaflets through the tendinous cords. Given the tight interdependence with the ventricular free wall and the unique arrangements of the different components, changes in ventricular geometry can have serious consequences for the mitral valve dynamics (19,20). Left ventricular free wall dyskinesia can change the orientation of the tertiary (basal) cords with a tethering effect on the valve leaflets. And yet more global left ventricular dilatation can displace the papillary muscles in an apical direction creating tenting of the mitral leaflets. The result will be a malcoaptation of the mitral leaflets and eventually mitral regurgitation.

Coronary Venous and Arterial Anatomy
It's not our aim to give a comprehensive review of the coronary venous and arterial circulation. Rather, we would present relevant anatomical data illustrating the complex relationship between the coronary vasculature and the mitral valve annulus.

In a venous system where there is plenty of interindividual variability, consistent entities are the anterior interventricular vein (AIV), the great cardiac vein (GCV) and the CS (20,21). In general, the AIV originates at the lower or middle third of the anterior interventricular groove (22). It follows the groove toward the base of the heart and then turns posterior at the atrioventricular groove to enter the GCV. The GCV wraps around the left atrioventricular groove to fuse with the oblique left atrial vein (remnant of the embryonic left superior vena cava) to become the CS. The middle cardiac vein (MCV) runs along the posterior interventricular groove to empty into the CS close to its orifice in the right atrium. The orifice of the CS in the right atrium is slightly posterior to the atrioventricular bundle and is guarded by a thin semicircular valve, the thebesian valve, which may have a cribriform, muscular, fibrous, or fibromuscular morphology and composition (Fig. 1.7) (20). The AIV and MCV are accompanied by the left anterior descending artery and posterior descending artery respectively (23). The CS and the GCV have a more unpredictable course relative to the left circumflex artery (LCX) and its marginal branches. There is a vast literature on the complex interrelation between the CS-GCV, the LCX and the mitral annulus (MA) (20,21,24–26). Several imaging modalities each with their pros and cons have proved to be useful in examining this particular anatomy: venography, 3D echocardiography, multislice CT, electron-beam CT, and cMRI. On top of this there is also valuable pathology data available (20).

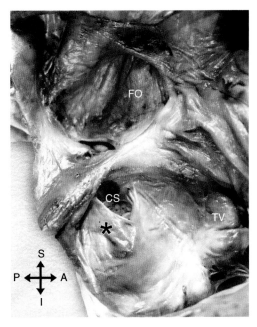

Figure 1.7 Right atrial view on the trial septum. The orifice of the coronary sinus (CS) in the right atrium is guarded by the Thebesian valve (asterisk). *Abbreviations*: FO, foramen ovale; TV, tricuspid valve.

Unfortunately, there is no standardized method of measuring or reporting, which makes it virtually impossible to extrapolate quantitative data from one study to the other and from one imaging technology to the other. Nonetheless, some general principles can be extracted.

The location of the CS relative to the MA changes along its course. In the majority of cases (90–100%), the body of the CS is adjacent to the posterior left atrial wall, well above and cranial to the deeper laying MA (Fig. 1.8) (21,24,27). It is closest to the lateral segment of the MA (at the corresponding P2 level) and furthest from the commissures. With significant mitral regurgitation (particularly in ischemic cardiomyopathy) the CS gets lifted away from the lateral MA segment, and conversely moves closer to the commissures (21,25). This coincides with the flattening of the "3D saddle shaped" annulus and the increase in the septal-to-lateral annular diameter (11). As the CS nears its ostium and accepts several branches, its caliber grows. The CS always runs in close vicinity to the LCX (distance CS-LCX 1.3 ± 1.0 mm (21) to 2.7 ± 1.0 mm (25)). The LCX is overcrossed by the CS/GCV in 60–80% of the time (Fig. 1.9). The crossing point relative to the CS ostium, the length of the overlapping segment, the length of the parallel course as well as the distance of the CS–LCX crossing point to the MA is highly variable. The AIV on its turn overcrosses a diagonal or ramus branch in up to 16% of cases according to the pathology study by Maselli (20).

CONCLUSIONS
The mitral valve is part of a broader mitral valvular complex. Normal valvular mechanics require a sophisticated interaction

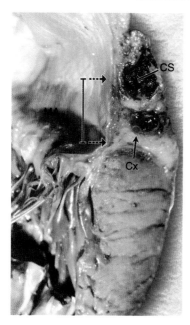

Figure 1.8 The coronary sinus (CS) is located well above and cranial to the deeper laying mitral annulus (MA). The distance is indicated by the dotted arrows. *Black arrow*: left circumflex artery (LCX).

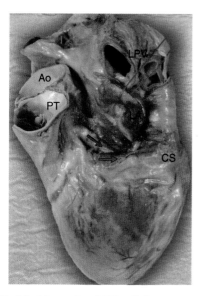

Figure 1.9 The left trial appendage (LA) is pulled away to expose the coronary sinus (CS)/great cardiac vein (*blue arrow*), which crosses the left circumflex artery (*red arrow*). *Abbreviations*: Ao, aorta; LPV, left pulmonary veins; PT, pulmonary trunk.

of the different valve components and the adjacent left ventricular and atrial myocardium.

ACKNOWLEDGMENTS

The authors thank L.J. Wisse for his expertise in preparing the anatomical illustrations.

REFERENCES

1. Edwards JE, Burchell HB. Endocardial and intimal lesions (jet impact) as possible sites of origin of murmurs. Circulation 1958; 18: 946–60.
2. Perloff JK, Roberts WC. The mitral apparatus. functional anatomy of mitral regurgitation. Circulation 1972; 46: 227–39.
3. Ho SY. Anatomy of the mitral valve. Heart 2002; 88(Suppl 4): iv5–10.
4. Nkomo VT, Gardin JM, Skelton TN, et al. Burden of valvular heart diseases: a population-based study. Lancet 2006; 368: 1005–11.
5. Van Mieghem NM, Piazza N, Anderson RH, et al. Anatomy of the mitral valvular complex and its implications for transcatheter interventions for mitral regurgitation. J Am Coll Cardiol 2010; 56: 617–26.
6. Angelini A, Ho SY, Anderson RH, et al. A histological study of the atrioventricular junction in hearts with normal and prolapsed leaflets of the mitral valve. Br Heart J 1988; 59: 712–16.
7. Levine RA, Handschumacher MD, Sanfilippo AJ, et al. Three-dimensional echocardiographic reconstruction of the mitral valve, with implications for the diagnosis of mitral valve prolapse. Circulation 1989; 80: 589–98.
8. Levine RA, Weyman AE, Handschumacher MD. Three-dimensional echocardiography: techniques and applications. Am J Cardiol 1992; 69: 121H–30H; discussion 31H–34H.
9. Anwar AM, Soliman OI, ten Cate FJ, et al. True mitral annulus diameter is underestimated by two-dimensional echocardiography as evidenced by real-time three-dimensional echocardiography and magnetic resonance imaging. Int J Cardiovasc Imaging 2007; 23: 541–7.
10. Muresian H. The clinical anatomy of the mitral valve. Clin Anat 2009; 22: 85–98.
11. Hutchins GM, Moore GW, Skoog DK. The association of floppy mitral valve with disjunction of the mitral annulus fibrosus. N Engl J Med 1986; 314: 535–40.
12. Timek TA, Miller DC. Experimental and clinical assessment of mitral annular area and dynamics: what are we actually measuring? Ann Thorac Surg 2001; 72: 966–74.
13. Flachskampf FA, Chandra S, Gaddipatti A, et al. Analysis of shape and motion of the mitral annulus in subjects with and without cardiomyopathy by echocardiographic 3-dimensional reconstruction. J Am Soc Echocardiogr 2000; 13: 277–87.
14. Burns AT, McDonald IG, Thomas JD, et al. Doing the twist: new tools for an old concept of myocardial function. Heart 2008; 94: 978–83.
15. Silbiger JJ, Bazaz R. Contemporary insights into the functional anatomy of the mitral valve. Am Heart J 2009; 158: 887–95.
16. Veronesi F, Corsi C, Sugeng L, et al. A study of functional anatomy of aortic-mitral valve coupling using 3D matrix transesophageal echocardiography. Circ Cardiovasc Imaging 2009; 2: 24–31.
17. Timek TA, Green GR, Tibayan FA, et al. Aorto-mitral annular dynamics. Ann Thorac Surg 2003; 76: 1944–50.
18. Sakai T, Okita Y, Ueda Y, et al. Distance between mitral anulus and papillary muscles: anatomic study in normal human hearts. J Thorac Cardiovasc Surg 1999; 118: 636–41.
19. Otto CM. Clinical practice evaluation and management of chronic mitral regurgitation. N Engl J Med 2001; 345: 740–6.
20. Maselli D, Guarracino F, Chiaramonti F, et al. Percutaneous mitral annuloplasty: an anatomic study of human coronary sinus and its relation with mitral valve annulus and coronary arteries. Circulation 2006; 114: 377–80.

21. Choure AJ, Garcia MJ, Hesse B, et al. In vivo analysis of the ana-tomical relationship of coronary sinus to mitral annulus and left circumflex coronary artery using cardiac multidetector computed tomography: implications for percutaneous coronary sinus mitral annuloplasty. J Am Coll Cardiol 2006; 48: 1938–45.

22. Van de Veire NR, Schuijf JD, De Sutter J, et al. Non-invasive visual-ization of the cardiac venous system in coronary artery disease patients using 64-slice computed tomography. J Am Coll Cardiol 2006; 48: 1832–8.

23. El-Maasarany S, Ferrett CG, Firth A, et al. The coronary sinus con-duit function: anatomical study (relationship to adjacent struc-tures). Europace 2005; 7: 475–81.

24. Tops LF, Van de Veire NR, Schuijf JD, et al. Noninvasive evaluation of coronary sinus anatomy and its relation to the mitral valve annulus: implications for percutaneous mitral annuloplasty. Cir-culation 2007; 115: 1426–32.

25. Chiribiri A, Kelle S, Kohler U, et al. Magnetic resonance cardiac vein imaging: relation to mitral valve annulus and left circumflex coronary artery. JACC Cardiovasc Imaging 2008; 1: 729–38.

26. Piazza N, Bonan R. Transcatheter mitral valve repair for functional mitral regurgitation: coronary sinus approach. J Interv Cardiol 2007; 20: 495–508.

27. Shinbane JS, Lesh MD, Stevenson WG, et al. Anatomic and electro-physiologic relation between the coronary sinus and mitral annu-lus: implications for ablation of left-sided accessory pathways. Am Heart J 1998; 135: 93–8.

2   The pathophysiology of mitral regurgitation
Blase A. Carabello

INTRODUCTION

Incompetence of the mitral valve allows a portion of left ventricular (LV) stroke volume to be regurgitated into the left atrium (LA), necessitating an increased volume output to make up for that lost to regurgitation. In addressing the pathophysiology of mitral regurgitation (MR) it is mandatory to distinguish between primary (organic) MR and secondary (functional) MR. In primary MR there is disease of one or more components of the mitral valve causing the valve to leak, allowing blood to flow back into the LA during systole. Regurgitation, in turn, places a hemodynamic overload upon the LV which, if severe and prolonged, leads to LV damage, heart failure, and eventual death. This pathophysiology is relatively straightforward. It is valve disease that leads to negative sequelae and restoration of valvular competence is curative if performed in a timely manner.

The pathophysiology of secondary or functional MR is far more complex. Here, it is the disease of the ventricle caused by myocardial infarction or cardiomyopathy that causes regional wall motion abnormalities, ventricular dilatation, papillary muscle displacement, and annular dilatation which in turn cause a normal mitral valve to leak. Thus, the main problem is not the MR itself but rather severe LV damage to which MR is added as a secondary pathology. Because restoration of mitral competence cannot cure the underlying ventricular pathology, the role of such therapy is much less clear than it is for primary MR.

PRIMARY MR
The Stages of Primary MR
Acute MR

Acute severe MR as might occur with the rupture of a chorda tendina or with leaflet destruction in infective endocarditis imparts a sudden volume overload on the LA and LV (Fig. 2.1A) (1). The volume overload on the LV increases preload (sarcomere stretch), maximizing utilization of the Frank–Starling mechanism (2) which increases LV's pumping ability and also causes a small increase in the end diastolic volume. At the same time the new low impedance pathway for ejection into the LA reduces LV afterload. The increased preload and decreased afterload, both act in concert with sympathetically increased contractility to increase the total LV stroke volume. However, because a large portion of the total stroke is ejected into the LA instead of the aorta, forward output falls. At the same time the small LA is overfilled, causing high LA filling pressure, resulting in pulmonary congestion. Thus, the patient with acute severe MR experiences heart failure, yet LV muscle function is normal or even increased.

Chronic Compensated MR

Many patients with acute MR require immediate surgery to relieve heart failure by correcting the leaking valve. However, if severe MR develops more gradually allowing for LV and LA adaptation, the patient may enter a chronic compensated phase (Fig. 2.1B). In this phase eccentric cardiac hypertrophy develops, leading to a large increase in LV end diastolic volume, allowing for increased LV total and forward stroke volume. Increased LV radius increases the systolic wall stress from its reduced level in the acute phase to normal in this phase. However, increased preload in conjunction with normal contractile function still maintains a higher-than-normal ejection fraction. In this phase the LA has also enlarged, allowing it to receive the regurgitant volume at a lower filling pressure. Thus, compensated with normal forward output and left-sided filling pressures, the patient may be entirely symptom free despite severe MR.

Chronic Decompensated MR

While chronic severe MR may be tolerated for several years, most patients progress to the decompensated stage in about five years (3,4). In this stage persistent severe MR has caused both substantial myocardial damage and pronounced LV remodeling leading to LV contractile dysfunction. The loss of contractile force impairs LV shortening so that the end systolic volume increases. This increase is compounded by abnormally high afterload. Although MR is often believed to unload the LV by way of the ejection pathway into the LA, this tendency is offset by the increase in the radius term of the Laplace equation for wall stress (σ, afterload): $\sigma = P \times r/2th$ where P = LV systolic pressure, r = LV radius, and th = LV thickness. Thus in decompensated MR, afterload is increased not decreased as is often held (5). In turn LV filling pressures are increased and forward stroke volume decreases. In most cases these adverse changes lead to heart failure symptoms. However, even though contractile dysfunction has occurred, increased preload may maintain LV ejection fraction in the "normal" range, potentially falsely reassuring the clinician that the patient is still compensated (6).

THE MECHANISMS OF LEFT VENTRICULAR DYSFUNCTION

An obvious question arises from the above discussion: What are the mechanisms that transit the LV from its compensated to the decompensated state? Are these mechanisms a property of the LV chamber, the myocytes comprising the chamber, or some combination of both?

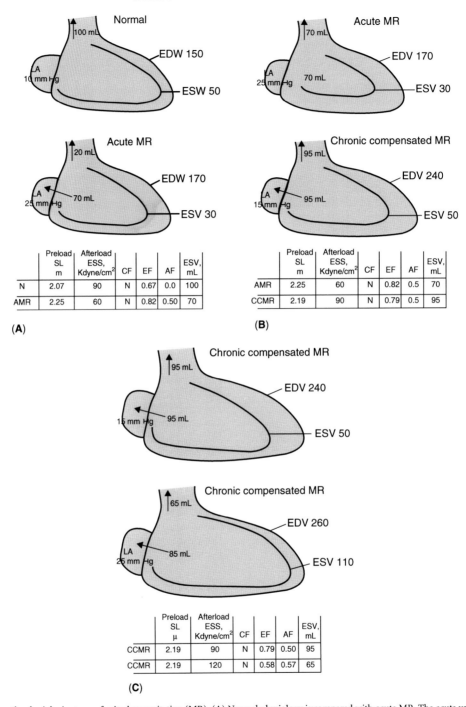

	Preload SL m	Afterload ESS, Kdyne/cm^2	CF	EF	AF	ESV, mL
N	2.07	90	N	0.67	0.0	100
AMR	2.25	60	N	0.82	0.50	70

(A)

	Preload SL m	Afterload ESS, Kdyne/cm^2	CF	EF	AF	ESV, mL
AMR	2.25	60	N	0.82	0.5	70
CCMR	2.19	90	N	0.79	0.5	95

(B)

	Preload SL μ	Afterload ESS, Kdyne/cm^2	CF	EF	AF	ESV, mL
CCMR	2.19	90	N	0.79	0.50	95
CCMR	2.19	120	N	0.58	0.57	65

(C)

Figure 2.1 The pathophysiologic stages of mitral regurgitation (MR). (A) Normal physiology is compared with acute MR. The acute volume overload of MR maximizes preload (sarcomere length, SL) and increases end diastolic volume (EDV) modestly. The extra pathway for ejection into the left atrium (LA) reduces afterload (end systolic stress, ESS) thereby further enhancing left ventricular (LV) ejection, reducing end systolic volume (ESV). Contractility is normal (N) or enhanced. These factors act in concert to increase ejection fraction (EF) and total stroke volume. However, regurgitation reduces forward stroke volume (FSV). The portion of total stroke volume regurgitated is referred to as the regurgitant fraction (RF). (B) Acute MR is compared to chronic compensated MR (CCMR). Eccentric cardiac hypertrophy has intervened in chronic compensated MR, increasing EDV and both total and forward stroke volume. Increased LV size increases its radius and also ESS in turn increasing ESV so that EF falls slightly. Increased LA size accommodates the RF at substantially lower filling pressure. (C) Chronic compensated MR is compared to chronic decompensated MR. In this stage LV contractile dysfunction has ensued causing a large increase in ESV and a fall in stroke volume and EF although EF may still be maintained in "normal" range by increased preload. Increased LV radius increases ESS leading to a further decline in LV function and further cardiac dilatation in turn increasing the RF. *Source:* From Ref. 1.

The Chamber: Geometry, Loading, and Coronary Blood Flow

Decades ago Grossman et al. proposed a schema by which hemodynamic load was translated into LVH (7). They suggested that systolic stress, increased by increased pressure in the numerator of the Laplace equation in some way informed the myocyte to add sarcomeres in parallel, increasing myocyte thickness in turn leading to concentric hypertrophy. In this way the increased LV pressure in the Laplace numerator was offset by an increase in thickness in the Laplace denominator, in turn maintaining normal afterload. Conversely, in volume overload, increased diastolic stress led to the replication of sarcomeres in series, leading to myocyte lengthening, resulting in an increase in chamber volume, allowing the LV to pump the additional volume required by the overload. In this context MR is nearly unique among LV volume overloads by being essentially a "pure" volume overload (8). In most other volume overloads such as anemia, aortic regurgitation, complete heart block etc., the extra volume is pumped into the relatively high pressure of the aorta where increased stroke volume also increases the systolic pressure. As such, most volume overloads are in fact combined pressure and volume overloads (9). In contrast, in MR the extra volume is pumped into the low pressure of the LA and systemic blood pressure is normal or even reduced. These hemodynamic factors lead to an enlarged thin-walled LV with the largest radius-to-thickness ratio and the smallest mass-to-volume ratio of adult valvular heart diseases (Table 2.1) (8). This pattern of LVH leads to a very unusual circumstance for cardiac disease, that of supernormal diastolic compliance (10,11). In most heart diseases diastolic dysfunction precedes systolic dysfunction. This is not true in MR where the thin-walled LV allows for rapid LV filling of a large volume at normal filling pressure. While this pattern of hypertrophy in MR is beneficial to diastolic function, it is disadvantageous to systolic function. The r/th ratio is central to the Laplace equation. As noted above, while the LV–LA systolic ejection pathway may tend to unload the LV, the high r/th ratio increases the systolic wall stress and actually increases the LV afterload, eventually restricting LV contraction when LV radius becomes markedly increased (5).

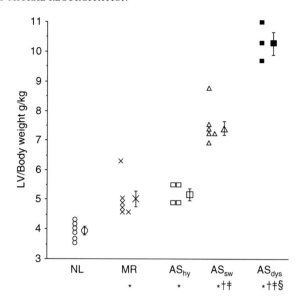

Figure 2.2 Left ventricular (LV) mass normalized to body weight is shown for normal dogs (NL), dogs with severe chronic mitral regurgitation (MR), dogs with aortic stenosis matched to have the same amount of hypertrophy as the MR dogs (AS$_{hy}$), dogs with AS matched to have the same stroke work as the MR dogs (AS$_{sw}$), and dogs with AS and LV dysfunction (AS$_{dys}$). LVs from dogs with MR performing the same amount of stroke work as the LVs from dogs with AS had far less hypertrophy. *Source:* From Ref. 12.

At the same time, this geometry leads to the smallest mass-to-volume ratio in valvular heart disease (8). Thus in MR, there is the least amount of mass to propel the volume requirements of the LV. Indeed when the stroke work increased from the pressure overload was matched to an equal increase in the stroke work from MR, LV mass was far less in MR than in aortic stenosis despite the similar workload (Fig. 2.2) (12). In summary, the LV in MR remodels in a way favorable to diastolic function, wherein the thin-walled LV can fill rapidly at a tolerable filling pressure. However, this same geometry is unfavorable to systole, "paradoxically" loading the LV while providing little increase in LV mass to accommodate the hemodynamic overload.

A chamber property implicated in the LV dysfunction of **pressure** overload is abnormal coronary blood flow which is especially reduced to the subendocardium (13–15). In pressure overload it appears that there is inadequate capillary ingrowth to supply the thickened LV wall (16). Inadequate coronary blood flow seems in part responsible for the LV dysfunction that occurs in pressure overload. However, in an experimental model of **volume** overload from MR, no such reduction in coronary blood flow was detected consistent with the thin wall architecture of the MR LV (17). Thus, ischemia is not a likely cause of LV dysfunction in MR in subjects with normal epicardial coronary arteries.

Table 2.1 Hypertrophy in Human Left-Sided Overload Valve Lesions

	Mass Index g/m² (n)	r/h (n)	m/v (n)
NL	86 (259)	3.05 (88)	1.25 (225)
MR	158 (146)	4.03 (64)	0.87 (117)
AR	230 (148)	3.52 (31)	1.00 (141)
AS	178 (302)	2.35 (93)	1.55 (296)

Abbreviations: AR, aortic regurgitation; AS, aortic stenosis; MR, mitral regurgitation; m/v, ratio of left ventricular mass to volume; n, number of subjects analyzed; NL, normal subjects; r/h, ratio of left ventricular radius to thickness.

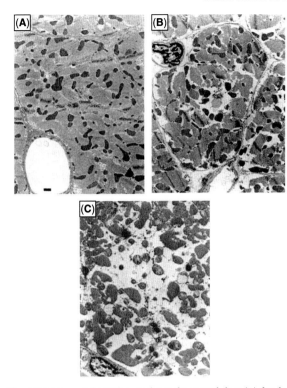

Figure 2.3 Myocardial histology is shown for normal dogs (A) for dogs with mitral regurgitation (MR) and preserved LV function (B) and for dogs with MR and LV dysfunction (C). With LV dysfunction there is an obvious loss of contractile elements. *Source*: From Ref. 18.

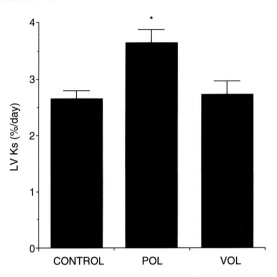

Figure 2.4 Myosin heavy chain synthesis rate (k_s) is shown for normal dogs, for dogs with severe acute pressure overload (POL) and for dogs with severe acute volume overload (VOL) from mitral regurgitation (MR). POL induced a 35% increase in myosin synthesis rate while MR caused no change in K_s. *Source*: From Ref. 24.

The Myocyte in MR

It is the myocyte the produces the driving force for LV contraction and thus it is logical that a portion of the LV dysfunction of MR will stem from the dysfunction of the myocyte itself. Indeed when the contractility of individual myocytes taken from MR LVs that had entered the decompensated phase was examined, myocyte contractility was reduced (18). Reduced contractility in turn stemmed from loss of contractile elements in myocytes taken from dogs with experimental MR (Fig. 2.3), a result also seen in the papillary muscles taken from MR patients (19). In addition, in muscle strips taken from patients with MR, the myocardial force–frequency relationship was altered such that the peak force occurred at low heart rates, followed by a fall in force as heart rate increased. These changes were reversible by addition of forskolin (20). Taken together these findings suggest that abnormalities in calcium handling also contribute to the contractile dysfunction of decompensated MR.

When MR is corrected in a timely fashion, chamber dysfunction and myocyte dysfunction are reversible coincident with a return to the normal cytoarchitecture of the myocyte (21–23).

The Cellular Process of Hypertrophy

As noted above, the LV in MR develops a characteristic pattern of LVH such that the ventricle transforms into a dilated thin-walled chamber. By definition, the term hypertrophy indicates that the LV has gained mass, mediated by an increase in chamber proteins. The myocardial proteins are in constant flux between synthesis and degradation. In order for LV mass to increase, synthesis rate must exceed degradation rate, either because synthesis rate increases or as degradation rate decreases. The contractile proteins turn over in approximately every 10 days so that even in six hours enough of a labeled amino acid is newly incorporated into the myocardium allowing the synthesis rate to be measured. As shown in Figure 2.4, following acute LV pressure overload created by aortic banding, myosin heavy chain synthesis rate (k_s) had increased by 35% (24). However, acute severe MR caused no such detectable increase in protein synthesis rate (24). Further, observations at two weeks, four weeks, and three months following the creation of severe MR never found an increase in myosin heavy chain k_s (25). Yet LV mass in severe MR did increase. Since K_s remained constant it is reasonable to hypothesize that LV mass in MR increased not by an increase in K_s but rather by a decrease in degradation rate (k_d). A similar observation was made in a rabbit model of MR (26). The obvious consequence of these changes in protein kinetics is that the contractile proteins in the MR ventricle become older than normal. It is possible that aging contractile proteins develop dysfunction more easily than normal and thus this process could be in part responsible for the LV dysfunction found in MR.

Systems Overload

The Adrenergic Nervous System in MR

The heart holds a wealth of complex cellular mechanisms yet simplistically its ability to respond to an overload is limited. It can utilize the Frank–Starling mechanism to increase the force of contraction. It can increase the LV mass (hypertrophy) to increase the pumping ability and/or it can make use of the adrenergic nervous system to increase inotropy. Hypertrophic compensation is limited (see above) and sarcomere stretch is maximized early after MR develops (2). Since these mechanisms provide only temporary compensation, it raises the hypothesis that adrenergic activation might play a central role in compensating the MR ventricle. However, while adrenergic stimulation may be initially compensatory, a wealth of data in heart failure support the premise that prolonged adrenergic myocardial stimulation damages the myocardium, worsening heart failure in the long run, and shortening life span. Thus, beta adrenergic blockade has become a key therapy in the treatment of heart failure, prolonging life, and chronically increasing systolic performance.

In MR, the adrenergic nervous system also appears to play a clear role. Starling and colleagues noted that norepinephrine release in patients with MR was well correlated to LV size and function (27). They found that catecholamine release progressively increased as LV ejection fraction decreased and as LV end systolic volume increased. Catecholamine excess persisted postoperatively if LV dysfunction also persisted (28). These data could be interpreted as the adrenergic system **supporting** a failing heart or as the adrenergic nervous system **causing** LV dysfunction (29). Some insight into this conundrum can be gleaned from experimental MR. In a canine model, severe MR was associated with a two- to threefold increase in serum norepinephrine release in dogs that had developed LV dysfunction. Beta blockade restored LV function at both the myocyte and chamber levels (Fig. 2.5) (30). Since beta blockade was the only intervention made, it seems highly likely that adrenergic overdrive was the cause rather than the result of the LV dysfunction observed.

The use of beta blockade in human MR is limited. In a short-term study, metoprolol increased forward stroke volume without affecting regurgitant volume and as such, improved the ventricular pumping efficiency (forward stroke volume/total stroke volume), implying a potentially salutary effect (31). In an observational study of 896 patients with severe MR, those receiving beta blockers had increased survival irrespective of the presence of coronary disease and/or hypertension (32). Obviously, a randomized trial of beta blockers in MR patients is required to establish whether they have a therapeutic role to play.

The Renin-Angiotensin System in MR
The renin-angiotensin system has long been implicated in the deleterious effects of remodeling in heart failure. It was natural then to wonder whether angiotensin-converting enzyme inhibitors (ACEIs) or angiotensin receptor blockers might be useful in treating the MR patient both by effecting remodeling and also because their vasodilator properties might allow for a preferential increase aortic outflow, simultaneously reducing the amount of MR. A table partially

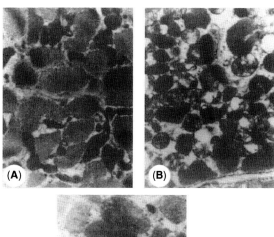

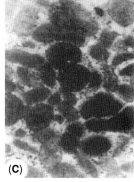

Figure 2.5 LV histology is shown for normal dogs (A), for dogs with severe mitral regurgitation (MR) and left ventricular (LV) dysfunction with loss of contractile elements (B), and for dogs with severe MR and LV dysfunction subsequently treated with a beta blocker (C). LV function improved with beta blockade coincident with improved histology. *Source*: From Ref. 30.

summarizing the effects of ACEIs and angiotensin receptor blockers in subjects with MR is shown (Table 2.2) (33–38). The totality of the data indicates that renin-angiotensin system blockade has not been effective in preventing the progression of MR or in forestalling the need for surgery. Thus, their use for that purpose has been rated class III (ineffective) by the American Heart Association (AHA)/American College Cardiology (ACC) guidelines for the treatment of patients with valvular heart disease (39). However, ACEIs may still be used to treat heart failure in MR patients not deemed to be candidates for surgery and also may be used to treat the MR patient with hypertension.

The Role of the Mitral Valve Apparatus
The mitral valve apparatus has often been viewed simply as a group of structures that prevent MR during systole, and therefore it used to be removed with impunity when a prosthetic valve was inserted to restore mitral competence. However, the mitral valve apparatus is also an integral part of the LV, helping to maintain LV shape while aiding in LV contraction. Destruction of the mitral valve apparatus during surgery results in permanent LV damage (40–49), LV dysfunction (Fig. 2.6) (47), and reduced postoperative prognosis. In recognition of these facts

Table 2.2 Effects of ACEIs and ARBs in Subjects with MR

References	n	Intervention	Duration	Results
(33)	32	Captoril	6 mo	No change in ESD or EF
(34)	12	Lisinopril 18	1 yr	No change in LV dimensions; RF fell 6.4%
(35)	28	Losartan 50	1 mo	13 cc reduction in RV
(36)	26	Ramapril	6 mo	No change in MR severity or symptoms
(37)	7 dogs	Irbesartan	3 mo	Worsened LV remodeling
(38)	11 dogs	Lisinopril	3 mo	Decreased filling pressure without improvement in LV function

Abbreviations: ACEIs, angiotensin-converting enzyme inhibitors; ARBs, angiotensin receptor blockers; EF, ejection fraction; ESD, end systolic dimension; LV, left ventricle; MR, mitral regurgitation; Pts, patients; RAS, renin-angiotensin system; RV, regurgitant volume.

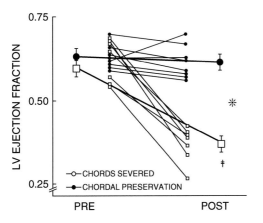

Figure 2.6 Left ventricular (LV) ejection fraction is shown for patients with severe mitral regurgitation (MR) before (preop) and after (postop) correction of MR by operations that did or did not preserve the mitral apparatus. Destruction of the MV apparatus led to a substantial fall in LV EF. *Source*: From Ref. 47.

mitral repair (when possible) instead of mitral replacement is the standard of care for treating primary MR (39).

Clinical Markers of Left Ventricular Dysfunction

As noted above, severe MR eventually causes LV damage, heart failure, and death if left untreated. Accordingly, the clinician needs markers that such damage is impending. The onset of symptoms of heart failure such as dyspnea on exertion, orthopnea, etc. indicates a change in the disease state and a reduced prognosis if MR is not treated at their onset (50). On the other hand, some patients develop LV dysfunction without symptoms. Markers showing that LV dysfunction is ensuing include

an ejection fraction falling toward 0.60 and an LV that fails to contract to 40 mm at end systole (39,51,52). Increasing LA size and pulmonary hypertension at rest or provoked with exercise are also worrisome developments and press the patient and his/her provider toward mitral valve repair (53,54).

FUNCTIONAL MR
Functional MR develops when ischemic or dilated cardiomyopathy results in severe LV dysfunction, regional wall motion abnormalities, papillary muscle displacement, and mitral annular dilatation. The changes in LV function and geometry restrict mitral valve motion and prevent leaflet coaptation. Further, the weakened LV generates less force to close the mitral valve tightly during systole. Thus, in functional MR the leak is the **result** of LV dysfunction rather than its **cause**, the direct opposite of organic MR where it is the MR that causes LV dysfunction. Thus, it is less certain that correction of functional MR will improve patient outcome since the underlying coronary disease or dilated cardiomyopathy still exists and treating the MR does not directly treat these conditions.

Correction of functional MR does have positive effects on the LV. There is clear reverse remodeling with a reduction in LV volume, reduced afterload, and increased ejection fraction (55). In addition, some patients report symptomatic improvement following MR surgery. However, despite these salutary effects there is no hard evidence that treating functional MR surgically after the appropriate therapies for heart failure have been applied improves survival or even leads to a long-term improvement in symptoms (56–59). Thus, mechanical treatment of functional MR is rated a 2b (possibly helpful) (39) in the AHA/ACC guidelines.

SUMMARY
Organic MR places a nearly unique hemodynamic overload upon the LV, that is, of a pure volume overload. Initially compensated by activation of the Frank–Starling mechanism, eccentric cardiac hypertrophy ensues permitting an increased LV volume pumping capacity. The remodeling that accompanies this hypertrophy is also particular to MR, leading to a thin-walled enlarged LV that enhances diastolic function but eventually impairs systolic function. When hypertrophy is no longer compensatory, activation of neurohumoral systems, especially the adrenergic nervous system, compounds the pathophysiology of the disease eventually worsening LV function. Timely mechanical correction of MR with mitral valve repair is "curative" and consistent with a normal lifespan.

Functional MR in many respects is a different disease than is organic MR because it must coexist with other serious heart diseases, diseases that by themselves are eventually fatal thus clouding the exact role that the MR plays in the patient's pathophysiology and also clouding the role of restoration of mitral competence in treating the patient. The issue of the proper therapy for functional MR can only be clarified by randomized controlled trials.

REFERENCES

1. Carabello BA. Mitral regurgitation: basic pathophysiologic principles. Mod Concepts Cardiovasc Dis 1988; 57: 53–8.
2. Ross J Jr, Sonnenblick EH, Taylor RR, Spotnitz HM, Covell JW. Diastolic geometry and sarcomere lengths in the chronically dilated canine left ventricle. Circ Res 1971; 28: 49–61.
3. Ling LH, Enrique-Sarano M, Seward JB, et al. Clinical outcome of mitral regurgitation due to flail leaflet. N Engl J Med 1996; 335: 1417–23.
4. Rosenhek R, Rader F, Klaar U, et al. Outcome of watchful waiting in asymptomatic severe mitral regurgitation. Circulation 2006; 113: 2238–44.
5. Corin WJ, Monrad ES, Murakami T, et al. The relationship of afterload to ejection performance in chronic mitral regurgitation. Circulation 1987; 76: 59–67.
6. Schuler G, Petersen KL, Johnson A, et al. Temporal response of left ventricular performance to mitral valve surgery. Circulation 1979; 59: 1218–31.
7. Grossman W, Jones D, McLaurin LP. Wall stress and patterns of hypertrophy in the human left ventricle. J Clin Invest 1975; 53: 332–41.
8. Carabello BA. The relationship of left ventricular geometry and hypertrophy to left ventricular function in valvular heart disease. J Heart Valve Dis 1995; 4(Suppl 2): S132–8; discussion S138-9.
9. Wisenbaugh T, Spann JF, Carabello BA. Differences in myocardial performance and load between patients with similar amounts of chronic aortic versus chronic mitral regurgitation. J Am Coll Cardiol 1984; 3: 916–23.
10. Zile MR, Tomita M, Nakano K, et al. Effects of left ventricular volume overload produced by mitral regurgitation on diastolic function. Am J Physiol 1991; 261(5 Pt 2): H1471–80.
11. Corin WJ, Murakami T, Monrad ES, Hess OM, Krayenbuehl HP. Left ventricular passive diastolic properties in chronic mitral regurgitation. Circulation 1991; 83: 797–807.
12. Carabello BA, Zile MR, Tanaka R, Cooper G 4th. Left ventricular hypertrophy due to volume overload versus pressure overload. Am J Physiol 1992; 263(4 Pt 2): H1137–44.
13. Rembert JC, Kleinman LH, Fedor JM, Wechsler AS, Greenfield JC Jr. Myocardial blood flow distribution in concentric left ventricular hypertrophy. J Clin Invest 1978; 62: 379–86.
14. Alyono D, Anderson RW, Parrish DG, Dai X-Z, Bache RJ. Alterations of myocardial blood flow associated with experimental canine left ventricular hypertrophy secondary to valvular aortic stenosis. Circ Res 1986; 58: 47–57.
15. Bache RJ, Vrobel TR, Arentzen CE, Ring WS. Effect of maximal coronary vasodilation on transmural myocardial perfusion during tachycardia in dogs with left ventricular hypertrophy. Circ Res 1981; 49: 742–50.
16. Breisch EA, Houser SR, Carey RA, Spann JF, Bove AA. Myocardial blood flow and capillary density in chronic pressure overload of the feline left ventricle. Cardiovasc Res 1980; 14: 469–75.
17. Carabello BA, Nakano K, Ishihara K, et al. Coronary blood flow in dogs with contractile dysfunction due to experimental volume overload. Circulation 1991; 83: 1063–75.
18. Urabe Y, Mann DL, Kent RL, et al. Cellular and ventricular contractile dysfunction in experimental canine mitral regurgitation. Circ Res 1992; 70: 131–47.
19. Mulieri LA, Tischler MD, Martin BJ, et al. Regional differences in the force-frequency relation of human left ventricular myocardium in mitral regurgitation: implications for ventricular shape. Am J Physiol Heart Circ Physiol 2005; 288: H2185–91.
20. Mulieri LA, Leavitt BJ, Kent RL, et al. Myocardial force-frequency defect in mitral regurgitation heart failure is reversed for forskolin. Circulation 1993; 88: 2700–4.
21. Starling MR. Effects of valve surgery on left ventricular function in patients with long-term mitral regurgitation. Circulation 1995; 92: 811–18.
22. Nakano K, Swindle MM, Spinale F, et al. Depressed contractile function due to canine mitral regurgitation improves after correction of the volume overload. J Clin Invest 1991; 88: 723.
23. Spinale FG, Ishihara K, Zile M, et al. Structural basis for changes in left ventricular function and geometry because of chronic mitral regurgitation and after correction of volume overload. J Thorac Cardiovasc Surg 1993; 106: 1147–57.
24. Imamura T, McDermott PJ, Kent RL, et al. Acute changes in myosin heavy chain synthesis rate in pressure versus volume overload. Circ Res 1994; 75: 418–25.
25. Matsuo T, Carabello BA, Nagatomo Y, et al. Mechanisms of cardiac hypertrophy in canine volume overload. Am J Physiol 1998; 275(1 Pt 2): H65–74.
26. Magid NM, Wallerson DC, Bent SJ, Borer JS. Hypertrophy and heart failure in experimental mitral regurgitation. JACC 1994; 23: 248A.
27. 27. Mehta RHJ, Supiano Ma, Oral H, et al. Relation of systemic sympathetic nervous system activation to echocardiographic left ventricular size and performance and its implications in patients with mitral regurgitation. Am J Cardiol 2000; 85: 1193.7.
28. Mehta RH, Supiano MA, Grossman PM, et al. Changes in systemic sympathetic nervous system activity after mitral valve surgery and their relationship to changes in left ventricular size and systolic performance in patients with mitral regurgitation. Am Heart J 2004; 147: 729–35.
29. Nagatsu M, Zile MR, Tsutsui H, et al. Native beta-adrenergic support for left ventricular dysfunction in experimental mitral regurgitation normalizes indexes of pump and contractile function. Circulation 1994; 89: 818–26.
30. Tsutsui H, Spinale FG, Nagatsu M, et al. Effects of chronic B-adrenergic blockade on the left ventricular and cardiocyte abnormalities of chronic canine mitral regurgitation. J Clin Invest 1994; 93: 2639–48.
31. Stewart RAH, Raffel OC, Kerr AJ, et al. Pilot study to assess the influence of B-blockade on mitral regurgitant volume and left ventricular work in degenerative mitral valve disease. Circulation 2008; 118: 1041–6.
32. Varadarajan P, Joshi N, Appel D, Duvvuri L, Pai RG. Effect of beta-blocker therapy on survival in patients with severe mitral regurgitation and normal left ventricular ejection fraction. Am J Cardiol 2008; 102: 611–15.
33. Wisenbaugh T, Sinovich V, Dullabh A, Sareli PI. Six month pilot study of captopril for mildly symptomatic, severe isolated mitral and isolated aortic regurgitation. J Heart Valve Dis 1994; 3: 197–204.
34. Marcotte F, Honos GN, Walling AD, et al. Effect of angiotensin-converting enzyme inhibitor therapy in mitral regurgitation with normal left ventricular function. Can J Cardiol 1997; 13: 479–85.
35. Dujardin KS, Enriquez-Sarano M, Bailey KR, Seward JB, Tajik AJ. Effect of losartan on degree of mitral regurgitation quantified by echocardiography. Am J Cardiol 2001; 87: 570–6.

36. Harris KM, Aeppli DM, Carey CF. Effects of angiotensin-converting enzyme inhibition on mitral regurgitation severity, left ventricular size, and functional capacity. Am Heart J 2005; 150: 1106.

37. Perry GJ, Wei CC, Hankes GH, et al. Angiotensin II receptor blockade does not improve left ventricular function and remodeling in subacute mitral regurgitation in the dog. JACC 2002; 39: 1374–9.

38. Nemoto S, Hamawaki M, De Freitas G, Carabello BA. Differential effects of the angiotensin-converting enzyme inhibitor lisinopril versus the beta-adrenergic receptor blocker atenolol on hemodynamics and left ventricular contractile function in experimental mitral regurgitation. JACC 2002; 40: 149–54.

39. Bonow R, Carabello BA, Kanu C, et al. ACC/AHA 2006 guidelines for the management of patients with valvular heart disease: a report of the American college of cardiology/American heart association task force on practice guidelines (writing committee to revise the 1998 guidelines for the management of patients with valvular hear disease): developed in collaboration with the society of cardiovascular aneshthesiologists: endorsed by the society of cardiovascular angiography and interventions and the society of thoracic surgeons. Circulation 2006; 114: e84.231.

40. Enriquez-Sarano M, Schaff HV, Orszulak TA, et al. Valve repair improves the outcome of surgery for mitral regurgitation analysis. Circulation 1995; 91: 1022–8.

41. Horskotte D, Schulte HD, Bircks W, Strauer BE. The effect of chordal preservation on late outcome after mitral valve replacement: a randomized study. J Heart Valve Dis 1993; 2: 158–8.

42. Jokinen JJ, Hippelainen MJ, Pitkanen OA, Hartikainen JE. Mitral valve replacement versus repair: propensity-adjusted survival and quality-of-life analysis. Ann Thorac Surg 2007; 84: 451–8.

43. David TE. Outcomes of mitral valve repair for mitral regurgitation due to degenerative disease. Semin Thorac Cardiovasc Surg 2007; 19: 116–20.

44. Lillehei CW, Levy MJ, Bonnabeau RC Jr. Mitral valve replacement with preservation of papillary muscles and chordate tendineae. J Thorac Cardiovasc Surg 1964; 47: 532–43.

45. Rushmer RF, Finlayson BL, Nash AA. Movements of the mitral valve. Circ Res 1956; 4: 337–42.

46. Carpentier A, Relland J, Deloche A, et al. Conservative management of the prolapsed mitral valve. Ann Thorac Surg 1978; 26: 294–302.

47. Rozich JD, Carabello BA, Usher BW, et al. Mitral valve replacement with and without chordal preservation in patients with chronic mitral regurgitation: mechanisms for differences in post-operative ejection performance. Circulation 1992; 86: 1718–26.

48. David TE, Burnes RJ, Racchus CM, Druck MN. Mitral valve replacement for mitral regurgitation with and without preservation of chordate tendineae. J Thorac Cardiovasc Surg 1984; 88: 718–25.

49. Sarris GE, Cahill PD, Hansen DE, et al. Restoration of left ventricular systolic performance after reattachment of the mitral chordate tendineae: the importance of valvular-ventricular interaction. J Thorac Cardiovasc Surg 1988; 95: 969–79.

50. Tribouilloy CM, Enriquez-Sarano M, Schaff HV, et al. Impact of preoperative symptoms on survival after surgical correction of organic mitral regurgitation: rationale for optimizing surgical indications. Circulation 1999; 99: 400–5.

51. Enriquez-Sarano M, Tajik AJ, Schaff HV, et al. Echocardiographic prediction of survival after surgical correction of organic mitral regurgitation. Circulation 1994; 90: 830–7.

52. Matsumura T, Ohtaki E, Tanaka K, et al. Echocardiographic prediction of left ventricular dysfunction after mitral valve repair for mitral regurgitation as an indicator to decide the optimal timing of repair. J Am Coll Cardiol 2003; 42: 458–63.

53. Crawford MH, Souchek J, Oprian CA, et al. Determinants of survival and left ventricular performance after mitral valve replacement. department of veterans affairs cooperative study on valvular heart disease. Circulation 1990; 81: 1173–81.

54. Rusinaru D, Tribouilloy C, Grigioni F, et al. Mitral regurgitation international database (MIDA) investigators. left atrial size is a potent predictor of mortality in mitral regurgitation due to flail leaflets: results from a large international multicenter study. Circ Cardiovasc Imaging 2011; 4: 473–81.

55. Acher Ma, Jessup M, Bolling SF, et al. Mitral valve repair in heart failure: five-year follow-up from the mitral valve replacement stratum of the acorn randomized trial. J Thorac Cardiovasc Surg 2011; 142: 569–74; 574.e1.

56. Wu AH, Aaronson KD, Billing SF, et al. Impact of mitral valve annuloplasty on mortality risk in patients with mitral regurgitation and left ventricular systolic dysfunction. J Am Coll Cardiol 2005; 45: 381–7.

57. Mihaljevic T, Lam BK, Rajeswaran J, et al. Impact of mitral valve annuloplasty combined with revascularization in patients with functional ischemic mitral regurgitation. J Am Coll Cardiol 2007; 49: 2191–203.

58. Diodato MD, Moon MR, Pasque MK, et al. Repair of ischemic mitral regurgitation does not increase mortality or improve long-term survival in patients undergoing coronary artery revascularization: a propensity analysis. Ann Thorac Surg 2004; 78: 794–9; discussion 794-9.

59. Kang DH, Kim MJ Kang SJ, Song JM, et al. Mitral valve repair versus revascularization alone in the treatment of ischemic mitral regurgitation. Circulation 2006; 114(Suppl I): I499–503.

3   Genesis of the surgical edge-to-edge repair
Ottavio Alfieri and Michele De Bonis

INTRODUCTION

The edge-to-edge (E2E) technique was introduced in the surgical armamentarium of mitral valve repair in the early 1990s and has been used progressively to restore mitral competence in the setting of degenerative, functional and, occasionally, postendocarditis mitral regurgitation (MR) (1,2). While the aim of traditional mitral repair techniques is to realize an anatomical reconstruction of the diseased valve, the original idea behind the E2E approach is that the competence of a regurgitant mitral valve can be effectively restored with a "functional" rather than an anatomical repair. Indeed, the key point of this surgical method is to identify by preoperative transesophageal echocardiography the precise location of the regurgitant jet. Exactly at that level, the free edge of the diseased leaflet is sutured to the corresponding edge of the opposing leaflet thereby eliminating mitral incompetence. When the regurgitant jet is in the central part of the mitral valve, the application of the E2E technique produces a mitral valve with a double-orifice configuration (double-orifice repair) (Fig. 3.1). Depending on the extension and location of the suture performed, the two orifices can have similar or different sizes. In case of commissural prolapse or flail, on the other hand, the jet of regurgitation is usually identified in correspondence with the commissural area and the application of the E2E technique leads to a surgical closure of the commissure ("paracommissural edge-to-edge repair"). Under these circumstances, the mitral valve will have a single orifice with a relatively smaller area compared with the preoperative value (Fig.3. 2).

Historical Note

The E2E technique was introduced into surgical practice by Dr Alfieri in 1991. At that time, in the presence of MR due to anterior or bileaflet prolapse, the conventional methods of mitral valve repair were often technically demanding, time consuming, and not easily reproducible by many surgeons. In addition, the results reported in these settings were certainly less gratifying compared with those observed in patients with posterior leaflet prolapse treated by quadrangular resection (3–6).

The first E2E repair was inspired by a young lady who underwent surgical correction of an atrial septal defect. She had the very rare, but well-described congenital double-orifice mitral valve which was perfectly competent. This finding provided the idea to Dr Alfieri of reproducing surgically a double-orifice shape to treat MR. Therefore, in a patient with severe MR due to anterior leaflet prolapse who was operated on the same day, the prolapsing portion of the anterior leaflet was sutured to the

facing part of the posterior leaflet and a double-orifice competent valve was obtained. Since then, because of its simplicity, effectiveness, and durability, the E2E technique has become a useful addition to the surgical armamentarium in mitral valve reconstruction with more than 1500 cases published worldwide and with the longest follow-up now approaching 20 years.

Surgical Technique

Despite its simplicity, the E2E technique needs to be performed following important technical details to be effective and durable. The procedure is carried out through a conventional median sternotomy or, in selected patients, through a small right anterior thoracotomy. Following aortic and bicaval cannulation, in normothermic cardiopulmonary bypass, the aorta is clamped and intermittent cold-blood cardioplegia is delivered into the ascending aorta to obtain cardioplegic arrest. The mitral valve is usually approached through the left atrium and is carefully inspected to recognize the type of lesion and the location of the regurgitant jet. The E2E suture has to be placed exactly at the site of origin of the regurgitant jet. Minimal technical modifications are adopted according to the single case anatomy and pathology. In Barlow's disease, for instance, although the entire valve is prolapsing, the segments with the most extensive pathologic involvement are usually the middle scallops of the anterior and posterior leaflets (A2 and P2) (Fig. 3.3). By using the subvalvular apparatus as a guide, the first stitch is positioned at the anatomical middle of the two leaflets. The symmetry of the two orifices created is checked and, if the correct position of the stitch is confirmed, a continuous mattress suture of 4-0 polypropylene is passed along the whole length of the middle scallop of the anterior and posterior leaflets (A2 and P2). A second over-and-over continuous suture is then added (Fig. 3.4). The shortest sutured apposition length that is able to eliminate MR without inducing stenosis is used. The distance of the suture bites from the free edges of the leaflets is variable according to the redundancy of the tissue. The more redundancy is present, the deeper the stitches should be. In Barlow's disease, big bites (approximately 0.5–1 cm deep) should be taken to reduce the height of the leaflets in the middle of the double-orifice valve and to eliminate the occurrence of postoperative systolic anterior motion (SAM). When a flail segment is found, the position of the stitch may be somewhat asymmetric, corresponding to the center of the flail portion of the leaflet. In this case, the size of the two orifices is likely to be different, one being larger than the other one. Finally, in patients with severe fibroelastic deficiency, a 5-0, rather than a 4-0, polypropylene suture should be preferred.

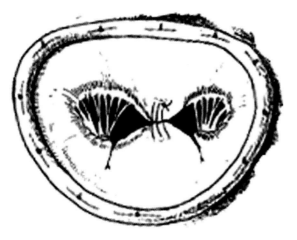

Figure 3.1 The edge-to-edge technique used as a double-orifice repair.

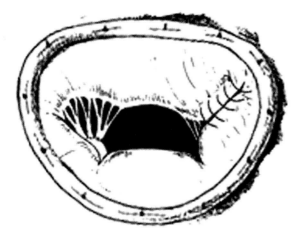

Figure 3.2 The edge-to-edge technique used as a paracommissural repair.

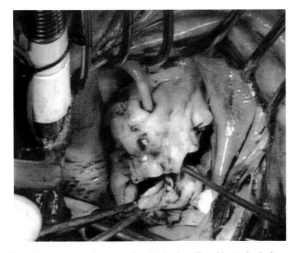

Figure 3.3 Intraoperative view of a mitral valve affected by Barlow's disease with significant redundancy of all the valve tissue and severe bileaflet prolapse.

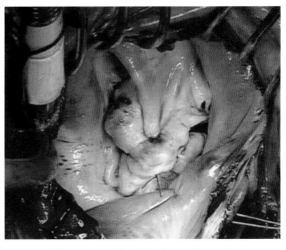

Figure 3.4 Double-orifice edge-to-edge repair.

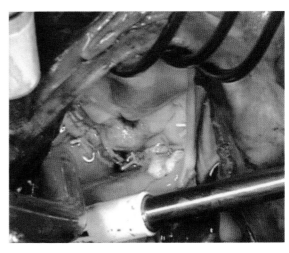

Figure 3.5 Saline test showing a competent mitral valve following double-orifice edge-to-edge repair and flexible ring annuloplasty.

A flexible or semi-rigid ring annuloplasty is regularly added to complete and stabilize the repair. The final competence of the two mitral orifices is evaluated by forceful saline filling of the left ventricle (Fig. 3.5) and the residual mitral area is assessed by direct inspection. In case of doubts, Hegar valve dilators are introduced into the orifices to be sure that a global valve area of at least 2.5 cm² has been left in normal-size patients. Transesophageal echo-Doppler reassessment of the valve is routinely performed after weaning from cardiopulmonary bypass. The valve area is commonly assessed by a planimetric method using the transgastric, short-axis view. Doppler methods can be used as well.

Indications for the E2E Technique

The E2E technique is a simple and versatile approach which has been effectively utilized for correction of MR due to different etiologies and mechanisms. Initially it was adopted mainly in patients with degenerative MR and anterior or bileaflet prolapse (Barlow's disease). With increasing experience, however, commissural prolapse and functional MR secondary to ischemic or idiopathic dilated cardiomyopathy have become common indications for this surgical option. Also patients with postendocarditis chordal rupture of the anterior leaflet have successfully been treated with the E2E repair.

Finally, the E2E method has been progressively adopted as a rescue procedure in case of suboptimal result of conventional mitral repair operations, to prevent or treat SAM of the anterior leaflet (7–10) and in other special situations, which are described later.

Bileaflet Prolapse of Facing Segments in Barlow's Disease

In patients with Barlow's disease, all the components of the mitral valve apparatus are affected by a severe myxomatous degeneration, which leads to generalized bileaflet prolapse, severe annular dilatation, and severe mitral insufficiency. In most of the cases, however, the prolapse involves mainly the facing segments of the central portions of the anterior and posterior leaflets (A2 and P2) making it possible the surgical correction of MR by the E2E technique. Indeed, by suturing the middle scallop of the anterior and posterior leaflet (A2–P2) followed by ring annuloplasty, the E2E technique restores valve competence and prevents postoperative SAM (11).

Segmental Anterior Leaflet Prolapse

The E2E technique is very effective in treating severe degenerative MR due to segmental prolapse of the anterior leaflet involving only one scallop (12). However, when the prolapsing or flailing lesions involve more than one scallop, the E2E repair alone may not be sufficient to obtain a perfectly competent valve since a long suture will be required with higher risk of inducing mitral stenosis. Under those circumstances, the implantation of artificial chordae may be required in order to eliminate incompetence without excessively reducing the mitral valve area.

Commissural Prolapse

In patients with prolapse or flail of the commissural area, mitral repair can be very challenging. The E2E technique can enable a rapid and durable mitral reconstruction in this setting and is probably the simplest and most reproducible method to repair isolated commissural prolapse or flail (13,14).

Functional Mitral Regurgitation

In functional or secondary MR the valve leaflets and chordae are structurally normal and the valve dysfunction is due to left ventricular remodeling with displacement of one or both papillary muscles. Tethering of the leaflets is the main mechanism responsible for secondary MR. Annular dilatation is often concomitantly present, particularly when the valve insufficiency is severe and long-standing and the left ventricle is remarkably dilated.

Undersized annuloplasty using a complete rigid ring is the standard operation, effective in most cases. To enhance the likelihood of a successful and durable repair, other procedures have been proposed to be added to annuloplasty including the E2E repair. In regard to the latter technique, the Cleveland Clinic group reported a disappointing 24% recurrence rate of moderately severe (3+) MR two years after E2E repair of functional MR (9). These results, however, can mainly be explained by the fact that, in that series, the E2E technique was always employed in association with a posterior flexible band, which may not prevent the recurrence of annular dilatation in the setting of advanced dilated cardiomyopathy. Indeed, the patients requiring reoperation almost invariably presented for re-dilatation of the mitral annulus. In our institution the "edge-to-edge" was associated with an undersized annuloplasty whenever substantial apical tenting was present (coaptation depth >1 cm). However, from a technical point of view, the concomitant annuloplasty was always performed with a complete rigid or semi-rigid ring and the site of leaflet approximation was literally guided by the echocardiographic findings. This approach significantly increased the durability of mitral repair in our series (15).

Rescue "Edge-to-Edge"

The E2E technique has also been used as a "rescue" procedure in patients with significant residual MR after conventional mitral repair. Under these circumstances, the original reconstruction is not taken down and the additional E2E suture is added at the location of the residual regurgitant jet. Satisfactory results (16) have been reported with this approach by some authors, whereas others have described suboptimal outcomes (17). This is not surprising considering, in this context, the added complexity of including the E2E technique to restore the competence of the mitral valve after a failed conventional repair. The efficacy of the procedure in this situation is extremely difficult to predict.

The "Edge-to-Edge" Technique to Prevent or Treat Systolic Anterior Motion

Systolic anterior motion of the anterior mitral leaflet causing left ventricular outflow tract obstruction remains one of the most common complications after mitral valve repair. It has been demonstrated that the use of the E2E technique might be an effective way to prevent or treat SAM occurring after mitral repair (18). Postoperative SAM can be completely eliminated without inducing mitral stenosis even in patients with hypertrophic obstructive cardiomyopathy and residual SAM after myectomy (9).

Special Situations

Infants and children with complex congenital heart disease associated with atrioventricular valve incompetence can occasionally take advantage of the E2E technique (19).

Moreover, when appropriate exposure of the mitral valve is extremely difficult, as in the presence of constraints like deep chest, small left atrium, severe left ventricular hypertrophy, or dilated aortic root, the simple E2E suture can be particularly convenient when compared with other complex reconstructive procedures, which will be extremely difficult to perform under conditions of suboptimal view.

Finally, in the presence of severe left ventricular dysfunction, the duration of the aortic cross-clamp time can have an impact on the outcome and the E2E technique can be again conveniently applied due to its simplicity and speed of execution.

Contraindications to the E2E Technique

Because of the risk of inducing stenosis, the E2E technique should not be used in patients with a small mitral valve area and rheumatic mitral regurgitation. In addition, its application is not indicated in case of degenerative MR whenever the mitral lesions involve not facing segments of the anterior and posterior leaflets.

The Role of Annuloplasty in E2E Repair

At the beginning of our experience, the E2E was used occasionally, without a concomitant ring annuloplasty in patients with calcified mitral annulus, in some cases of functional MR, or whenever the mitral annulus appeared to be not significantly dilated. With increasing experience, however, it has become progressively evident that a concomitant annuloplasty represents an important factor for the long-term durability of the E2E repair. Indeed, in the absence of annuloplasty, further dilatation of the mitral annulus can take place after surgery leading to recurrent MR. Timek and co-workers (20) have demonstrated that the tension on the E2E suture is dependent on the mitral annulus size. This means that if a further dilatation of the mitral annulus takes place after surgery, MR is likely to recur. Therefore, a ring annuloplasty should be added to the E2E repair whenever possible. In our clinical experience, freedom from reoperation has been less when annuloplasty was omitted for whatever reasons (21).

Double-Orifice E2E Repair and Hemodynamics

When the E2E technique is adopted as a double orifice repair, the morphology of the mitral valve becomes that of a valve with two orifices. The possible hemodynamic effects of such an unusual configuration have been a matter of concern since we started using the technique. This important issue has been addressed using computational model studies which have demonstrated that the hemodynamic performance of a double-orifice mitral valve depends exclusively on the total valve area as well as the cardiac output (22) and not on the double orifice shape. In double-orifice valve configuration, the velocity of the flow through each orifice is similar to the one observed through a single-orifice valve of area equal to the sum of the areas of the two orifices. Moreover, the flow velocities through the two orifices are exactly the same, even when the orifice sizes are significantly different, which means that the Doppler

sampling of any of the two orifices is sufficient to assess the hemodynamic of the mitral valve. Indeed, in our clinical practice, patients previously submitted to double-orifice repair demonstrated at Doppler examination blood flow velocities comparable in the two orifices.

E2E Repair and the Risk of Functional Mitral Stenosis

The potential restrictive effect at rest and during exercise of a valve submitted to the E2E repair has also been postulated shortly after its introduction. In our experience the gradients measured at rest across the mitral valve after E2E repair have always been very low, both immediately after surgery and at follow-up (2). Moreover, to assess whether the E2E technique could be a limiting factor for exercise tolerance, we performed an exercise echocardiographic study in patients previously submitted to central double-orifice mitral repair (23). This study demonstrated that during physical exercise the mean transmitral gradient after double-orifice mitral valve repair remains below 5 mmHg and the peak transmitral gradient does not exceed 10 mmHg. Moreover, the pulmonary pressure does not increase to pathologic levels. Finally, the mean planimetric mitral valve area at the peak of stress is more than 4 cm², this being coupled with hemodynamic physiologic response involving a significant increase in stroke volume. These findings support that the artificially created double-orifice valves follow a physiologic behavior under stress conditions, with a good valvular reserve in response to the increased cardiac output. Functional mitral stenosis does not develop either at baseline or under exercise conditions even with a concomitant ring annuloplasty. Similar findings have been reported by other authors who have demonstrated that the E2E repair is no more restrictive at peak exercise than conventional repairs (24).

CONCLUSIONS

Twenty years after its introduction, the E2E technique remains an effective and versatile method to treat mitral regurgitation. Simplicity, reliability, and effectiveness are the main advantages of this method and these have led to its increasingly widespread application in the surgical community. Precise patient selection criteria are mandatory, and the well-established technical aspects of the procedure have to be respected. The E2E concept of mitral valve repair is the basis for the current, most widespread percutaneous method of correcting MR, which has opened a new age in the fascinating field of reconstructive mitral valve surgery.

REFERENCES
1. Fucci C, Sandrelli L, Pardini A, et al. Improved results with mitral valve repair using new surgical techniques. Eur J Cardiothorac Surg 1995; 9: 621–6.
2. Maisano F, Torracca L, Oppizzi M, et al. The edge-to-edge technique: a simplified method to correct mitral insufficiency. Eur J Cardiothorac Surg 1998; 13: 240–6.

3. Gillinov AM, Cosgrove DM, Blackstone EH, et al. Durability of mitral valve repair for degenerative disease. J Thorac Cardiovasc Surg 1998; 111: 734–43.

4. Braunberger E, Deloche A, Berrebi A, et al. Very long-term results (more than 20 years) of valve repair with carpenter's techniques in nonrheumatic mitral valve insufficiency. Circulation 2001; 104(12 Suppl 1): I8–11.

5. Mohty D, Orszulak TA, Schaff HV, et al. Very long-term survival and durability of mitral valve repair for mitral valve prolapse. Circulation 2001; 104: I1–I.7.

6. Flameng W, Herijjers P, Bogaerts K, et al. Recurrence of mitral valve regurgitation after mitral valve repair in degenerative valve disease. Circulation 2003; 107: 1609–13.

7. Kuduvalli M, Ghotkar SV, Grayson AD, et al. Edge-to-edge technique for mitral valve repair: medium-term results with echocardiographic follow-up. Ann Thorac Surg 2006; 82: 1356–61.

8. Brinster DR, Unic D, D'Ambra MN, et al. Midterm results of the edge-to-edge technique for complex mitral valve repair. Ann Thorac Surg 2006; 81: 1612–17.

9. Bhudia SK, McCarthy PM, Smedira NG, et al. Edge-to-edge (alfieri) mitral repair: results in diverse clinical settings. Ann Thorac Surg 2004; 77: 1598–606.

10. Kherani AR, Cheema FH, Casher J, et al. Edge-to-edge mitral valve repair: the Columbia Presbyterian experience. Ann Thorac Surg 2004; 78: 73–6.

11. Maisano F, Schreuder JJ, Oppizzi M, et al. The double-orifice technique as a standardized approach to treat mitral regurgitation due to severe myxomatous disease: surgical technique. Eur J Cardiothorac Surg 2000; 17: 201–5.

12. De Bonis M, Lorusso R, Lapenna E, et al. Similar long-term results of mitral valve repair for anterior compared with posterior leaflet prolapse. J Thorac Cardiovasc Surg 2006; 131: 364–8.

13. Gillinov AM, Shortt KG, Cosgrove DM 3rd. Commissural closure for repair of mitral commissural prolapse. Ann Thorac Surg 2005; 80: 1135–6.

14. Lapenna E, De Bonis M, Sorrentino F, et al. Commissural closure for the treatment of commissural mitral valve prolapse or flail. J Heart Valve Dis 2008; 17: 261–6.

15. De Bonis M, La penna E, La Canna G, et al. Mitral valve repair for functional mitral regurgitation in end-stage dilated cardiomyopathy: the role of the "edge-to-edge" technique. Circulation 2005: 112 (Suppl I): I 402–8.

16. Gatti G, Cardu G, Trane R, et al. The edge-to-edge technique as a trick to rescue an imperfect mitral valve repair. Eur J Cardiothorac Surg 2002; 22: 817–20.

17. Brinster DR, Unic D, D'Ambra MN, et al. Midterm results of the edge-to-edge technique for complex mitral valve repair. Ann Thorac Surg 2006; 81: 1612–17.

18. Mascagni R, Al Attar N, Lamarra M, et al. Edge-to-edge technique to treat post-mitral valve repair systolic anterior motion and left ventricular outflow tract obstruction. Ann Thorac Surg 2005; 79: 471–3.

19. Ando M, Takahashi Y. Edge-to-edge repair of common atrioventricular or tricuspid valve in patients with functionally single ventricle. Ann Thorac Surg 2007; 84: 1571–6.

20. Timek TA, Nielsen SL, Lai DT, et al. Mitral annular size predicts Alfieri stitch tension in mitral edge-to-edge repair. J Heart Valve Dis 2004; 13: 165–73.

21. Alfieri O, Maisano F, De Bonis M, et al. The double-orifice technique in mitral valve repair: a simple solution for complex problems. J Thorac Cardiovasc Surg 2001; 122: 674–81.

22. Maisano F, Redaelli A, Pennati G, et al. The hemodynamic effects of double-orifice valve repair for mitral regurgitation: a 3D computational model. Eur J Cardiothorac Surg 1999; 15: 419–25.

23. Agricola E, Maisano F, Oppizzi M, et al. Mitral valve reserve in double-orifice technique: an exercise echocardiographic study. J Heart Valve Dis 2002; 11: 637–43.

24. Frapier JM, Sportouch C, Rauzy V, et al. Mitral valve repair by alfieri's technique does not limit exercise tolerance more than carpentier's correction. Eur J Cardiothorac Surg 2006; 29: 1020–5.

4 Outcomes from surgical edge-to-edge repair
Francesco Maisano

The edge-to-edge (E2E) technique was developed by Alfieri in 1991 to treat mitral valve regurgitation in patients with complex anatomy, not suitable for repair with conventional techniques (1–5). The inspiration for the technique came from nature: it is not uncommon to observe well-functioning natural double-orifice mitral valves in otherwise healthy individuals. Alfieri noted such a congenital anomaly in a patient undergoing ostium secundum atrial septal defect surgical closure, who had a completely functioning mitral valve. The following day, he applied the double-orifice concept on a patient with complex anatomy not amenable for repair with conventional techniques. The E2E is technically simpler than other techniques. It can be used to treat various forms of organic and functional mitral regurgitation (MR). The surgical technique consists in the suturing of the free edge of the leaflets at the site of regurgitation, resulting in a valve with two orifices when the regurgitation originates from the middle scallops. For this reason E2E is also known as the "double-orifice" technique (Figs. 4.1, 4.2). In cases where the lesions involve one commissure, the suture of the leaflets determines the reduction of a valve area, but with single-orifice configuration (paracommissural repair). The E2E technique has been demonstrated safe, effective, and durable, even when applied in the most complex settings.

Initially the technique was applied selectively, often without annuloplasty, because of the fear of inducing mitral valve stenosis. As safety, effectiveness, and durability data became available, gradually the adoption of E2E technique was expanded and its application peaked in the year 2000 when it was used in about one-third of the patients undergoing mitral valve repair at San Raffaele Hospital, Italy. The most common indications were anterior and bileaflet disease and functional MR.

HEMODYNAMICS OF THE DOUBLE-ORIFICE REPAIR
The main concerns related to the E2E technique are the risk of mitral valve stenosis and the risk of suture dehiscence. Hemodynamic and structural effects of the E2E procedure have been evaluated with computational (6,7) and clinical studies, specifically addressing the issue of impairment of diastolic flow, and the stresses acting on the E2E suture. As a general rule, although mitral stenosis is a potential complication of the technique, this is rare in patients with pliable leaflets. In these patients, valve area reduction is clinically irrelevant if the sum of the area of the two orifices is above 1.5 cm²/m². Moreover, computational models have suggested that mitral valve hemodynamic behavior is not affected by the double-orifice configuration, even in the case of uneven orifices. The hemodynamics

of a double-orifice valve is comparable to that of a single-orifice valve with an area equal to the sum of the two orifice areas. In addition, a computer-model analysis suggested that a Doppler-derived analysis of the hemodynamics from one orifice flow closely represents the whole valve function (Fig. 4.1). Clinical echocardiographic studies confirmed these preliminary findings. Agricola et al. (8) reported normal response to exercise echocardiography in patients treated with the E2E technique. Interestingly, during exercise, planimetric valve area increases significantly (3.2 ± 0.6 cm² vs. 4.3 ± 0.7 cm², p < 0.00001), compared with baseline, suggesting that resting valve area may overestimate the reduction of valve area observed after the procedure. Subsequently, Hori et al. (9) observed that the response to exercise of patients treated with E2E repair is equal to those treated with conventional repairs with Carpentier techniques.

The risk of dehiscence of the E2E suture has not been common in our clinical experience. Computational studies have clarified that, particularly in case of nondilated annulus, the forces acting on the leaflets at the level of the suture are low and maximal in diastole, when the leaflets open, while in systole forces are distributed along the coaptation surface (7) and are not affecting the suture.

THE BASIC RULES OF A SUCCESSFUL SURGICAL E2E REPAIR
The ideal E2E surgical repair should completely incorporate the diseased segments, in order to close the origin of the regurgitant jet, an example being in the case of a redundant prolapsing leaflet, a long suture is necessary. Computational models suggest that a longer suture is associated with a reduced structural stress on the leaflets (7,10), although it determines a significant reduction of effective orifice area (40–50% reduction from baseline if the suture is positioned in the middle of the valve (11)). In addition to the suture length, valve area is determined by leaflet pliability. In case of fibrotic tissue (e.g., in the case of rheumatic disease), transmitral gradients are increased and the procedure is affected by limited durability (3). An eccentric position of the E2E suture, producing two uneven orifices, is not deleterious from a hemodynamic perspective. However, it is associated with a smaller decrease of the valve area and potentially facilitates improved structural stress distribution (10). All of these findings could possibly also apply to percutaneous clip-based E2E repair. Another important requirement for effective and durable E2E repair is with respect to valve symmetry. Asymmetric suturing leads to leaflet distortion with limited efficacy and potential for later dehiscence.

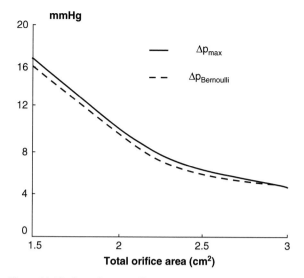

Figure 4.1 The hemodynamic effects of the double-orifice repair: total valve area and prediction of transvalvular gradient. Influence of the total orifice area (sum of the areas of the two orifices) on the transvalvular pressure gradients at diastolic peak flow (11 l/min). Δp_{max} = peak gradient calculated by fluid dynamic computational models. $\Delta p_{bernoulli}$ = peak pressure gradient calculated by the simplified Bernoulli formula ($\Delta p = 4V^2 max$). *Source*: From Ref. 31.

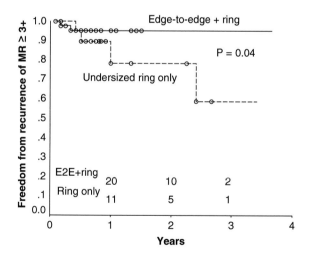

Figure 4.2 The role of the edge-to-edge (E2E) repair as an adjunct to undersized annuloplasty in the treatment of functional mitral regurgitation (MR). Freedom from recurrence of MR grade 3+ or more in the E2E plus annuloplasty and in the annuloplasty-only group. *Source*: From Ref. 26.

Suture depth (the amount of tissue incorporated in the suture bites) varied in our surgical experience: in patients with redundant tissue (e.g., with Barlow's disease), deeper suture bites were used to reduce the excess of tissue while in ischemic and functional MR, suture bites were superficial, to minimize loss of coaptation surface. Originally, the E2E sutures were reinforced with felt pledgets, but continuous sutures have been used in the majority of patients, with the same durability.

CLINICAL OUTCOMES IN DEGENERATIVE MITRAL REGURGITATION

The first relatively large series of patients treated with the E2E technique was reported in 1998 (5): the analysis included 121 patients operated between 1991 and 1997 (out of 432 mitral valve repairs performed in the same period). Patients included in this series suffered primarily from complex anatomic pathology and, at the time would be otherwise corrected with valve replacement. Most patients had degenerative disease with anterior or bileaflet disease, but the series also included patients with endocarditis, and rheumatic and ischemic disease. A double-orifice repair versus paracommissural E2E was done in 60% and 40%, respectively. Annuloplasty was performed in 93% of patients. Annuloplasty was intentionally not performed in the presence of a small mitral annulus (six patients) or rheumatic disease (two patients). Excluding annuloplasty, the E2E was effective as a stand-alone repair technique in 73% of cases, even in the case of complex or multiple lesions. Hospital mortality was 1.6% and six-year actuarial survival was $92 \pm 3.1\%$. Freedom from reoperation was $95 \pm 4.8\%$ for the overall group. No patients with isolated posterior leaflet prolapse required reoperation during the follow-up period, whereas $98 \pm 1.6\%$ of patients with isolated anterior leaflet prolapse were free from reoperation. Echocardiographic follow-up showed a mean degree of MR of 0.4 ± 0.83 with 91% of patients having no or trivial MR, and a mean valve area of 3.0 ± 1 cm^2.

One of the main current indications for the E2E technique is complex Barlow's disease with bileaflet prolapse. We published a series of studies on 82 patients with Barlow's disease and bileaflet prolapse treated with the E2E technique with a standardized approach (4): in all cases with multisegment prolapse a central E2E suture incorporating about 1–2 cm of the free edge of the A2 and P2 region was associated with complete ring annuloplasty (annuloplasty was not performed in eight patients with calcified annulus). The combination of ring annuloplasty and central E2E technique was sufficient to treat the majority of patients even in the presence of multiple regurgitant jets. Only eight patients received quadrangular resection of the posterior leaflet in addition to the E2E, four patients had subcommissure closure and three patients had additional commissural E2E.

The main value of the E2E technique was the possibility of treating anterior leaflet lesions with a simple and reproducible technique. In the 1990s, most patients with anterior lesions would undergo mitral valve replacement (2). Later, we demonstrated that the E2E technique has been the first repair technique neutralizing the presence of anterior leaflet lesions as risk factor for repair failure. De Bonis et al. (12) compared the long-term outcomes of 122 patients with anterior leaflet (13) prolapse treated by the E2E repair to 605 patients with posterior leaflet prolapse disease treated with conventional quadrangular resection. In all patients concomitant annuloplasty was used to complete the repair. No hospital deaths occurred in the E2E group while two (0.3%) patients treated by quadrangular resection died prior to discharge. At 10 years, overall survival was $91 \pm 4\%$ for anterior leaflet prolapse (treated with the E2E technique) and 93 ± 2% for posterior leaflet prolapse (treated by quadrangular resection, p = 0.18). Freedom from reoperation was 96 ± 2% and 96 ± 1% in the E2E and quadrangular resection group, respectively (P = 0.37). Echocardiographic follow-up showed comparable freedom from moderate or severe MR for the two techniques (14,15) clearly supporting the conclusion that the E2E technique abolishes the effect of anterior leaflet prolapse as a risk factor for shorter durability of repair.

Adding to the conclusions of our series, other international groups reported their experience with the E2E technique in the setting of degenerative disease, confirming the above-mentioned results (16–20). In most occasions, the technique was used in challenging environments such as in the presence of complex anatomy, a minimally invasive or robotic surgery (21,22). The E2E repair has been successfully used to treat postsurgical systolic anterior motion of the anterior leaflet, a challenging complication following mitral valve repair with conventional techniques (more commonly after quadrangular resection of the posterior leaflet and annuloplasty).

The E2E technique has been used also as a "magic tool" in an attempt to correct residual MR following a failed previous repair with conventional techniques. The reported data suggest that although early results of the E2E repair used as a bailout can be satisfactory (23), long-term results are suboptimal (24). It has to be noted that most of the detractors of the technique have applied the E2E technique mainly with this application, further contributing to the aura of skepticism associated with the procedure. On the other hand, if a previous attempt of repair has failed, the cause of the failure of the E2E repair could be lack of understanding of the mechanism of the regurgitation or technical mistakes related to the previously performed techniques (e.g., restricted motion due to excessive tissue resection or tissue distortions).

The E2E repair has been successfully applied to treat commissural lesions (25), both as an isolated and as an associated procedure, and also both in the case of degenerative or functional MR. In the situation of commissural prolapse, the E2E technique is both more reproducible and simpler than other techniques, while carrying very little risk of mitral stenosis. Therefore it has become the technique of choice in our practice for all commissural prolapse cases.

CLINICAL OUTCOMES IN FUNCTIONAL MITRAL REGURGITATION

Undersized annuloplasty has been, for many years, the gold standard technique to treat functional mitral valve regurgitation. However, this technique is associated with suboptimal durability in some patients, particularly those with more pronounced left ventricular remodeling. In an attempt to improve the outcomes of isolated undersized annuloplasty, the Alfieri technique has been effectively used to treat functional MR (5,16,26). The E2E suture was positioned in the center of the valve or at the commissure, according to the position of the regurgitant orifice on preoperative echocardiography. The E2E

repair has been usually performed in selected patients, with more advanced remodeling, and particularly in those with a coaptation depth longer than 10 mm. This threshold of coaptation depth has been associated with a shorter durability of undersized annuloplasty (27). In a retrospective analysis, the addition of the E2E repair has been identified as the only predictor of repair durability (26) in patients undergoing undersized annuloplasty to treat functional MR: 77 patients (51 ischemic), were treated either with undersized annuloplasty alone (in 23 patients) or in association with the E2E suture (in 54 patients). The combination of E2E and annuloplasty was selectively used in patients with a coaptation depth greater than 10 mm. Although patients receiving the E2E in addition to annuloplasty had more advanced ventricular and valve remodeling compared with those receiving annuloplasty alone, mitral repair failure (defined as recurrence of MR greater than or equal to 3/4) was documented in two patients in the E2E (3.7%) and in 5 (21.7%) in the isolated annuloplasty group (P = 0.03). Freedom from repair failure at 1.5 years was 95 ± 3% and 77 ± 12% (P = 0.04), respectively (Fig. 4.2).

The edge-to edge repair has also been used in combination with left ventricular remodeling, often as a stand-alone procedure without annuloplasty, to treat concomitant MR (28). However, isolated surgical E2E without annuloplasty has not been always effective to treat functional MR in our personal experience. Indeed it was surprising to learn that, on the contrary, the isolated MitraClip® (Abbott Vascular Inc, Santa Rosa CA, USA) procedure can be very effective in the treatment of functional MR. The different behavior is probably related to the difference in the mechanism of action of the suture-based to the clip-based E2E technique.

THE EDGE-TO-EDGE TECHNIQUE IN OTHER SETTINGS

The E2E repair has been successfully used in other uncommon settings. Several patients have been treated with the technique to correct systolic anterior motion in the context of hypertrophic cardiomyopathy (29). The technique has been used to treat secondary MR in patients undergoing aortic valve surgery, to reduce the operative times and control the operative risk, usually with a transaortic approach. Although we have been using the technique to treat rheumatic disease patients, we discontinued to do so, due to poor long-term outcomes and owing to the intrinsic risk of high transvalvular gradients in the presence of leaflets with limited pliability (3).

EDGE-TO-EDGE WITHOUT ANNULOPLASTY

The addition of annuloplasty at the end of leaflet repair is a standard practice in surgical mitral repair, due to the evidence of better early and long-term results in the overall population (15). Annuloplasty is known to reduce the stress acting on valve structures following repair, mainly due to the increase of coaptation. In addition, in cases of new lesions occurring after repair, the presence of a ring annuloplasty is thought to be protective by limiting the amount of recurrent regurgitation. The same concepts apply to the E2E technique: in the overall population, the absence of the annuloplasty has been associated with shorter durability and higher risk of reintervention following the Alfieri technique (3). Initially, several patients were treated without annuloplasty because of the fear of creating a stenotic valve. When initial clinical data excluded a meaningful risk of mitral stenosis, a ring has been routinely implanted in nearly all patients. It was still omitted in selected cases. In the presence of severe annular calcification, annuloplasty was omitted due to the technical challenge of suturing the ring into the calcified tissue, and in the hope that no further dilatation would occur (although it has to be noted that usually the calcified annulus is also dilated). Annuloplasty was also omitted in the early experience of minimally invasive and robotic interventions (to reduce operative times), in the presence of endocarditis (for the risk of prosthesis infection), and in patients with rheumatic disease due to the relatively small valve area and the intrinsic risk of creating mitral stenosis. Finally, the ring was often removed when the E2E technique was used as a bailout, following a failed attempt of repair. This was again perceived as a mandatory step to avoid mitral stenosis in a patient who had received leaflet resections and or annular plications. We reported the mid-term results of 81 patients treated with the E2E repair without annuloplasty, in an attempt to clarify the role of the isolated E2E concept. The majority of patients had degenerative and functional disease but the series also included six patients with rheumatic disease, four with endocarditis (active in one), and two with hypertrophic cardiomyopathy and systolic anterior motion. The series was characterized by an overall short survival. This outcome was probably related to the challenging case mix (85% ± 7% survival at four years). The overall freedom from reoperation was 89% ± 3.9% at four years. The main predictors of residual or recurrent MR were annular calcification and residual MR at the end of the procedure. Reoperation rate was 77% ± 22% versus 95% ± 4.6% in the calcified (Fig. 4.3) versus noncalcified annulus (p = 0.03) and late failure was predicted by the early suboptimal result assessed either by intraoperative saline testing or by transesophageal echocardiography soon after the discontinuation of cardiopulmonary bypass (24). Although the overall results were suboptimal, selected patients who received the isolated E2E repair without annuloplasty in the absence of annular calcification or other high-risk-specific conditions (e.g., rheumatic disease, endocarditis, rescue repair, etc.) had a mid-term durability comparable with that observed in patients undergoing repair with annuloplasty. Since we felt that the option of not implanting a ring after the E2E repair was not intentional in most cases, but was mainly driven by complex conditions, a post-hoc analysis of the long-term outcomes of a subgroup of patients in whom the decision to avoid annuloplasty was intentional was carried out. The study showed that the isolated E2E procedure, in selected patients with relatively preserved annular size and function, has the same efficacy and durability as conventional repair techniques with annuloplasty (30). Hospital mortality in this subset of patients was 3.4% (due to one patient with functional MR who died of postoperative low-cardiac output syndrome and multiorgan failure). There was one late death (sudden death four years after the operation) in a patient with functional MR and left ventricular dysfunction. Cause of death in this patient was not related to recurrent MR (trivial at the last examination before death). Two patients had uneventful mitral valve replacement four years after isolated E2E repair because of recurrent MR. There was one readmission for heart failure in a patient who had E2E repair and left ventricular restoration. At the latest follow-up, 19 patients (68%) were in New York Heart Association (NYHA) class I, 8 (28%) in class II, and 1 (4%) in class III. No patients were in NYHA class IV.

At early postoperative assessment, 28 patients (97%) had at least a 2 grade MR reduction compared with baseline. One patient with preoperative moderate MR (of ischemic origin) had no early improvement, but MR remained stable during follow-up. The patient with the longest follow-up (12 years) showed trace MR at the latest follow-up, similar to the pre-discharge MR severity. Compared with the pre-discharge echocardiographic examination, about one-third of patients (11/28) showed a tendency of recurrence of MR over time. However at the latest follow-up, only two patients (7%) had progressed to moderate MR and two (7%) to severe MR. Both patients required reoperation. At a median follow-up of 6.3 years, 86% (24/28) of patients had an MR grade ≤2+. Freedom from the combined endpoint of reoperation and recurrence of MR >2+ was 90 ± 5% at 5 years (Fig. 4.4).

Although the small size of the patient cohort is a major limitation of this study, these findings were the clinical proof of concept for the isolated percutaneous treatment. Today the MitraClip® procedure is effectively performed as an isolated procedure with meaningful MR reduction in most patients. It is

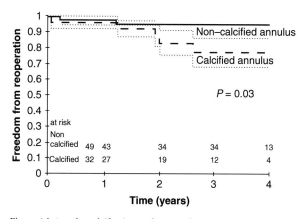

Figure 4.3 Annular calcification as the main determinant of repair failure in patients undergoing standalone edge-to-edge (E2E) repair without annuloplasty. Freedom from reoperation in patients undergoing stand-alone E2E repair without annuloplasty: the role of annular calcification. *Source*: From Ref. 24.

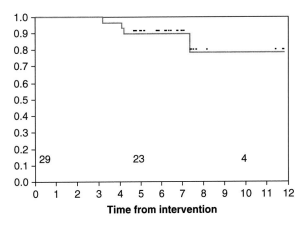

Figure 4.4 The proof of concept of isolated edge-to-edge repair without annuloplasty. Freedom from combined endpoint of reoperation and recurrence of mitral regurgitation greater than 2+ in selected patients undergoing isolated E2E repair without annuloplasty. *Source*: From Ref. 30.

probable that the addition of a percutaneous annuloplasty will improve in selective patients the ability of the MitraClip® to reduce MR and expand the applicability of the procedure. How much this will translate into a meaningful improvement in clinical benefit remains to be determined.

CONFLICTS OF INTEREST
F. Maisano is a consultant for Abbott Vascular.

REFERENCES

1. Alfieri O, De Bonis M, Lapenna E, et al. "Edge-to-edge" repair for anterior mitral leaflet prolapse. Semin Thorac Cardiovasc Surg 2004; 16: 182–7.
2. Alfieri O, Maisano F. An effective technique to correct anterior mitral leaflet prolapse. J Card Surg 1999; 14: 468–70.
3. Alfieri O, Maisano F, De Bonis M, et al. The double-orifice technique in mitral valve repair: a simple solution for complex problems. J Thorac Cardiovasc Surg 2001; 122: 674–81.
4. Maisano F, Schreuder JJ, Oppizzi M, et al. The double-orifice technique as a standardized approach to treat mitral regurgitation due to severe myxomatous disease: surgical technique. Eur J Cardiothorac Surg 2000; 17: 201–5.
5. Maisano F, Torracca L, Oppizzi M, et al. The edge-to-edge technique: a simplified method to correct mitral insufficiency. Eur J Cardiothorac Surg 1998; 13: 240–5; discussion 5–6.
6. Redaelli A, Guadagni G, Fumero R, Maisano F, Alfieri O. A computational study of the hemodynamics after "edge-to-edge" mitral valve repair. J Biomech Eng 2001; 123: 565–70.
7. Votta E, Maisano F, Soncini M, et al. 3-D computational analysis of the stress distribution on the leaflets after edge-to-edge repair of mitral regurgitation. J Heart Valve Dis 2002; 11: 810–22.
8. Agricola E, Maisano F, Oppizzi M, et al. Mitral valve reserve in double-orifice technique: an exercise echocardiographic study. J Heart Valve Dis 2002; 11: 637–43.
9. Hori H, Fukunaga S, Arinaga K, et al. Edge-to-edge repair for mitral regurgitation: a clinical and exercise echocardiographic study. J Heart Valve Dis 2008; 17: 476–84.
10. Dal Pan F, Donzella G, Fucci C, Schreiber M. Structural effects of an innovative surgical technique to repair heart valve defects. J Biomech 2005; 38: 2460–71.
11. Gaillard E, Eng LK, Durand LG. A simple non-invasive method to predict the mitral valve geometric orifice area after edge-to-edge repair. J Heart Valve Dis 2011; 20: 1–4.
12. De Bonis M, Lorusso R, Lapenna E, et al. Similar long-term results of mitral valve repair for anterior compared with posterior leaflet prolapse. J Thorac Cardiovasc Surg 2006; 131: 364–70.
13. Brinster DR, Unic D, D'Ambra MN, Nathan N, Cohn LH. Midterm results of the edge-to-edge technique for complex mitral valve repair. Ann Thorac Surg 2006; 81: 1612–17.
14. Mohty D, Orszulak TA, Schaff HV, et al. Very long-term survival and durability of mitral valve repair for mitral valve prolapse. Circulation 2001; 104(12 Suppl 1): I1–7.
15. Gillinov AM, Cosgrove DM, Blackstone EH, et al. Durability of mitral valve repair for degenerative disease. J Thorac Cardiovasc Surg 1998; 116: 734–43.
16. Bhudia SK, McCarthy PM, Smedira NG, et al. Edge-to-edge (Alfieri) mitral repair: results in diverse clinical settings. Ann Thorac Surg 2004; 77: 1598–606.
17. Raman J, Shah P, Seevanayagam S, Cheung J, Buxton B. Mitral regurgitation: comparison between edge-to-edge repair and valve replacement. Asian Cardiovasc Thorac Ann 2003; 11: 131–4.
18. Kuduvalli M, Ghotkar SV, Grayson AD, Fabri BM. Edge-to-edge technique for mitral valve repair: medium-term results with echocardiographic follow-up. Ann Thorac Surg 2006; 82: 1356–61.
19. Oc M, Doukas G, Alexiou C, et al. Edge-to-edge repair with mitral annuloplasty for barlow's disease. Ann Thorac Surg 2005; 80: 1315–18.
20. Kherani AR, Cheema FH, Casher J, et al. Edge-to-edge mitral valve repair: the Columbia Presbyterian experience. Ann Thorac Surg 2004; 78: 73–6.
21. Lapenna E, Torracca L, De Bonis M, et al. Minimally invasive mitral valve repair in the context of barlow's disease. Ann Thorac Surg 2005; 79: 1496–9.
22. Chitwood WR, Jr. Rodriguez E, Chu MW, et al. Robotic mitral valve repairs in 300 patients: a single-center experience. J Thorac Cardiovasc Surg 2008; 136: 436–41.
23. Gatti G, Cardu G, Trane R, Pugliese P. The edge-to-edge technique as a trick to rescue an imperfect mitral valve repair. Eur J Cardiothorac Surg 2002; 22: 817–20.
24. Maisano F, Caldarola A, Blasio A, et al. Midterm results of edge-to-edge mitral valve repair without annuloplasty. J Thorac Cardiovasc Surg 2003; 126: 1987–97.
25. Lapenna E, De Bonis M, Sorrentino F, et al. Commissural closure for the treatment of commissural mitral valve prolapse or flail. J Heart Valve Dis 2008; 17: 261–6.
26. De Bonis M, Lapenna E, La Canna G, et al. Mitral valve repair for functional mitral regurgitation in end-stage dilated cardiomyopathy: role of the "edge-to-edge" technique. Circulation 2005; 112(Suppl 9): I402–8.

27. Calafiore AM, Di Mauro M, Gallina S, et al. Mitral valve surgery for chronic ischemic mitral regurgitation. Ann Thorac Surg 2004; 77: 1989–97.

28. Sartipy U, Albage A, Mattsson E, Lindblom D. Edge-to-edge mitral repair without annuloplasty in combination with surgical ventricular restoration. Ann Thorac Surg 2007; 83: 1303–9.

29. Pereda D, Topilsky Y, Nishimura RA, Park SJ. Asymmetric Alfieri's stitch to correct systolic anterior motion after mitral valve repair. Eur J Cardiothorac Surg 2010.

30. Maisano F, Vigano G, Blasio A, et al. Surgical isolated edge-to-edge mitral valve repair without annuloplasty: clinical proof of the principle for an endovascular approach. EuroIntervention 2006; 2: 181–6.

31. Maisano F, Redaelli A, Pennati G, et al. The hemodynamic effects of double-orifice valve repair for mitral regurgitation: a 3D computational model. Eur J Cardiothorac Surg 1999; 15: 419–25.

5 An overview of the literature on surgical mitral valve repair
Sophie Jones, Michael Argenziano, and Allan Schwartz

INTRODUCTION

Mitral valve disease affects an estimated 2.5 million people in the United States, a number that is expected to double by 2030 (1). With this disease prevalence, mitral valve surgery constitutes up to one-third of all cardiac procedures. When evaluating mitral disease, regurgitation and stenosis are considered separately. For the purposes of this text, the focus will be on mitral regurgitation (MR). MR can be subdivided into categories based on the underlying pathology. Primary or "degenerative" disease broadly defines pathology affecting the valve leaflets and chordae. This is also referred to as "structural" mitral valve disease. Primary MR affects approximately 2% of the population and is the most common type of MR encountered in the surgical setting. Secondary or "functional" disease results from valve misalignment caused by a shift in the geometry of the left ventricle. Changes in the left ventricular geometry occur with either local remodeling of the ventricle due to an infarct or global remodeling due to dilated cardiomyopathy. In particular, MR is often observed after an inferior or posterior infarct causing malalignment of the papillary muscles and tethering of the mitral leaflets. Changes in the ventricular geometry also result in annular dilation, which exacerbates MR.

The most common method of classifying MR is the Carpentier Classification System. This system categorizes disease by leaflet activity on echocardiography. MR is divided into three categories: normal leaflet motion with annular dilation, increased leaflet motion, or restricted leaflet motion (2,3). Considerations for surgical repair utilize this classification as an adjunct to considerations based on disease causality.

SURGICAL RISK ASSESSMENT

When considering surgical correction of mitral valve pathology, risks and benefits to the patient must be carefully considered. Medical management of MR is limited to symptom control and treatment of the consequences of MR—atrial fibrillation and congestive heart failure in structural disease, and control of underlying left ventricular disease in the case of functional MR (4,5). In structural MR, surgical correction, if initiated early, prevents irreversible left ventricular dysfunction and symptoms of heart failure (6). In severe MR, no medical therapy is known to favorably alter the natural history of this disease (7,8). Thus, surgical therapy is indicated with the presence of symptoms (usually dyspnea and fatigue) or, in the absence of symptoms, evidence of severe MR with or without left ventricular enlargement, pulmonary hypertension, or atrial fibrillation. Functional disease, on the other hand, cannot be corrected through an isolated valve intervention without concomitant therapy targeted at controlling the underlying ventricular disease. Further, the impact of correction on prognosis is not so well defined, which further obfuscates the decision-making process.

Echocardiography serves as the gold standard for evaluation of the valve, as well as surgical planning. Transthoracic echocardiography is recommended for all adult patients suspected of having mitral valve disease, with or without the presence of symptoms (9). Echocardiography allows for a comprehensive evaluation of valvular structure, mechanism of regurgitation, and degree of compensatory change resulting from volume overload. An accurate assessment of mitral regurgitant severity can be obtained through measurements of the valve orifice area, regurgitant jet area, jet volume, regurgitant fraction, and the width of the vena contracta—the narrowest portion of a jet that occurs at or just downstream from the orifice (10).

In all-comers, valvular surgery poses an increased risk in perioperative mortality in comparison with other cardiac surgeries, exclusive of the aorta. One bedside assessment tool to aid physicians and patients in the decision-making process is the European System for Cardiac Operative Risk Evaluation, the EuroSCORE, first introduced in 1999. It is primarily reflective of the impact of comorbidities and New York Heart Association (NYHA) functional class (11,12). There have been several other attempts at classifying patients' surgical risk specific to mitral valve surgery. One such score developed in the United States by Norwicki et al. evaluated short-term mortality in patients undergoing either mitral or aortic valve surgery (13). While this score is more specific to valvular disease assessment, it focuses on patient comorbidities as a guide to risk assessment, just as the EuroSCORE does. At the present time, there is no universal bedside score that has demonstrated wide applicability. Instead, best-practice guidelines have been developed by the American College of Cardiology/American Heart Association Task Force on Practice Guidelines. While these guidelines are highly involved, they are currently the only reference that adequately addresses the nature of the disease—structural versus functional—as well as the state of the valve and ventricle on echocardiography, in the overall assessment of surgical risk (14–16). Finally, while the nature of the disease itself is paramount in the evaluation of surgical risk, multiple studies including one large series by Bolling et al. (2010) have demonstrated that surgeon's experience (17,18), as well as institutional volume (19) also play key roles, and must be taken into account when assessing a patient's overall surgical risk.

Mitral Valve Replacement vs. Mitral Valve Repair

It has been demonstrated that patients with severe structural MR benefit from early repair, before the occurrence of irreversible left ventricular dysfunction, fixed pulmonary hypertension, or atrial fibrillation (20). The advantage of repair over replacement is multifaceted. First, repair carries a lower operative risk. Second, it does not expose the patient to the risks associated with a prosthetic mitral valve, namely long-term anticoagulation requirement, thromboembolism, and in the case of tissue valves, degeneration (21). Repair of the native valve also allows for a return to the native physiologic construction of the heart. Papillary attachments to the valve have been shown to shape the ventricle in a way that prosthetic valves have been unable to replicate. Thus, a native valve repair potentially acts on both the valve as well as the ventricle. As a result, the ventricular function improves (22,23).

In general, mitral valve replacement is performed when mitral valve repair is not reasonable. This is particularly true in primary MR. Some high-volume centers report greater than 90% of mitral valve surgeries being completed in this way (24). In the case of functional MR, whether the procedure of choice is repair or replacement is the subject of debate. Replacement may also be indicated in patients with either structural or functional pathologies, when the nature of the disease makes repair unfeasible. This can be seen in end-stage Barlow's disease, severe and progressive rheumatic disease, or in the case of extensive and surgically limiting valvular calcifications. Although, as noted above, surgical experience as well as institutional factors lead to wide variations, it is the extent of pathology that is deemed repairable (25). Overall, surgical techniques focus on retaining as much of the apparatus as possible, while correcting malcoaptation and restoring the annulus.

Techniques for Mitral Valve Repair

Patients with more complex pathologies may require different approaches. Although anterior leaflet prolapse occurs less frequently than posterior leaflet prolapse, it requires specific surgical consideration. When anterior leaflet abnormalities are due to chordal rupture, a chordal transfer procedure should be performed to reapproximate the leaflets. In this technique, a healthy primary or secondary posterior chorda and its corresponding leaflet segment are detached with papillary connections maintained intact. The segment is then transferred to the prolapsed anterior leaflet with the chordal rupture and attached onto the ventricular side. The resulting gap in the posterior leaflet is repaired by reapproximation of the leaflets with a simple running suture.

Chordal replacement is also a viable option that may result in a more physiologic repair than the classic quadrangular repair (27,28). Polytetrafluoroethylene (PTFE) neochordae are the preferred material and have shown favorable outcomes in patients undergoing repair with this procedure. The PTFE is anchored in the fibrous area of the papillary muscle and then attached to the free, prolapsed leaflet segment. Of particular importance is avoidance of the midline and contact with other chordae. This technique requires the surgeon to measure out an appropriate chordal length, presenting a challenge that is avoided in chordal transfer. An appropriate length is one that restores the line of coaptation and resolves the prolapse.

The edge-to-edge or Alfieri technique has been utilized for more complex pathologies (29). The technique involves suturing of the labile leaflet to its leaflet counterpart thereby artificially coapting the two leaflets. This is particularly useful in patients with high surgical risk, as this repair allows for shorter cross-clamp and operative times. Also, those patients with significant annular calcification who may not be candidates for other forms of repair may do well with the Alfieri approach, because involvement of the annulus in the repair is not necessary. Patients with posterior annular calcification and anterior chordal rupture may also be unsuitable for traditional resection. In this situation, the Alfieri technique stabilizes the anterior leaflet while avoiding the complexities of repairing a calcified posterior leaflet. This presents a controversial solution, as a double orifice valve is created. However, this technique has been shown to have satisfactory freedom from complication and reoperation, as well as reduction in cross-clamp times.

Along with repair of the mitral valve, most patients require annuloplasty to correct for pathologic annular dilation. Patients with severe MR generally have some degree of annular enlargement, usually occurring along the posterior annulus. There is a wide range of prosthetic annular rings/bands and all have been shown to be effective in correcting dilation, realigning the plane of coaptation, and preventing future annular dilation. Interrupted sutures are secured in the firm annular tissue and secured to the prosthetic, with care taken to ensure an even alignment with the native annulus. Patients with a calcified annulus may require debridement before annuloplasty.

Current Surgical Outcomes in Mitral Valve Repair
Structural Mitral Valve Disease
Surgical outcomes after mitral valve repair should be considered in two categories: repairs for structural disease and repairs for functional MR. Surgical correction of structural MR has widely demonstrated repair to be superior to replacement. Durability of repairs has also significantly increased over the past two decades. One study by Suri et al. (2006) evaluated 1411 patients undergoing mitral valve repair or replacement for leaflet prolapse. This study found repair to be superior in long-term survival with long-term reoperation rates similar to those who underwent replacement (30).

In another study by Gillinov et al. (2008) in which 3286 patients undergoing mitral valve replacement or repair during the years 1985–2005 were evaluated. This study sought to identify patient factors associated with repair versus replacement. Overall, patients who underwent replacement were older, had more complex valvular pathology, and had more severe left ventricular dysfunction. This study showed that survival at 5, 10, and 15 years was 95%, 87%, and 68% after repair and 80%, 60%, and 44% after replacement. However, when the analysis was performed among propensity-matched patients, survival trended more toward similar results—86% after repair versus

83% for replacement (p = 0.8) at 5 years, 63% versus 62% at 10 years, and 43% versus 48% at 15 years. Further, freedom from reoperation revealed similar trends among propensity-matched patients—94% at 5 and 10 years after repair and 95% and 92% at 5 and 10 years after replacement (p = 0.6). It follows from this study that repair is indicated over replacement in most circumstances. However, among selected patients with complex valvular pathologies it is likely that replacement is a safe and durable procedure. It should also be noted the risk of reoperation was elevated when patients did not undergo ring annuloplasty at the time of initial operation (31).

More recently, Flameng (2008) reviewed recurrence rates after surgical correction of structural valve disease. In a series of 348 patients with serial echocardiographic evaluation, freedom from reoperation at 10 years remained 94%. However, only 65% of patients were free of MR recurrence of greater than 2/4+. There was a linear recurrence rate of 8.3% per year for MR greater than 1/4, and a recurrence of 3.2% per year for MR greater than 2/4. Similar trends were demonstrated by David (2007) in a review of 649 patients undergoing isolated mitral valve repairs for structural MR. However, this series notably revealed a recurrence rate of 30% at 15 years for MR greater than 2/4. These studies demonstrate that, while patients appear to do well from the standpoint of symptom minimization and freedom from reoperation, current surgical management is only able to achieve a modest long-term rate of freedom from recurrence.

Functional Mitral Valve Disease

The possible goals of surgical valve correction in the treatment of functional MR are to halt ventricular remodeling, improve NYHA functional class, decrease hospitalizations for congestive heart failure exacerbations, and improve survival. Functional disease is most often treated with reduction annuloplasty in order to restore valve coaptation. One study by Bolling (2002) described 140 patients with refractory MR and end-stage cardiomyopathy undergoing mitral valve repair. All repairs utilized an undersized flexible annuloplasty ring to allow for appropriate valve coaptation. This study demonstrated that first, operative risk was reasonable given the number and perioperative mortality in these patients were similar to that of patients undergoing mitral valve repair for structural disease. Further, two-year follow-up demonstrated significant symptom improvement. Namely, the entire cohort went from NYHA class III/IV to NYHA class I/II, with improvements in ejection fraction, cardiac output, end-diastolic volumes, sphericity index, and regurgitant volumes (32). Badhwar and Bolling (2002) further evaluated these data and were able to demonstrate that mitral valve reconstruction with annuloplasty provided an appropriate first-line management strategy for patients with severe MR and end-stage heart failure (33). That being said, the propensity analysis of Bolling's data showed no surgical mortality benefit and other studies have failed to demonstrate a decrease in mortality after coronary artery bypass

grafting for ischemic heart disease when concurrent mitral valve surgery was performed (34). Recent data published as part of the "Acorn Trial" (Acker et al. 2011) evaluated cardiac function after mitral valve repair including application of a CorCap cardiac support device (Acorn Cardiovascular, St. Paul, Minnesota, USA)—a mesh wrap around the ventricle that was shown to improve the ventricle shape in heart failure patients. Specifically, of the 193 patients who underwent mitral valve repair, 30-day mortality was 1.6%. However, the patient population was largely made up of patients with non-ischemic-dilated cardiomyopathy, and is not generalizable to patients with ischemic disease. Further, only 59% of patients in this trial had severe MR at the time of surgery due to achievement of maximal medical management prior to surgery in this controlled study population. Also, while the study did demonstrate positive ventricular remodeling in the MR group, it is unclear what contributions the CorCap device provided in this regard. Thus, this study is in ultimately unable to provide clear evidence that valvular intervention in functional disease offers long-term benefit in the more heterogeneous population of patients with functional MR (35).

Among patients undergoing mitral repair for functional disease, there has been a notable rate of recurrent MR among patients undergoing annuloplasty for end-stage heart failure. One study by McGee et al. (2004) evaluated 585 patients who underwent annuloplasty over the years 1985–2002. This study demonstrated a decrease in patients with 0 or 1+ MR from 71% to 41%, whereas the proportion with 3+ or 4+ regurgitation increased from 13% to 28% over the first six post-operative months. In spite of the high recurrence rate, freedom from reoperation remained 97% at five years. Of note, these conclusions must be considered in the setting of a large proportion of patients lost to follow-up after their initial postoperative visits, with only 17% of patients having echocardiography greater than a year out. This may have falsely elevated the percentage of patients with recurrent disease, as symptom-free patients self-selected out of the study (36).

Another study by Lee et al. (2009) sought to address the causes of recurrent MR through echo evaluation of cardiac structure. Recurrence was defined as ≥2+ regurgitation on echocardiography. Of the 104 patients undergoing ring annuloplasty for end-stage heart failure, 24% developed recurrence. Patients with recurrence showed evidence of an exaggerated distal mitral anterior leaflet angle (ALAtip) and basal mitral anterior leaflet angle, greater coaptation depth, larger left ventricular volumes, and worse left ventricular ejection fraction. On regression analysis, ALAtip was specifically shown to be the major determinant of recurrent MR (37).

Relation of Surgeon Volume to Outcome

As demonstrated in the above studies, the safety and outcomes of mitral valve repair have proven to be excellent in terms of perioperative mortality and long-term rates of freedom from reoperation in spite of the only modest ability to prevent recurrence of disease. Notably, high volume surgeons as well as hospitals specializing in valvular disease have shown the best outcomes. Gammie et al. (2006) demonstrated procedural outcomes with an unadjusted mortality rate of 3% in the lowest-volume centers (performing 20–30 cases per year), compared with 1% in the highest-volume centers (performing 400+ mitral valve procedures per year), with the number of successful repairs versus replacements almost double in high-volume centers (38,39). Bolling et al. (2010) demonstrated in a review of patients in 639 institutions that increased surgeon volume was an independent predictor of successful valve repair, with the rate of repair increasing in an exponential pattern in surgeons performing greater than 20 mitral valve operations per year.

Barriers to Treatment and Guideline Adherence
While current best-practice guidelines encourage early surgical referral in patients with structural mitral valve disease, it has been repeatedly demonstrated that multiple barriers prevent referral from a cardiologist to a surgeon. Amongst those barriers, are patient age and comorbidities, as well as a commonly held tenet by both patients and physicians that surgery is a late-stage resort that should be avoided if alternatives exist (40–42). However, as options for valve repair have expanded rapidly in recent years, so too has the potential to definitively treat a broader category of patients. At the present time, reparative surgery is still considered the gold standard, but newer interventions—both minimally invasive as well as percutaneous procedures such as the MitraClip®—are potentially allowing a wider range of patients to become candidates for mitral valve intervention. Further trials are clearly needed to define the role of mitral valve repair for functional MR, where surgical therapy has not been able to demonstrate a survival benefit in the face of elevated surgical risk.

SUMMARY

Surgical repair for degenerative MR has been highly successful with excellent outcomes. Repair is clearly superior to replacement in this setting. While annuloplasty for functional MR may reduce MR, recurrences are common and mortality benefits are nil, because the underlying left ventricular disease is not treated. Surgical outcomes are significantly related to surgeon and site mitral surgery volumes. Referral of patients with degenerative MR when the LV ejection fraction falls below 60%, even in the absence of symptoms, is a critical step in patient management.

REFERENCES

1. Nkomo V\T, Gardin JM, Skelton TN, et al. Burden of valvular heart diseases: a population-based study. Lancet 2006; 368: 1005–11.
2. i Carpentier A, Chauvaud S, Fabiane al. Reconstructive surgery of mitral valve incompetence: ten-year appraisal. J Thorac Cardiovasc Surg 1980; 79: 338–48.
3. de Marchena E, Badiye A, Robalino G, et al. Respective prevalence of the different carpentier classes of mitral regurgitation: a

stepping stone for future therapeutic research and development. J Card Surg 2011; 26: 385–92.
4. Stevenson LW, Bellil D, Grover-McKay M, et al. Effects of afterload reduction (diuretics and vasodilators) on left ventricular volume and mitral regurgitation in severe congestive heart failure secondary to ischemic or idiopathic dilated cardiomyopathy. Am J Cardiol 1987; 60: 654–8.
5. Rosenhek R, Iung B, Tornos P, et al. ESC working group on valvular heart disease position paper: assessing the risk of intervention in patients with valvular heart disease. Eur Heart J 2012; 33: 822–8, 828a, 828b.
6. Carabello BA. The current therapy for mitral regurgitation. J Am Coll Cardiol 2008; 52: 319–26.
7. Ling LH, Enriquez-Sarano M, Seward J, et al. Clinical outcome of mitral regurgitation due to flail leaflet. N Engl J Med 1996; 335: 1417–23.
8. Kang D, Kim J, Rim J, et. al. Comparison of early surgery versus conventional treatment in asymptomatic severe mitral regurgitation. Circulation 2009; 119: 797–804.
9. Bonow RO, Carabello BA, Chatterjee K, et al. 2006 Writing committee members; American college of cardiology/American heart association task force. 2008 focused update incorporated into the ACC/AHA 2006 guidelines for the management of patients with valvular heart disease: a report of the American college of cardiology/American heart association task force on practice guidelines (writing committee to revise the 1998 guidelines for the management of patients with valvular heart disease): endorsed by the society of cardiovascular anesthesiologists, society for cardiovascular angiography and interventions, and society of thoracic surgeons. Circulation 2008; 118: e523–661.
10. Zoghbi WA, Enriquez-Sarano M, Foster E, et al. Recommendations for evaluation of the severity of native valvular regurgitation with two-dimensional and Doppler echocardiography. J Am Soc Echocardiogr 2003; 16: 777–802.
11. Nashef SAM, Roques F, Michel P, et al. European system for cardiac operative risk evaluation (EuroSCORE). Eur J Cardiothorac Surg 1999; 161: 9–13.
12. Roques F, Michel P, Goldstone AR, Nashef SA. The logistic Euro SCORE. Eur Heart J 2003; 24: 882–3.
13. Nowicki ER, Birkmeyer NJO, Weintraub RW, et al. Multivariable prediction of in-hospital mortality associated with aortic and mitral valve surgery in northern new England. Ann Thorac Surg 2004; 77: 1966–77.
14. Bonow RO, Carabello BA, Chatterjee K, et al. 2006 Writing committee members; American college of cardiology/American heart association task force. 2008 focused update incorporated into the ACC/AHA 2006 guidelines for the management of patients with valvular heart disease: a report of the American college of cardiology/American heart association task force on practice guidelines (writing committee to revise the 1998 guidelines for the management of patients with valvular heart disease): endorsed by the society of cardiovascular anesthesiologists, society for cardiovascular angiography and interventions, and society of thoracic surgeons. Circulation 2008; 118: e523–661.
15. Matsumura T, Ohtaki E, Tanaka K, et al. Echocardiographic prediction of left ventricular dysfunction after mitral valve repair for mitral regurgitation as an indicator to decide the optimal timing of repair. J Am Coll Cardiol 2003; 42: 458–63.

16. Tribouilloy C, Grigioni F, Avierinos JF, MIDA Investigators. Survival implication of left ventricular end-systolic diameter in mitral regurgitation due to flail leaflets a long-term follow-up multicenter study. J Am Coll Cardiol 2009; 54: 1961–8.

17. Matsunaga A, Shah PM, Raney AA Jr. Impact of intraoperative echocardiography/surgery team on successful mitral valve repair: a community hospital experience. J Heart Valve Dis 2005; 14: 325–30; discussion 330–1.

18. Bolling SF, Li S, O'Brien SM, et al. Predictors of mitral valve repair: clinical and surgeon factors. Ann Thorac Surg 2010; 90: 1904–11; discussion 1912.

19. Gammie JS, O'Brien SM, Griffith BP, Ferguson TB, Peterson ED. Influence of hospital procedural volume on care process and mortality for patients undergoing elective surgery for mitral regurgitation. Circulation 2007; 115: 881–7.

20. Nardi P, Pellegrino A, Scafuri A, et al. Survival and durability of mitral valve repair surgery for degenerative mitral valve disease. J Card Surg 2011; 26: 360–6.

21. Gammie JS, Sheng S, Griffith BP, et al. Trends in mitral valve surgery in the United States: results from the society of thoracic surgeons adult cardiac surgery database. Ann Thorac Surg 2009; 87: 1431–7; discussion 1437-9.

22. Enriquez-Sarano M, Schaff HV, Orszulak TA, et al. Valve repair improves the outcome of surgery for mitral regurgitation. a multivariate analysis. Circulation 1995; 91: 1022–8.

23. Gillinov AM, Blackstone EH, Nowicki ER, et al. Valve repair versus valve replacement for degenerative mitral valve disease. J Thorac Cardiovasc Surg 2008; 135: 885–93; 893 e881–882.

24. 24. Gammie JS, Bartlett ST, Griffith BP. Small-incision mitral valve repair: safe, durable, and approaching perfection. Ann Surg 2009; 250: 409–15.

25. Bolling SF, Li S, O'Brien SM, et al. Predictors of mitral valve repair: clinical and surgeon factors. Ann Thorac Surg 2010; 90: 1904–11; discussion 1912.

26. Landoni G, Crescenzi G, Zangrillo A, et al. Validation of a decision-making strategy for systolic anterior motion following mitral valve repair. Ann Card Anaesth 2011; 14: 85–90.

27. Bizzarri F, Tudisco A, Ricci M, Rose D, Frati G. Different ways to repair the mitral valve with artificial chordai: a systematic review. J Cardiothorac Surg 2010; 5: 22; Review.

28. Lange R, Guenther T, Noebauer C, et al. Chordal replacement versus quadrangular resection for repair of isolated posterior mitral leaflet prolapse. Ann Thorac Surg 2010; 89: 1163–70. discussion; 1170.

29. Alfieri O, De Bonis M. The role of edge-to-edge repair in the surgical treatment of mitral regurgitation. J Card Surg 2010; 25: 536–41.

30. Suri RM, Schaff HV, Dearani JA, et al. Survival advantage and improved durability of mitral repair for leaflet prolapse subsets in the current era. Ann Thorac Surg 2006; 82: 819–26.

31. Gillinov AM, Blackstone EH, Nowicki ER, et al. Valve repair versus valve replacement for degenerative mitral valve disease. J Thorac Cardiovasc Surg 2008; 135: 885–93; 893 e881–882.

32. Bolling SF. Mitral reconstruction in cardiomyopathy. J Heart Valve Dis 2002; 11(Suppl 1): S26–31.

33. Badhwar V, Bolling SF. Mitral valve surgery: when is it appropriate? Congest Heart Fail 2002; 8: 210–13.

34. Benedetto U, Melina G, Roscitano A, et al. Does combined mitral valve surgery improve survival when compared to revascularization alone in patients with ischemic mitral regurgitation? a meta-analysis on 2479 patients. J Cardiovasc Med (Hagerstown) 2009; 10: 109–14.

35. Acker MA, Jessup M, Bolling SF, et al. Mitral valve repair in heart failure: five-year follow-up from the mitral valve replacement stratum of the acorn randomized trial. J Thorac Cardiovasc Surg 2011; 142: 569–74; 574.e1.

36. McGee EC, Gillinov AM, Blackstone EH, et al. Recurrent mitral regurgitation after annuloplasty for functional ischemic mitral regurgitation. J Thorac Cardiovasc Surg 2004; 128: 916–24.

37. Lee AP, Acker M, Kubo SH, et al. Mechanisms of recurrent functional mitral regurgitation after mitral valve repair in nonischemic dilated cardiomyopathy: importance of distal anterior leaflet tethering. Circulation 2009; 119: 2606–14.

38. McCarthy PM. When is your surgeon good enough? when do you need a 'referent surgeon'? Curr Cardiol Rep 2009; 11: 107–13.

39. Gammie JS, O'Brien SM, Griffith BP, Ferguson TB, Peterson ED. Influence of hospital procedural volume on care process and mortality for patients undergoing elective surgery for mitral regurgitation. Circulation 2007; 115: 881–7.

40. Detaint D, Iung B, Lepage L, et al. Management of asymptomatic patients with severe non-ischaemic mitral regurgitation. are practices consistent with guidelines? Eur J Cardiothorac Surg 2008; 34: 937–42.

41. Bach DS, Awais M, Gurm HS, Kohnstamm S. Failure of guideline adherence for intervention in patients with severe mitral regurgitation. J Am Coll Cardiol 2009; 54: 860–5.

42. Adams DH, Anyanwu AC. The cardiologist's role in increasing the rate of mitral valve repair in degenerative disease. Curr Opin Cardiol 2008; 23: 105–10.

6 Development of percutaneous edge-to-edge repair: The MitraClip® story
Frederick St Goar

Innovative concepts for disruptive, paradigm-shifting medical technologies are rarely hatched as lightning bolt revelations. More commonly they develop through an interactive, methodical process involving extensive collaborative work. Such is the story of the MitraClip® (Evalve, Abbott Vascular).

THEORETICAL BACKGROUND

The foundation for the development of the MitraClip® device was laid in Silicon Valley in the early 1980s. In 1979, John Simpson, a Stanford cardiology fellow, pioneered the technique for over-the-wire balloon angioplasty and went on to found Advanced Cardiovascular Systems (ACS), later to become part of Guidant Group. He, along with the well-known innovator, Tom Fogarty, followed then by Simon Stertzer (first U.S. angioplasty) and Paul Yock (innovator of rapid exchange percutaneous transluminal coronary angioplasty and intravascular ultrasound), established a tradition of successful cardiovascular innovators. These were the people, and this was the creative, innovative environment that cardiology trainees at Stanford were exposed to in the early and mid-1980s. It was a community ripe with engineers coming out of biomedical programs and an active venture capital community. If someone had a good idea, the supportive "ecosystem" was there to assist in its development and move toward commercialization. Stanford fellows and Silicon Valley cardiologists were the idea generators. Besides ACS, in the cardiovascular space alone, there were companies like Devices for Vascular Intervention, Cardiovascular Imaging Systems, Perclose, LocalMed, Transvascular, and LuMens to name just a few. Thanks to this environment in 1991, it was only natural that cardiology fellow Fred St Goar was approached by John Stevens, then a cardiovascular surgeon in training, to become involved with his endeavor for developing a catheter-based system for percutaneously delivering a replacement aortic valve. The project, originally called Stanford Surgical Technologies, subsequently changed its name to HeartPort and embarked on a different pathway, specifically to develop surgical tools for performing less invasive (Port Access) coronary artery bypass graft and valve surgery. The HeartPort transaortic valve replacement intellectual property was acquired by Percutaneous Valve Technologies which subsequently developed the Cribier valve, the precursor to the current Edwards Life Sciences Sapien valve. St Goar served as a cardiovascular consultant to HeartPort helping to develop the catheter system for ascending aortic balloon cardiopulmonary bypass. He was also provided limited support to investigate the feasibility of either catheter-based mitral valve replacement or a technique for catheter-based annuloplasty. This work was performed in conjunction with Jan Komtebadde, a forward

thinking Doctor of Veterinary Medicine and one of the creative minds behind the development of the HeartPort technology. They both appreciated the challenges and issues of the mitral valve. At the same time HeartPort chose to abandon their mitral valve project. The development of percutaneous mitral technology thus moved to be independent of HeartPort.

Fortuitously, while trying to come up with a method for catheter-based annuloplasty, St Goar referred one of his patients to a Stanford cardiothoracic surgeon, Scott Mitchell, for a combined aortic and mitral valve surgical intervention. Mitchell replaced the patient's aortic valve and placed a ring on her mitral annulus. When he took her off cardiopulmonary bypass, she still had significant MR. Mitchell put the patient back on bypass and placed a simple pledgeted suture between the A2 and P2 scallops creating a successful Alfieri edge-to-edge repair. After the procedure, he called up St Goar and described what he had done. St Goar, having never heard of the edge-to-edge repair technique, was intrigued by the procedure and was impressed with its simplicity and elegance. This was the fall of 1998, when there were only two published reports of the Alfieri repair, both in the European literature (1,2). While tracking down the two articles, St Goar sketched ideas for performing the catheter-based edge-to-edge repair in a lab book. These original concepts set out to reproduce the surgical paradigm, that is, a suture-based approach (Fig. 6.1). In the meantime, the first article in the United States describing the technique was published by Mehmet Oz, MD (3). Not only did he document its successful use in 10 patients, but he also modeled the horizontal and vertical systolic forces on the A2-P2 apposition point, showing that it was a low stress point and the fulcrum of the mitral valve/ventricular apparatus. It was an elegant description of the scientific basis for the success of a mitral valve edge-to-edge repair. Follow-up publications by Drs Maisano and Alfieri provided further clinical validation (4,5). More sophisticated modeling and in vivo testing have shown low forces exerted on the suture in an edge-to-edge repair (6,7).

INCUBATOR ACCELERATION

St Goar presented his edge-to-edge ideas to a medical device intellectual property lawyer who confirmed that there were, as of yet, no significant patents in this space. St Goar then approached the team at The Foundry, a new Silicon Valley medical device incubator, with the concept of the catheter-based mitral valve edge-to-edge repair. The Foundry entrepreneurs, Hanson Gifford and Allan Will, both quickly appreciated the possible value of the catheter-based valve repair technology and that the edge-to-edge approach had great potential as a way to accomplish such a repair. Under the guidance of the Foundry,

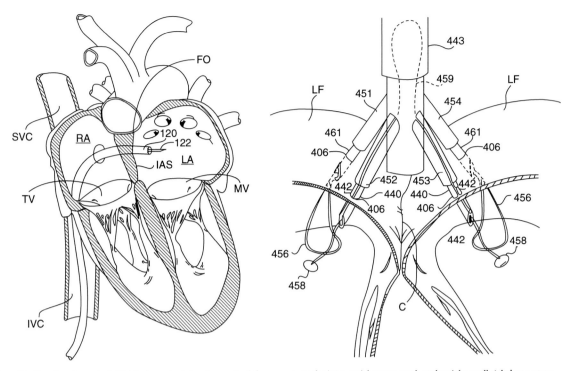

Figure 6.1 Drawings from the initial Evalve patent showing on the *left* access across the intra-atrial septum and on the *right* needle/pledget system.

the intellectual property was consolidated including the acquisition of an early methodology patent from Mehmet Oz, MD and another surgical approach created by Jacques Suigin, MD. A highly skilled engineering team was pulled together to further the "proof of concept" process and a business plan was developed. The team then embarked on the process of raising funds to support the project.

As a litmus test for the validity and potential of the project, Gifford and St Goar arranged to present the idea first to John Simpson, followed by Tom Fogarty, two well-established medical technology innovators in Silicon Valley. Both responded positively, fueling the venture capital fund raising process. Next was a poignant visit to the prominent venture firm, NEA, where one of the senior founding partner's wives had unfortunately died from complications of mitral valve surgery. At the end of the presentation, the partner commented in a heart-felt manner about the overwhelming need for a less invasive technology for mitral valve repair, and funding followed. This commitment, along with support from Three Arch Capital, secured the funding necessary to launch Evalve, Inc.

One of the major contributions to the project by the Foundry was pulling together a superb management team. Ferolyn Powell, a bright, energetic leader who came in with an engineering and operations background after having worked at Devices for Vascular Intervention and then was running operations at General Surgical Innovations, took on the role of president and CEO. Her understanding of device development and manufacturing operations proved invaluable. Her vision and comprehension

of the complexity of development of complex medical devices provided the fundamental foundation for the success of the project. Troy Thornton, who had worked at the training ground for many cardiovascular device engineers, ACS, and then Prograft Medical, joined as the director of R&D. Liz McDermott, who also had extensive product development and regulatory affairs experience at ACS, was brought in to tackle the extremely challenging issues surrounding the clinical trial and regulatory processes of a novel, paradigm-shifting technology. These three insightful, inspiring leaders have directed the MitraClip® device endeavor throughout its 11-year existence. Without their long-range vision, resilient commitment, and dogged determination to always keep patient safety and benefit as the highest priority, the project would likely have failed on numerous occasions.

DESIGN DEVELOPMENT

The initial development of the clip and its delivery system was far from linear. To assist in the process, the Evalve engineering team created a clever and extremely valuable bench-testing system. The left atrium was trimmed off a porcine heart and the ventricle was placed in a saline-filled Lucite tub. A polyethylene tube was advanced through the apex of the left ventricle in which the pressure was varied comparable to a cardiac cycle. This demonstrated the competency of the mitral valve. When one or more chordae was transected, the valve leaked. Various methods for repairing the leaky valve were tested on the model. The initial approaches involved reproducing a suture-based surgical approach. A major challenge was developing a method

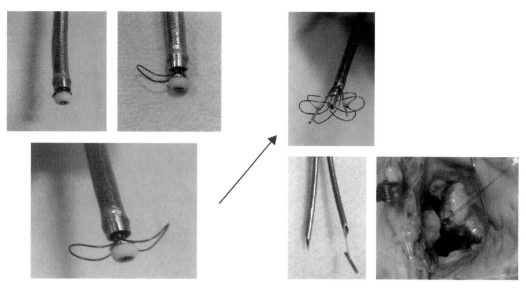

Figure 6.2 Early grasping prototype with retractable atrial and ventricular stabilizing wires, hollow bore needles with "T" pledgeted sutures and deployment in a porcine model.

to stabilize the leaflets prior to placement of sutures. Approaches from both the atrial and the ventricular sides of the leaflets were evaluated. It was difficult to avoid snaring the chordae when entering retrograde through the aortic valve. Arriving at the valve from an ante grade approach across the intra-atrial septum was feasible, but devising an atraumatic method for stabilizing the leaflets to place the sutures from the atrial side posed additional challenges. A prototype that appeared to be feasible had retractable wire loops on the ventricular aspect with a second set of loops advanced from the atrial side, thus stabilizing the leaflets such that one or more pledgeted sutures could be inserted (Fig. 6.2). The concept of sutures being advanced through the leaflets and the associated potential for damaging the leaflets dampened the enthusiasm for this design. During the testing of the stabilizing loop system, it was noted that the leaflets could be coapted by the opposing loops, thus resolving the MR. With the belief that the loop system could be left in place and the evidence that it may be less traumatic than sutures, combined with the added benefit that it was repositionable, the deployable loop system became the next design iteration.

The loop system subsequently evolved into a device with rigid grasping arms (Fig. 6.3). This facilitated more robust tissue-to-tissue apposition and is the foundation for the MitraClip® system that is in use today. Once the mechanisms for deploying the two grippers from the atrial aspect, and for opening, closing, inverting, and releasing the implant were perfected, it was covered with polyester to enhance tissue healing. The rigid ventricular arms and the atrial tissue stabilizing grippers were a tremendous engineering breakthrough as the device then modeled a "cinching-annuloplasty" versus a simple edge-to-edge repair. This premise has since been supported by

medium-term echocardiogram studies which demonstrate that the MitraClip® interrupts the progressive annular dilatation seen in patients suffering from chronic MR.

In parallel to the development of the MitraClip® implant, a separate team of engineers worked on a complex triaxial catheter delivery system. This consisted of a guiding catheter and a MitraClip® delivery catheter system, both of which are steerable and provide multiple planes of movement. The implant and the delivery system were tested in vivo in the animal laboratory prior to human studies. The MitraClip® device, using a shortened delivery system, initially was placed in porcine subjects via direct access through the dome of the left atrium. These studies demonstrated both the acute success of the ability to place the MitraClip® on the beating heart and successfully grasp and coapt the leaflets, and also the chronic healing response with tissue incorporation of the device similar to what is observed after surgical edge-to-edge repair. The porcine subject provided for a challenging model as the left atrium is small, the left and right atria are at times slightly offset, and the heart lies in a very different orientation relative to the vena cava than in humans. Maneuvering the guiding catheter and Mitra-Clip® delivery system from the groin to across the septum to access the valve was challenging with devices designed for human anatomy. It was only through extensive trial and error, patience and perseverance, that the team mastered the procedure. With feasibility studies completed, tests on a series of animals were performed and reported (8). This described creating an edge-to-edge repair in 14 normal adult pigs. Direct epicardial echocardiographic guidance was used as a substitute for transesophageal echocardiogram to place the MitraClip® device on the valve. A double orifice was created in all 14 animals, sometimes requiring several grasps. There was no echocardiographic

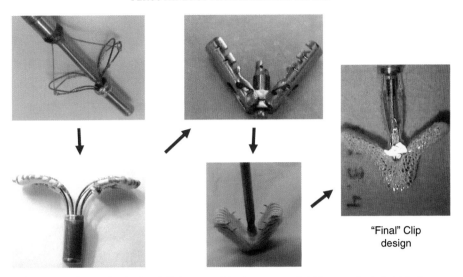

"Final" Clip
design

Figure 6.3 Evolution of a wire-based clip into one with polyester covered rigid arms and raised atrial grippers.

evidence of mitral stenosis after deployment of the device. In two animals, the MitraClip® device released from the anterior leaflet, retrospectively determined to be related to grasping technique with the device not properly configured for grasping. Acute postmortem analysis confirmed a double orifice in the remaining 12 pigs with device deployment perpendicular to the line of coaptation. This highlighted a key step of the procedure of confirming optimal tissue insertion prior to deployment of the implant from the delivery catheter. The challenges addressed in the early animal experience were invaluable for gaining expertise and confidence as it was much more challenging than what was eventually required in man.

In parallel Fann et al. described the healing response of the MitraClip® device in chronic animal studies (9). At four weeks, the entire implant was encapsulated in a layer of tissue. There was evidence of tissue deposition and leaflet-to-leaflet healing. At 12 weeks, tissue encapsulation was further developed with leaflet-to-leaflet bridging between the arms of the device. At 24 weeks, development of mature solid tissue bridging was present. Scanning electron microscopy of three mitral valves (one each at 4 weeks, 12 weeks, and 24 weeks) showed complete tissue encapsulation of the implant with endothelial cells on the surface. The device became well incorporated into the valve leaflets with no significant tissue growth beyond the edges of the implant or evidence of tissue necrosis between the device arms. These chronic animal findings mimicked what was observed after surgical suture approximation. Privitera et al. described the pathology of a patient who received isolated surgical edge-to-edge repair and then four years later underwent cardiac transplantation for progressive heart failure in spite of a competent nonstenotic mitral valve (10). The point of suture apposition of the anterior and posterior mitral leaflets was shown to be encapsulated with

endothelial tissue surrounding a fibrous tissue bridge comparable to the MitraClip® porcine results.

FIRST-IN-HUMAN USE
In conjunction with the animal work, extensive cycle fatigue testing and in vivo bench testing were performed to establish that the implant would be functioning and durable in excess of the stresses that it would be subjected to in the human. The voluminous data of bench and animal testing were submitted to the FDA in order to gain permission to proceed with an initial safety and feasibility trial. Given the unpredictability of the time required to initiate a feasibility trial in the United States, a parallel pathway for an overseas first-in-man experience was pursued. Interestingly, the opportunity to proceed with initial clinical testing overseas (OUS) and in US occurred simultaneously. In the last week of June 2003, a group of physicians, including Fred St Goar and Patrick Whitlow from The Cleveland Clinic Foundation, traveled to Caracas, Venezuela. The first patient treated had severe MR from bileaflet prolapse. The case, performed by Dr Jose Condado, went well with the reduction of MR to a mild status after deployment of a single clip (Fig. 6.4). It was an exciting moment when the first clip was placed. As soon as it was deployed and the MR resolved, the patient's heart rate and systolic blood decreased. On the transesophageal echo it was noted that her left ventricle had increased in size. Then over the course of several minutes, without inotropic support, the blood pressure increased. Measured forward cardiac output improved significantly as compared to just prior to the clip placement. The operators appreciated that they were witnessing a dramatic example of what was, at the time, a novel hemodynamic challenge, to which the left ventricle transiently complained and then robustly recovered. The operators reported the details of the case as well as the patient's

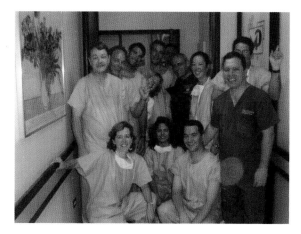

Figure 6.4 The Caracas team that performed the first-in-man case which included Pat Whitlow, Ferolyn Powell, Jan Komtebedde, Eric Goldfarb, Fred St Goar, Brian Martin, Harry Acquatella, Leonardo Rodriguez, Sylvia Fann, Jose Condado, and Troy Thornton.

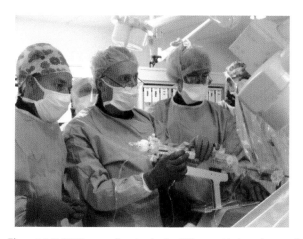

Figure 6.5 Ted Feldman performing the first U.S. case with the assistance of Jan Komtebedde and Tim Sanborn.

two-year follow-up echo which showed 1+ MR (11). Clinically the patient had done very well with no return of her pre-procedure symptoms. An echo performed, now eight years after the procedure, showed a durable result with mild/moderate MR (Condado, personal communication). A photo taken at the end of these first procedure shows all the involved participants and illustrates the group effort required to achieve success (Fig. 6.5). A week after the Caracas trip, Ted Feldman, performed the first case in the United States in the Endovascular Valve Edge-to-edge REpair STudy (EVEREST) I trial. The success of the first two cases was not simply fortuitous, but represented an enormous amount of hard work by a large group of dedicated individuals.

SUMMARY

Development of the MitraClip® has been a long and demanding endeavor. The pivotal IDE (FDA defined Investigational Device Exemption pathway) trial was called EVEREST for good reason; the process was, and continues to be, quite a climb. The number of people who have put their hearts and souls into making the device a therapeutic reality is both remarkable and humbling. On the clinical front, the early investigators including Feldman, Block, Herrmann, Whitlow, and Gray to name but a few, demonstrated phenomenal confidence, courage, and thoughtful expertise. Behind the scenes, which cannot be easily appreciated, has been the extraordinary dedication and determination of the development and operations teams. The creativity and dogged determination of the engineers, the large quantities of data accumulated and organized by the regulatory group, and the focused and inspiring leadership of the senior managers, all have added up to a remarkably successful project and the creation of a therapy from which patients will benefit for years to come.

REFERENCES

1. Fucci C, Sandrelli L, Pardini A, et al. Improved results using new surgical techniques. Eur J Cardiothorac Surg 1995; 9: 621–7.
2. Maisano F, Torracca L, Oppizzi M, et al. The edge-to-edge technique: a simplified method to correct mitral insufficiency. Eur J Cardiothorac Surg 1998; 13: 240–5.
3. Umana JP, Salehizadeh B, DeRose JJ, et al. "Bow-tie" mitral valve repair: an adjuvant technique for ischemic mitral regurgitation. Ann Thorac Surg 1998; 66: 1640–6.
4. Alfieri O, Maisano F, DeBonis M, et al. The edge-to-edge technique in mitral valve repair: a simple solution for complex problems. J Thoracic Cardiovasc Surg 2001; 122: 674–81.
5. Maisano F, Vigano G, Blasio A, et al. Surgical isolated edge-to-edge mitral valve repair without annuloplasty: clinical proof of the principle for an endovascular approach. Euro Interv 2006; 2: 181–6.
6. Nielsen SL, Timek TA, Lai DT, et al. Edge-to-edge mitral repair: tension on the approximating suture and leaflet deformation during acute ischemic regurgitation. Circulation 2001; 104: I29–35.
7. Votta E, Maisano F, Soncini M, et al. 3-D computational analysis of the stress distribution on the leaflets after edge-to-edge repair of mitral regurgitation. J Heart Valve Dis 2002; 11: 810–22.
8. St. Goar FG, James FI, Komtebedde J, et al. Endovascular edge-to-edge mitral valve repair: acute results in a porcine model. Circulation 2003; 108: 1990–3.
9. Fann JI, St. Goar FG, Komtebedde J, et al. Off pump edge-to-edge mitral valve technique using a mechanical clip in a chronic model. Circulation 2003; 108: 17: IV–493.
10. Privitera S, Butany J, Cusimano RJ, et al. Alfieri mitral valve repair: clinical outcome and pathology. Circulation 2002; 106: e173–4.
11. Condado JA, Acquatella H, Rodriguez Whitlow P, Velez-Gimo M, St Goar F. Percutaneous edge-to-edge mitral valve repair: 2-year follow-up in the first human case. Catheter Cardiovasc Interv 2006; 67: 323–5.

7 MitraClip® system design and history of development
Troy Thornton and Liz McDermott

OVERVIEW OF THE MITRACLIP® SYSTEM

The MitraClip® system consists of four major components: (*i*) the delivery catheter, (*ii*) the steerable sleeve, (*iii*) the Mitra-Clip® device, and (iv) the steerable guiding catheter (Fig. 7.1).

The MitraClip® system is composed of a triaxial catheter delivery system. The outermost catheter is a steerable guiding catheter (guide), which includes a tapered dilator and a knob on the handle that controls deflection of the distal tip. The clip delivery system is inserted into the guide and has an outer steerable sleeve with two knobs that control the medial-lateral (ML) and anterior-posterior (AP) deflection of the sleeve. The MitraClip® device is attached to the distal end of the innermost catheter called the delivery catheter, which has controls on its handle that enable opening, closing, and deployment of the device. The MitraClip® device (Clip) is a cobalt/chromium implant with two arms that are opened and closed via controls on the delivery catheter handle. The Clip includes a gripper adjacent to each arm to secure the leaflets as they are captured during grasping and while closing the arms of the Clip. Each leaflet is therefore independently secured between an arm and a gripper. Once the leaflets are grasped and the Clip arms are closed, the leaflets are permanently coapted at the location of the regurgitant flow resulting in the reduction of the mitral regurgitation. The Mitra-Clip® device has a locking mechanism to maintain the implanted Clip in a closed position, and the arms and grippers are covered with a polyester fabric to promote tissue ingrowth.

STEERABLE GUIDING CATHETER

The steerable guiding catheter (Fig. 7.2) serves as a conduit for the introduction of the clip delivery system and consists of a distal shaft (22 French) and a proximal shaft (24 French). The length of the catheter is constructed with braided stainless steel wire to provide axial stiffness and torque transmission. A radiopaque ring on the distal tapered tip allows fluoroscopic alignment with radiopaque markers on the steerable sleeve catheter and provides an echogenic atraumatic tip. The steerable guide catheter is delivered over a tapered dilator, which also has echogenic markings at the distal tip. A knob on the guide handle allows the distal tip to be straightened during introduction into the femoral vein and, once positioned in the left atrium, the rotation of the knob provides substantial curvature of the distal end to precisely position the MitraClip® device. The central lumen of the steerable guide catheter allows for aspiration of air and the infusion of fluids through a hemostasis valve located on the handle.

CLIP DELIVERY SYSTEM
Steerable Sleeve
The steerable sleeve aids in positioning and orienting the MitraClip® device above the mitral valve leaflets. The steerable

sleeve provides the physician with the means to position the Clip along the AP and ML axes, relative to the mitral valve anatomy.

The steerable sleeve is a long, flexible multilumen catheter with a handle at the proximal end (Fig. 7.3). The shaft has one central thru-lumen surrounded by six smaller lumens designed to house cables that are used to steer the distal tip. The steerable sleeve is designed to provide a mechanism for translation and rotation of the Clip delivery catheter, which lies within the thru-lumen. Three pairs of control cables lie within the six smaller lumens and serve to deflect the distal end of the steerable sleeve. The distal tip of the steerable sleeve is radiopaque to provide for visualization under fluoroscopy. An introducer on the shaft of the sleeve is used to introduce the MitraClip® implant into the steerable guide catheter.

The handle on the steerable sleeve has two control knobs for ML and AP steering (Fig. 7.4). Two control knobs allow the operator to adjust the curvature of the distal end of the steerable sleeve by applying tension to the control cables located inside the shaft.

A hemostasis valve facilitates air management of the thru-lumen of the steerable sleeve and provides a flush port for the introduction of fluids during the implant procedure.

The system includes a mechanism for alignment of the steerable sleeve within the steerable guide (Fig. 7.5). A stainless steel key near the distal end of the steerable sleeve mates with channels on the inner wall of the steerable guide catheter to maintain the two catheters in a fixed rotational orientation. This prevents the steerable sleeve from rotating relative to the guide and maintains its stability during deflection. A longitudinal alignment marker on the proximal shaft of the steerable sleeve ensures proper alignment with a corresponding mark on the steerable guide catheter.

The distal region of the steerable sleeve is deflectable to facilitate the precise position of the MitraClip® device. A stainless steel radiopaque tip ring at the distal tip provides the attachment point for the control cables. When tension is applied to the control cables via the control knobs, the radiopaque tip ring is pulled, which deflects the distal region of the sleeve in the desired direction. Two additional radiopaque alignment markers are embedded into the distal shaft to allow the positioning of the steerable sleeve relative to the distal tip of the steerable guide (Fig. 7.6).

Delivery Catheter
The delivery catheter consists of a handle and a multilumen shaft and provides the operator with the means to actuate and deploy the MitraClip® device. The delivery catheter resides inside the steerable sleeve thru-lumen and is free to translate

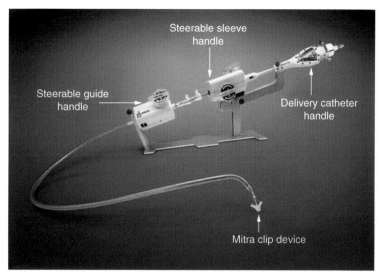

Figure 7.1 MitraClip® system: major components.

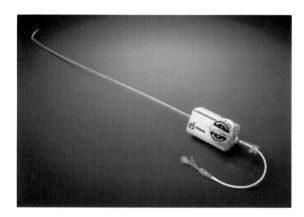

Figure 7.2 Steerable guiding catheter.

and rotate. The MitraClip® device is located at the distal tip of the delivery catheter. The delivery catheter handle consists of a fastener, lock lever, actuator knob, arm positioner, release pin, gripper lever, and two flush ports (Fig. 7.7). The fastener is used to temporarily secure the delivery catheter position relative to the sleeve, to prevent inadvertent manipulation of the MitraClip® device once the leaflets have been grasped. The lock lever is used to lock and unlock the locking mechanism of the MitraClip® device and the gripper lever is used to repeatedly raise and lower the grippers. The arm positioner opens, closes, and inverts the clip arms by advancing and retracting the actuator mandrel which is threaded onto the clip. Rotation of the arm positioner causes translation of the actuator mandrel, which controls the opening and closing of the clip arms. The flush ports allow for aspiration of air and infusion of liquids (e.g., heparinized saline) into the thru-lumens of the delivery catheter.

At the completion of the implant procedure, the double-length lock line and gripper line are removed from the delivery catheter. The release pin is removed; then the actuator knob is rotated to unthread the actuator from the clip, resulting in the deployment of the clip from the delivery catheter.

The delivery catheter's multilumen shaft (Fig. 7.8) consists of a stainless steel braided polymer jacket; a support coil that encapsulates the four gripper and lock line lumens; a compression coil that holds the actuator mandrel, and a tension cable to prevent elongation.

MitraClip® Device

The MitraClip® device is a percutaneously implanted, mechanical clip designed to reduce mitral regurgitation (Fig. 7.9). The MitraClip® device grasps and coapts the mitral valve leaflets, resulting in fixed approximation of the mitral leaflets throughout the cardiac cycle and a functional double-orifice mitral valve.

MitraClip® Components and Material

The MitraClip® device is made of cobalt-chromium and nickel-titanium metallic components and covered with polyester fabric to enhance the healing response. Each component has been carefully designed to complement the overall function and integrity of the MitraClip® device.

MitraClip® Functions

The MitraClip® device performs three primary functions:

1. Arm control: opening, closing, and inverting the arms for MitraClip® device to grasp and release the mitral valve leaflets.
2. Arm locking: locking of the clip arms in a closed position to coapt the leaflets and prevent opening of the MitraClip® device.

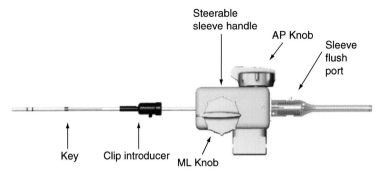

Figure 7.3 Steerable sleeve catheter assembly.

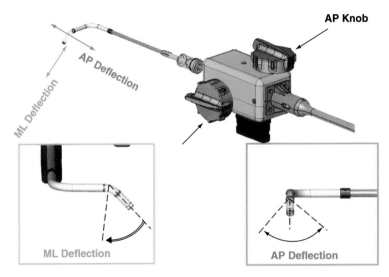

Figure 7.4 Steerable sleeve handle assembly. AP, anterior posterior, ML, medial lateral.

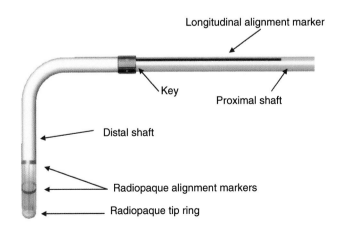

Figure 7.5 Distal end of the steerable sleeve.

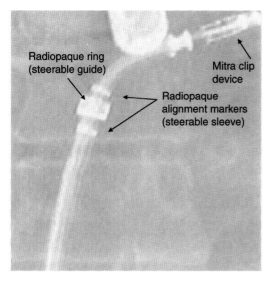

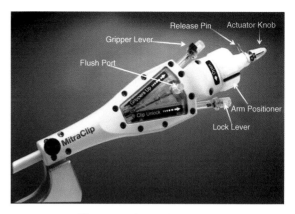

Figure 7.7 Delivery catheter handle.

Figure 7.6 Fluoroscopic image of steerable sleeve inside the steerable guide.

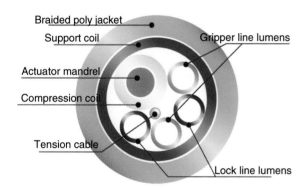

Figure 7.8 Delivery catheter, multi-lumen shaft cross-section.

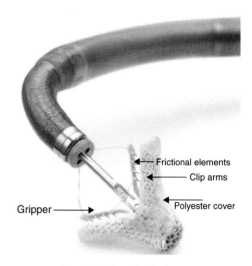

Figure 7.9 MitraClip® device.

3. Gripper control: raising and lowering of the grippers relative to the arms to secure the valve leaflets in the MitraClip® device.

The MitraClip® device arms can be adjusted to various positions (Fig. 7.10) such as closed, open, and inverted. These positions are designed to allow the MitraClip® device to grasp and approximate the leaflets of the mitral valve, using controls on the Delivery Catheter Handle. The MitraClip® device can be unlocked using the Lock Lever on the delivery catheter handle. The MitraClip® device can be repeatedly opened and closed using the Arm Positioner. The gripper can be raised or lowered repeatedly using the Gripper Lever.

Locking Mechanism
The MitraClip® device is locked by default. In this condition, the Binding Plate binds between the Threaded Stud and the

Connector. Pressure from the Leaf Spring initiates the wedging of the binding plate onto the threaded stud. The threaded stud can always be retracted, even though the MitraClip® device is locked, allowing the MitraClip® arms to close. However, advancement of the threaded stud is restricted when the MitraClip® device is locked. Therefore, the arms of the device cannot open when the device is locked (Fig. 7.11).

To unlock the MitraClip® device and allow the arms to open, tension is applied to the lock line by retracting the lock lever on the delivery catheter handle. This action raises the harness and the binding plate. The lifting binding plate compresses the leaf spring, unwedging the binding plate. The threaded stud is now able to move freely in both directions, allowing the arms to be opened and closed.

Deployment of the MitraClip® device from the delivery catheter requires three separate steps. First, the lock lines are

39

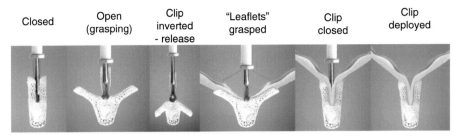

Closed | Open (grasping) | Clip inverted - release | "Leaflets" grasped | Clip closed | Clip deployed

Figure 7.10 Various arm positions of the MitraClip® device.

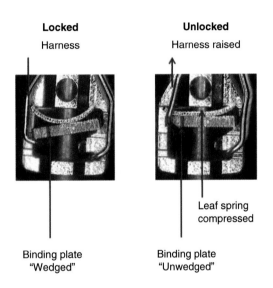

Locked
Harness

Unlocked
Harness raised

Leaf spring compressed

Binding plate "Wedged"

Binding plate "Unwedged"

Figure 7.11: Locked vs. unlocked MitraClip® device.

removed by removing the lock lever cap exposing both ends of the double-length lock line, then pulling on one end to remove the lock line. Second, the release pin is removed and the actuator is unthreaded from the clip by turning the actuator knob, which decouples the distal tip of the delivery catheter from the clip. The third step is the removal of the gripper line.

HISTORY OF DEVELOPMENT AND KEY DESIGN FEATURES

Mitral Valve Access

Devising a method to grasp the mitral leaflets on a beating heart proved to be a challenge. Early prototype device concepts were developed to accomplish grasping of the leaflets from the inferior (ventricular) side, but the desire to minimize manipulations within the ventricle to avoid the chordae tendinae resulted in the decision to approach the mitral valve from the superior (atrial) side of the leaflets. Subsequent designs approached the mitral valve via femoral vein access to the right atrium then transseptal access to the left atrium. This pathway allowed grasping of the mitral leaflets "from above" the valve.

Suture Design

The early concepts for replicating the surgical edge-to-edge mitral valve repair using a percutaneous catheter system involved placing sutures in the leaflets (Fig. 7.12). Early prototypes of grasping catheters used retractable, angled wire loops, positioned perpendicular to the line of coaptation to immobilize the leaflets from the ventricular side. Once grasped, a hollow needle was advanced to puncture each leaflet. A pledget made of a loop of nitinol wire was then advanced through the needle. A second catheter was used to fasten the sutures together using a "suture lock." Because of the risk of the suture cutting through the leaflet, as well as the inability of this design to allow multiple, atraumatic grasping attempts, the design complexity increased significantly and therefore alternate design concepts were pursued.

Butterfly Design

The creation of the suture prototypes with angled wire loops led to a breakthrough concept: The same component of the device that was used for grasping could also be used to coapt the leaflets as a permanent implant. This led to the butterfly design concept (Fig. 7.13), where a pair of nitinol wire loops was used to independently grasp and hold each leaflet. The superior loop included frictional elements to increase the grip of each leaflet. Once the leaflets were grasped, the loops were retracted into a barrel on the inferior side of the leaflets to bring the loops together to coapt the leaflets. This design concept was important in that it resulted in the invention of "grippers" with "frictional elements" and "arms" used to grasp the leaflets, which are key features of the final MitraClip® device design.

Final MitraClip® Design

Early animal studies indicated that an optimal design would include rigid arms, ability to close the clip to a low profile, and polyester covering to enhance the healing response. This resulted in the development of a clip with rigid arms that could be opened to a grasping position and closed to a low profile position multiple times. This design was implanted surgically onto porcine mitral valves to test the feasibility of this clip design. The clips were implanted using a short, rigid delivery catheter via direct access into the left atrium. These feasibility studies provided the first evidence that a mechanical clip could be safely attached to the beating mitral valve to permanently

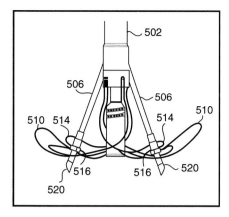
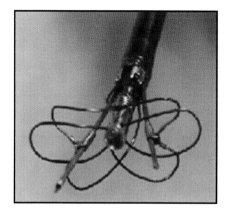

Figure 7.12 Early concept and prototype of the suture design.

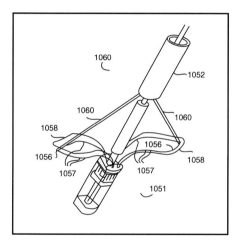
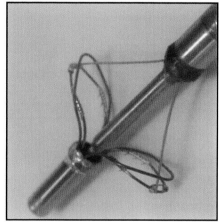

Figure 7.13 Early concept and prototype of the butterfly design.

coapt the mitral leaflet with a benign healing response. Further development and refinement of the clip concept resulted in two key changes. First was refinement of the "frictional elements" located on the "grippers" as integrated narrow pointed elements to engage and hold on to the leaflets while closing the clip arms. The geometry of the "frictional elements" was designed to not only partially penetrate the thickness of the leaflets to achieve atraumatic grasping, but also secure grasping of the leaflets. Also the frictional elements were angled in a direction that secured the leaflets when the clip was opened, the grippers raised, and the clip was retracted into the left atrium. Second was an important design addition that allowed the arms of the clip to be fully opened to an inverted state to allow for retraction from the ventricle back into the left atrium. These design features allowed atraumatic grasping and releasing of the leaflets multiple times, allowing for optimal clip placement. Another key design feature developed for the final design was a means of locking the clip arms once placed on the leaflets. The locking mechanism required the ability to be cycled between

the locked and unlocked state multiple times to allow repositioning of the clip to optimize the reduction of mitral regurgitation. The first-generation lock mechanism was limited to allowing the clip to be locked at only three angles. The final design of the steerable guide (Fig. 7.14) was improved to allow the lock to hold the clip at any arm angle.

IN VIVO CHRONIC ANIMAL STUDIES

Prior to the development of the femoral vein access catheter delivery system, animal studies were performed in a healthy porcine model using direct access into the left atrium to evaluate the chronic healing response. Dr Fann et al. (1) reported progressive healing of the clips with fibrous tissue and collagen over the surface of the clip and evidence of tissue deposition between the arms of the clip by week 4. By week 24 a mature, continuous tissue bridge had formed between the anterior and posterior leaflets between the arms of the clip. Scanning electron microscopy showed full encapsulation of the clip with complete endothelialization of the surface (Fig. 7.15).

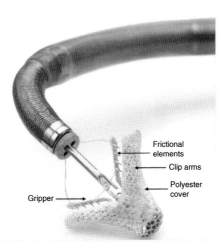

Figure 7.14 Final MitraClip® device design.

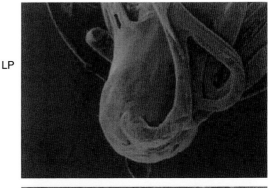

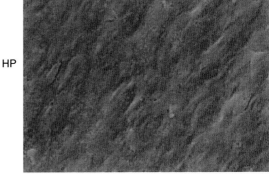

24-Week

Figure 7.15 Low-power (LP) and high-power (HP) scanning electron microscopy of clip incorporated by surrounding tissue and endothelialization at 12 and 24 weeks.

These early findings in the porcine model were later corroborated by Dr Ladich et al. (2), who reported on the pathologic healing response of MitraClip® devices that had been explanted from humans. Histopathologic analysis of long-term human implants showed fibrous encapsulation with extension over the adjacent mitral leaflets and tissue bridge formation between the clip arms and the presence of type I collagen (Fig. 7.16).

Durability Testing and Finite Element Analysis
To develop a permanent implant that is reliable and durable, it was critical to understand the forces acting on the device throughout its lifetime. Forces acting on an edge-to-edge mitral valve repair have been studied and reported in the literature. Nielsen et al. (3) utilized direct measurement of force by attaching a miniature C-ring force transducer to the leaflets in an acute ovine model. The peak load was reported to be 0.46 Newtons. An in vitro model that also used a miniature C-ring transducer was used by Jimenez et al. (4), who reported a peak load of 0.072 Newtons, and a finite element model was developed by Avanzini et al. (5) which showed a resulting peak load of 0.39 Newtons.

A large safety factor was added to the highest of these reported load values in order to perform accelerated durability testing at loads significantly exceeding these values. Testing was conducted by fixturing clips in an EnduraTEC 3200 fatigue tester and exerting diastolic and systolic loads on the clip arms immersed in a saline bath at 37°C (Fig. 7.17). Accelerated durability testing has been performed on the MitraClip® device representing over 15 years of life time, and the results show no fracture, damage, or clip lock failure.

A finite element analysis model (Fig. 7.18) was also developed in order to understand the theoretical fatigue safety factor for each component of the clip. This finite element model was validated by subjecting clips to "dynamic load to failure," where the loads are increased incrementally until a component fracture occurs. The predictions determined from the finite element model for which component would be first to fail concurred with the "dynamic load to failure" test results. The load at which the first failure occurred during "dynamic load to failure" testing was more than seven times the predicted in vivo load.

CATHETER DEVELOPMENT
To deliver, actuate, and deploy the clip on the mitral leaflets required the development of sophisticated steerable delivery and guiding catheters. Development of these catheter systems was very challenging. In order to approach the mitral valve from the left atrium and accurately position the clip perpendicular to the plane of the mitral valve, a two-part steerable catheter system was developed: a 16 French steerable sleeve catheter within a 24 French steerable guiding catheter.

The steerable guiding catheter must be straight for femoral vein introduction, yet must curve up to a 90° angle within the left atrium to allow for a wide range of expected transseptal puncture locations and to accommodate anatomical variability. This required a multilayered catheter design incorporating

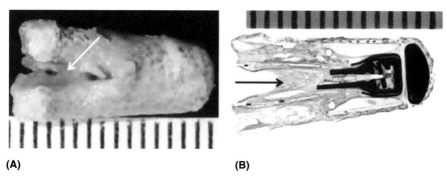

Figure 7.16 Chronic human explantation group (91–300 days). (A) Gross image demonstrating fibrous tissue bridging the area between the device arms (atrial tissue bridge, arrow). (B) Photomicrograph of the histological section of a MitraClip® device explanted after 283 days demonstrating the tissue bridge (arrows).

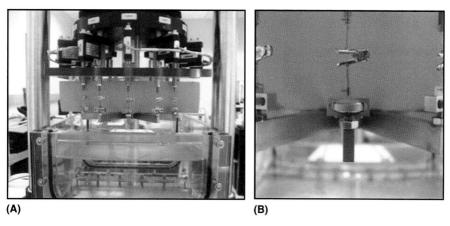

Figure 7.17 Accelerated durability testing.

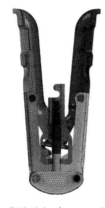

Figure 7.18 Finite element analysis model.

tension cables to actuate the curves. The steerable sleeve catheter must be able to maintain a plane of curvature roughly 90 degrees to the plane of curvature on the steerable guiding catheter. To maintain the curves of the two catheters in orthogonal planes, a rotational alignment system was devised with a metallic key feature on the steerable sleeve that is mated with channels on the inner wall of the steerable guide. The requirement for steerability

in multiple planes to accurately place the MitraClip® device was discovered during early animal studies. This led to the final steerable sleeve catheter design with three sets of tension cables incorporated into the wall of catheter. The tension cables allowed the steerable sleeve to be curved in three distinct directions. The final design of the steerable guide and steerable sleeve allow for a wide range of steerability to accommodate significant anatomical variation and provided precision and accuracy for positioning the clip on the mitral leaflets.

The catheter designed to actuate and deploy MitraClip® device has multiple functions: opening and closing the arms of the clip, raising and lowering the grippers, locking and unlocking the clip locking mechanism, and deploying the clip. The delivery catheter design also must perform with minimal elongation, minimal axial compressibility, and must maintain straightness when extended from the curved guide and sleeve. These multiple and, in some cases, conflicting design requirements were achieved by developing a composite delivery catheter using several stainless coils, a tension cable inside a braided outer shaft with differential stiffness along its length, and a novel clip deployment mechanism.

Preclinical animal studies in an acute porcine model were used to refine and optimize the steerable guide catheter, the

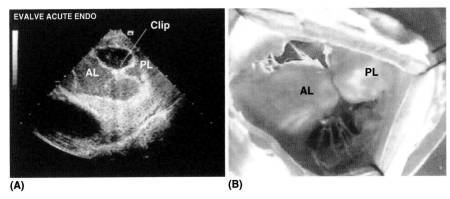

Figure 7.19 (A) Echo short axis of double orifice after clip deployment. AL indicates anterior leaflet PL, posterior leaflet. (B) Ex vivo picture from a similar angle showing well-apposed anterior and posterior mitral valve leaflets viewed from the atrium.

steerable sleeve, and the clip delivery catheter. Dr St Goar et al. (6) reported on 12 postmortem examinations of 12 acute porcine implants, where the clip was able to create a double-orifice mitral valve. In all cases the clip was located in the desired central location on the valve with the clip arms perpendicular to the line of leaflet coaptation (Fig. 7.19).

No clinically significant inferior vena cava, right atrial, atrial septum, left atrial, leaflet, left ventricle, or chordal trauma was observed in any animal. They concluded that the MitraClip® device was able to successfully approximate the middle scallops of the anterior and posterior leaflets, creating a functional double-orifice mitral valve.

During the early human feasibility study (EVEREST I, Feldman et al.) (7), several product enhancements and ease of use improvements were identified. For example, the initial angle between the steerable sleeve and steerable guide curve planes was adjusted by rotating the key on the steerable sleeve. Doing this resulted in an insertion position that was closer to the nominal position required for the human anatomy resulting in an easier clip positioning. Also, the steerable guide catheter was simplified by removing one of the steering knobs that was needed for the porcine model but was not necessary for placement of the clip in humans. In addition, the dilator tip was redesigned to be more echogenic to more easily visualize the tip relative to the interatrial septum. Also, the clip-locking mechanism was redesigned to provide greater flexibility in locking the clip at any desired angle. This final MitraClip® device and multicatheter system was utilized in the EVEREST II randomized clinical trial and the results of this trial have been reported by Feldman et al. (8).

In summary, the development of the MitraClip® system including designing three catheters and the implantable MitraClip® device was a significant engineering endeavor. The three catheters had many unique and challenging design requirements to allow accurate positioning of the clip on the mitral valve leaflets of a beating heart. The MitraClip® implant also posed many design challenges to ensure atraumatic grasping of the leaflets with a secure locking mechanism to ensure permanent attachment to coapt the leaflets. The final result has been studied in multiple human clinical trials demonstrating a high rate of safe MR reduction that has translated to clinical benefits for patients. These results demonstrate successful achievement of the design requirements for the MitraClip® device.

ACKNOWLEDGMENTS

We thank Jan Komtebedde, DVM, Brian Martin, Eric Goldfarb, Sylvia Erickson, Alfred Raschdorf, Jaime Sarabia, Larry Rogers, Kent Dell, Sandra Saenz, Sylvester Lucatero, Francisco Valencia, Steve Dang, Pedro Lucatero, Jessie Garcia, Mheng Heflin, and Rudy Arechiga for their excellent contributions in development of the MitraClip® therapy.

REFERENCES

1. Fann JI, St Goar FG, Komtebedde J, et al. Beating heart catheter-based edge-to-edge mitral valve procedure in a porcine model. efficacy and healing response. Circulation 2004; 110: 988–93.
2. Ladich E, Michaels MB, Jones RM, et al. Pathological healing response of explanted mitraclip® devices. Circulation 2011; 123: 1418–27.
3. Nielsen SL, Timek TA, Lai DT, et al. Edge-to-edge mitral repair: tension on the approximating suture and leaflet deformation during acute ischemic mitral regurgitation in the ovine heart. Circulation 2001; 104(Suppl 1): I-29–35.
4. Jimenez JH, Forbess J, Croft LR, et al. Effects of annular size, transmitral pressure, and mitral flow rate on the edge-to-edge repair: an in vitro study. Ann Thorac Surg 2006; 82: 1362–8.
5. Avanzini A, Donzella G, Libretti L. Functional and structural effects of percutaneous edge-to-edge double-orifice repair under cardiac cycle in comparison with suture repair. Proc IMechE 2011; 225: 959–71.
6. Goar FG, St Fann JI, Komtebedde J, et al. Endovascular edge-to-edge mitral valve repair: short-term results in a porcine model. Circulation 2003; 108: 1990–3.
7. Feldman T, Wasserman HS, Herrmann HC, et al. Percutaneous mitral repair using the edge-to-edge technique. six-month results of the EVEREST phase 1 clinical trial. JACC 2005; 46: 2134–40.
8. Feldman T, Foster E, Glower DG, et al. Percutaneous repair or surgery for mitral regurgitation. N Engl J Med 2011; 364: 1395–406.

8   The EVEREST trial results
Alice Perlowski and Ted Feldman

INTRODUCTION/TRIAL RATIONALE

The current standard of care for patients with symptomatic severe mitral regurgitation (MR) or asymptomatic severe MR with evidence of left ventricular (LV) dysfunction or dilation is surgical intervention (1). A sizable proportion of patients with severe symptomatic MR are not referred for an operation due to elevated surgical risk. Patients with previous coronary artery bypass graft surgery, multiple comorbidities, and older age constitute the majority of this group. Endovascular therapies for the treatment of severe mitral regurgitation have been developed as an alternative approach to surgical repair in high-risk patients.

The MitraClip® system (Abbott Vascular, Santa Clara, California, USA) involves an implantable clip applied to the mitral leaflets via a transseptal approach, replicating a surgical procedure in which the free edges of the mitral leaflets are sutured together to create a double-orifice mitral opening (Fig. 8.1) (2–6). The MitraClip® is the only percutaneous therapy for MR which has been compared with surgical intervention in a randomized trial, and is the most widely applied percutaneous therapy for MR worldwide.

Outcomes of therapy with the MitraClip® device in the United States have been evaluated in the Endovascular Valve Edge-to-edge REpair STudy (EVEREST) registry, EVEREST II Randomized trial, and EVEREST II High-Risk Registry (HRR). Patients continue to be enrolled in Real World ExpAnded MuLtIcenter Study of the MitraClip® System REALISM, the continued-access registry of EVEREST II. The total number of patients enrolled in these trials has exceeded 1000, rendering the Mitra-Clip® the most well-investigated percutaneous device for the treatment of MR.

EVEREST TRIAL DESIGN

The EVEREST trials enrolled anatomically suitable symptomatic patients with moderate to severe (3+) or severe (4+) MR meeting the recommendations of the American Heart Association/American College of Cardiology guidelines for surgical mitral valve repair (1). All subjects were acceptable candidates for mitral valve surgery and cardiopulmonary bypass. Study sites were chosen based on interventional investigator expertise in catheter-based valve therapies and experience with transseptal puncture, and involvement of a surgeon co-investigator performing more than 25 mitral valve surgeries yearly. Study candidates were evaluated by the principal investigator at each of the study sites to determine whether inclusion criteria for the study were met (Table 8.1) (7).

Prospective qualification of patients occurred based on strict predefined anatomic criteria.

A detailed pre-procedure transthoracic and transesophageal echocardiogram was performed on each patient to ensure that appropriate mitral valve anatomy was present. Degree of calcification in the grasping area, flail width, flail gap, coaptation length, coaptation depth, and leaflet thickness were assessed in detail. A parasternal short axis view with color Doppler was performed to identify the location of the mitral regurgitant jet origin along the line of leaflet coaptation. The ideal MR jet for treatment with MitraClip® is discrete, and originates within the central two-thirds of the line of leaflet coaptation.

Extensive training was provided to technicians and interpreting physicians at all sites to ensure standardization of MR assessment. All echocardiograms were carefully reviewed in an echocardiographic core laboratory (University of California, San Francisco) to determine if the study subjects met strict anatomic criteria required for trial eligibility.

The use of an echocardiographic core laboratory was a unique feature of the EVEREST trials, and likely contributed to the success of the initial experience with the device. In centers continuing to perform MitraClip® therapy, a clear communication must be present between interventionalists, noninvasive cardiologists, and echo technologists to ensure that screening echocardiograms are performed and evaluated with these criteria in mind to ensure that patient selection is optimal.

In the initial feasibility cohort (EVEREST I) was a prospective, multicenter, single arm study that included the initial 55 patients treated with the MitraClip® in the phase I trial, along with 52 roll-in nonrandomized patients treated in EVEREST II. The randomized trial (EVEREST II) was a prospective, multicenter, nonblinded study that randomized patients in a 2:1 fashion to MitraClip® device versus surgery. The HRR was a nonrandomized arm of EVEREST II where patients with high predicted surgical risks received MitraClip® therapy.

All procedures in the EVEREST trials were performed under general anesthesia with TEE and fluoroscopic guidance. Acute procedural success was defined as immediate reduction in MR to ≤2 + by ≥1 clip. Placement of a second clip for severe residual MRs occurred at the discretion of the operator. All patients received heparin for intraprocedural anticoagulation, and were treated with aspirin 325 mg daily for six months and clopidogrel 75 mg daily for 30 days.

The primary efficacy endpoint in EVERST II was the composite of freedom from surgery for mitral valve dysfunction, 3 or 4+ MR, and death at 12 months. The primary safety endpoint was defined as a composite of death, myocardial infarction, reoperation for failed mitral valve surgery, nonelective cardiovascular surgery for adverse events, renal failure, stroke, deep wound infection, prolonged mechanical ventilation, gastrointestinal

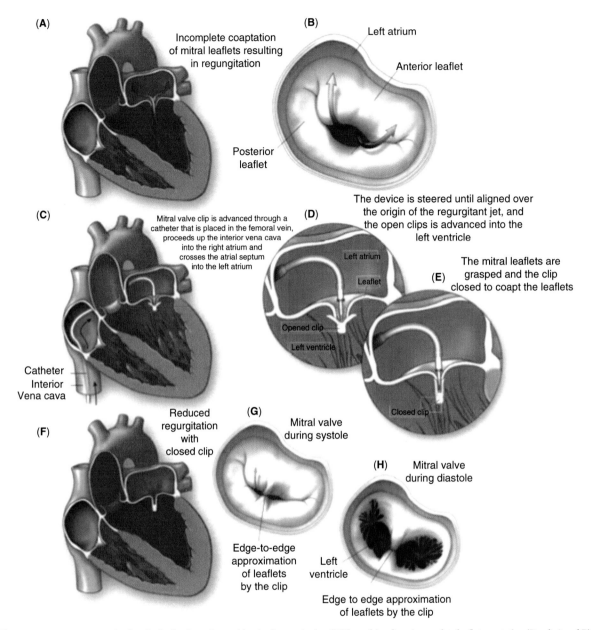

(A) Incomplete coaptation of mitral leaflets resulting in regungitation

(B) Left atrium

Anterior leaflet

Posterior leaflet

(C) Mitral valve clip is advanced through a catheter that is placed in the femoral vein, proceeds up the interior vena cava into the right atrium and crosses the atrial septum into the left atrium

Catheter
Interior
Vena cava

(D) The device is steered until aligned over the origin of the regurgitant jet, and the open clips is advanced into the left ventricle

Left atrium

Leaflet

Opened clip

Left ventricle

(E) The mitral leaflets are grasped and the clip closed to coapt the leaflets

Closed clip

(F) Reduced regurgitation with closed clip

(G) Mitral valve during systole

Edge-to-edge approximation of leaflets by the clip

(H) Mitral valve during diastole

Left ventricle

Edge to edge approximation of leaflets by the clip

Figure 8.1 Percutaneous repair of a mitral valve. In patients with mitral regurgitation (MR) resulting from incomplete leaflet coaptation (Panels A and B), percutaneous mitral valve repair is performed by means of femoral venous and transseptal access to the left atrium to steer the device toward the origin of the regurgitant jet (Panel C). A mitral clip is passed through the mitral orifice from the left atrium to the left ventricle and pulled back to grasp the leaflet edges (Panels D and E). If reduction of the mitral regurgitation is satis factory, the device can be locked and then released (Panel F). A double orifice is created in conjunction with reduction in MR (Panels G and H). *Source*: From Ref. 6.

complication requiring surgery, septicemia, new-onset permanent atrial fibrillation, and transfusion of two units or more of blood at 30 days. Clinical, laboratory, and echocardiographic follow-ups were performed prior to discharge and at 1, 6, 12, 18, and 24 months, and yearly up to 5 years.

An external, independent Data and Safety Monitoring Board composed of at least two interventional cardiologists, a cardiac surgeon, and a statistician monitored the trial progress. Interim analyses of safety were made, as were recommendations regarding study modification or termination.

TRIAL RESULTS
EVEREST I

The initial EVEREST cohort was a prospective, phase I trial designed to evaluate the safety and feasibility of the MitraClip® procedure (5). Symptomatic patients with moderate to severe

Table 8.1 Major Inclusion and Exclusion Criteria (7)

Major Inclusion Criteria

- Moderate to severe (3+) or severe (4+) chronic MR and symptomatic with >25% LVEF and LVESD ≤55 mm or
- Asymptomatic with one or more of the following:

i. LVEF 25–60%
ii. LVESD ≥40 mm
iii. New onset of atrial fibrillation
iv. Pulmonary hypertension defined as pulmonary artery systolic pressure >50 mmHg at rest or >60 mmHg with exercise

- Candidate for MV repair or replacement surgery, including cardiopulmonary bypass
- The primary regurgitant jet originates from malcoaptation of the A2 and P2 scallops of the MV. If a secondary jet exists, it must be considered clinically insignificant

Major Exclusion Criteria

- Acute myocardial infarction in the prior 12 weeks of the intended treatment
- The need for any other cardiac surgery
- Any endovascular therapeutic interventional or surgical procedure performed within 30 days prior
- Ejection fraction 25% and/or end-systolic dimension ≥55 mm
- MV orifice area <4.0 cm²
- If leaflet flail is present:

Width of the flail segment ≥15 mm or flail gap ≥10 mm

- If leaflet tethering is present

Coaptation depth >11 mm, or vertical coaptation length is <2 mm

- Severe mitral annular calcification
- Leaflet anatomy that may preclude clip implantation, proper clip positioning on the leaflets, or sufficient reduction in MR. This may include the following:

Evidence of calcification in the grasping area of the A2 and/or P2 scallops. Presence of a significant cleft of A2 or P2 scallops

More than 1 anatomic criterion dimensionally near the exclusion limits

Bileaflet flail or severe bileaflet prolapse

Lack of both primary and secondary chordal support

- Prior MV surgery or valvuloplasty or any currently implanted mechanical prosthetic valve or currently implanted VAD
- Echocardiographic evidence of intracardiac mass, thrombus, or vegetation
- History of or active endocarditis or rheumatic heart disease
- History of atrial septal defect or PFO associated with clinical symptoms

Abbreviations: LVEF, left ventricular ejection fraction; LVESD, left ventricular end-systolic diameter; MR, mitral regurgitation; MV, mitral valve; PFO, patent formen ovale; VAD, ventricular assist device.

(3+) or severe (4+) MR meeting the recommendations of the American Heart Association/American College of Cardiology guidelines (1) for surgical mitral valve repair were enrolled whether predefined anatomic criteria were met.

The initial cohort enrolled a total of 107 patients. Mean MR grade was 3.3 ± 0.7 at baseline. Degenerative or combined degenerative and functional MRs were present in 79% of patients, with the remainder having pure functional MR. Successful clip placement occurred in 90% of patients; 61% received one clip and 29% received two clips.

Acute procedural success (≥1 clip resulting in ≤2 + MR) was 74%. Of those who had achieved acute procedural success, 77%

had <2+ MR (either mild, or mild to moderate MR) at discharge. Of the 107 registry patients, 96 (90%) achieved a reduction in MR from the clip or mitral valve surgery performed after a clip attempt. Improvement in clinical symptoms occurred in approximately three quarters of patients. New York Heart Association (NYHA) class III/IV symptoms decreased from 55% at baseline to 8% at 12 months. At a median follow-up of 680 days, 70% of patients remained free of surgical intervention.

Surgical options were preserved after the placement of the MitraClip®. Surgical repair with clip removal was performed up to 18 months after percutaneous mitral repair. Eighty four percent of the surgical procedures performed post clip placement turned out to be successful.

The overall major adverse event rate was 9%. Blood transfusions ≥2 units represented the majority of these events. Postprocedure death, periprocedural stroke, and prolonged mechanical ventilation represented less common adverse events, each affecting less than 1%. Partial clip detachment (detachment of a single leaflet from the clip) occurred in 9%, the majority of which were asymptomatic, detected on 30-day echocardiography, and successfully treated with mitral valve surgery. There were no clip embolizations.

The EVEREST I registry provided the initial evidence that MitraClip® therapy was efficacious and safe. Reduction in MR severity to ≤2+ could be was achieved in the majority of patients and was accompanied by significant clinical improvements. There were no intraprocedural complications, minimal periprocedural complications, and low rates of major and minor adverse events. The procedure was well tolerated, with no hemodynamic fluctuations occurring with manipulation of the device in the mitral orifice with a beating heart. Extubation was possible within the first 24 hours in most patients, and hospitalizations were brief, with the majority of patients discharged to home with self-care.

EVEREST II Randomized Trial

The EVEREST I registry provided phase I evidence for percutaneous mitral valve repair, but did not address how the catheter-based approach compared with surgical intervention. EVEREST II was a multicenter, randomized controlled trial designed to evaluate the safety and efficacy of percutaneous mitral repair with the MitraClip® versus conventional surgical repair or replacement for MR (6,7). Patients in the United States and Canada with moderate-to-severe (3+) or severe (4+) MR who were candidates for mitral valve surgery were enrolled. Randomization occurred in a ratio of 2:1 between MitraClip® therapy and mitral surgery (repair or replacement). The primary safety and efficacy endpoints were identical to those of EVEREST I.

A total of 279 patients were enrolled and randomized. The demographics of the two groups were nearly identical with two exceptions (Table 8.2). Peripheral vascular disease was more prevalent in the surgical group versus the MitraClip® group (12% vs. 7%). In addition, there was a higher incidence of congestive heart failure in the MitraClip® group versus the surgical group (91% vs. 78%).

Table 8.2 Baseline Characteristics of the Patients

Characteristic	Percutaneous repair (N = 184)	Surgery (N = 95)	P Value
Age			
Mean (yr)	67.3 ± 12.8	65.7 ± 12.9	0.32
>75yr(no.; %)	55 (30)	26 (27)	0.68
Male sex—(no.; %)	115 (62)	63 (66)	0.60
Coexisting condition (no./total no. ;%)			
Congestive heart failure	167/184 (91)	74/95 (78)	0.005
Coronary artery disease	86/183 (47)	44/95 (46)	0.99
Previous myocardial infraction	40/183 (22)	20/94 (24)	0.99
Atrial fibrillation	59/175 (34)	35/89 (39)	0.42
Diabetes	14/184 (8)	10/95 (11)	0.50
Chronic obstructive pulmonary disease	27/183 (15)	14/95 (19)	0.99
Previous coronary artery bypass grafting	38/184 (21)	18/95 (19)	0.87
Previous percutaneous intervention	44/183 (24)	15/95 (16)	0.12
Left ventricular ejection fraction(%)	60.0 ± 10.1	60.6 ± 11.0	0.65
New York Heart Association functional class(no. %)'			0.16
I	17 (9)	19 (20)	
II	73 (40)	31 (33)	
III	82 (45)	41 (43)	
IV	12 (7)	4 (4)	
Severity of mitral regurgitation (no., %)			0.38
1+ to 2+ (mild to moderate)	0	1 (1)	
2+ (moderate)	8 (4)	6(6)	
3+ (moderate to severe)	130 (71)	67 (71)	
4+ (severe)	46 (25)	21 (22)	
Regurgitant volume (ml/beat)	42.0 ± 23.3	45.2 ± 26.6	0.31
Regurgitant orifice area (cm²)	0.56 ± 0.38	0.59 ± 0.35	0.55
Cause of mitral regurgitation (no. , %)			0.81
Functional	49 (27)	26 (27)	
Degenerative			
With anterior or bileaflet flail or prolapse	58 (32)	25 (26)	
With posterior flail or prolapse	72 (39)	42 (44)	
With no flail and no prolapse	5 (3)	2 (2)	

Source: From Ref. 6.

Table 8.3 Primary Efficacy Endpoint at 12 Months and Major Adverse Events at 30 Days in the Intention-to-Treat Population

Event	Percutaneous repair (no., %)	Surgery	P Value
Primary efficacy endpoint			
Freedom from death, from surgery for mitral valve dysfunction, and from grade 3+ or 4+ mitral regurgitation	100 (55)	65 (73)	0.007
Death	11 (6)	5 (6)	1.00
Surgery for mitral valve dysfunction	37 (20)	2 (2)	<0.001
Grade 3+ or 4+ mitral regurgitation	38 (21)	18 (20)	1.00
Major adverse event at 30 days			
Any major adverse event	27 (15)	45 (48)	<0.001
Any major adverse event excluding transfusion	9 (5)	9 (10)	0.23
Death	2 (1)	2 (2)	0.89
Myocardial infraction	0	0	NA
Reoperation for failed surgical repair or replacement	0	1 (1)	0.74
Urgent or emergency cardiovascular surgery for adverse event	4 (2)	4 (4)	0.57
Major stroke	2 (1)	2(2)	0.89
Renal failure	1 (<1)	0	1.00
Deep wound infection	0	0	NA
Mechanical ventilation for >48 hr	0	4 (4)	0.02
Gastrointestinal complication requiring surgery	2 (1)	0	0.78
New onset of permanent atrial fibrillation	2 (1)	0	0.78
Septicemia	0	0	NA
Transfusion of ≥2 units of blood	24 (13)	42 (45)	<0.001

Source: From Ref. 6.

difference in this composite endpoint: the need for subsequent surgery was 20% in the MitraClip® group at 12 months, compared with 2.2% for repeat mitral valve surgery in the surgical group. Nearly 80% of the MitraClip® recipients avoided surgery in the first 12 months, and the frequency of death and MR grade 3 to 4+ was not different in the device versus the surgical group.

The efficacy endpoint for noninferiority of the device was met at two years (p = 0.04), with surgery being superior for better reduction in MR grade. The difference in composite endpoint was again heavily influenced by the increased need for surgery for valve dysfunction post procedure in the percutaneous group (22% versus 4% in the surgical group). At two years' follow-up, the number of patients receiving MitraClip® therapy who avoided surgical intervention remained close to 80%.

Substantial clinical improvements were achieved in both the percutaneous and surgical groups. At one year, 98% of the MitraClip® patients and 87% of the surgical patients were NYHA class I/II. Both groups had significant reductions in LV

The safety and efficacy endpoint results of the EVEREST II trial are depicted in Tables 8.3 and 8.4. The efficacy endpoint for noninferiority of the MitraClip® therapy versus surgical intervention was met at 12 months. The device group achieved the primary efficacy endpoint (composite freedom from death, surgery for mitral valve dysfunction, or 3 or 4+ MR) in 55% compared with 73% in the surgical group (p = 0.0007) in an intention-to-treat analysis. The increased rate of surgical referral after MitraClip® therapy drove the

Table 8.4 Secondary Endpoints at 12 Months in the Intention-to-Treat Population

Endpoint	Percutaneous repair (N = 184)			Surgery (N = 95)			P Values for comparison between study groups
	No. of patients	Value	P Value for comparison between baseline and 12 mo	No. of patients	Value	P Value for comparison between baseline and 12 mo	
Change from Baseline in Left Ventricular Measurement							
End-diastolic volume (ml)	144	-25.3 ± 28.3	<0.001	66	-40.2 ± 35.9	<0.001	0.004
End-diastolic diameter (cm)	148	-0.4 ± 0.5	<0.001	67	-0.6 ± 0.6	<0.001	0.04
End-systolic volume (ml)	144	-5.5 ± 14.5	<0.001	66	-5.6 ± 21.0	0.04	0.97
End-systolic diameter (cm)	146	-0.1 ± 0.6	0.06	67	-0.0 ± 0.6	0.86	0.38
Ejection fraction (%)	144	2.8 ± 7.2	<0.001	66	-6.8 ± 10.1	<0.001	0.005
Change from Baseline in Quality-of-Life score							
30 days							
Physical component summary	147	3.1 ± 9.4	<0.001	64	-4.9 ± 13.3	0.004	<0.001
Mental component summary	148	4.4 ± 11.3	<0.001	64	1.8 ± 13.4	0.29	0.14
12 Months							
Physical component summary	132	4.4 ± 9.8	<0.001	60	4.4 ± 10.4	0.002	0.98
Mental component summary	133	5.7 ± 9.9	<0.001	60	3.8 ± 10.3	0.006	0.24
Severity of Mitral Regurgitation at 12 mo (no., %)	153			69			<0.001
0+ (none)		9 (6)	NA		13 (19)	NA	
1+ (mild)		57 (37)	NA		39 (57)	NA	
1+ to 2+ (mild to moderate)		18 (12)	NA		5 (7)	NA	
2+ (moderate)		41 (27)	NA		9 (13)	NA	
3+ (moderate to severe)		21 (14)	NA		3 (4)	NA	
4+ (severe)		7 (5)	NA		0	NA	

Source: From Ref. 6 .

and end diastolic and end systolic volumes and dimensions. Quality-of-life improvements were seen in both groups at 12 months, yet surgery was associated with a transient decrease in quality of life at 30 days.

Major adverse event rates at 30 days were 48% in the surgical repair group versus in 15% in the percutaneous repair group (p = 0.001) in an intent-to-treat analysis. Three times the amount of blood transfusions occurred in the surgical group compared with the percutaneous repair group (45% vs. 13%, p < 0.001), which drove the primary safety endpoint. When transfusions were excluded, the rate of major adverse events at 30 days continued to be lower in the device group versus the surgery group (5% vs. 10%, P = 0.23), although the difference was not significant.

Subgroup analysis for the primary efficacy endpoint at 12 months showed a significant interaction favoring percutaneous therapy in patients older than 75 years, with functional rather than degenerative MR, and with LVEF <60% (Fig. 8.2). No significant subgroup interactions were identified regarding the rate of major adverse events at 30 days.

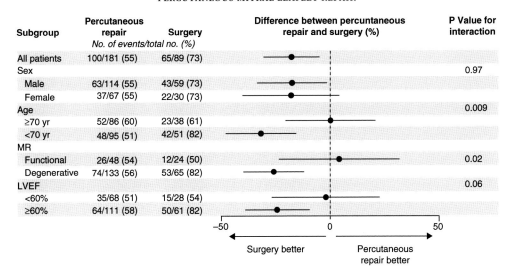

Subgroup	Percutaneous repair	Surgery	Difference between percuntaneous repair and surgery (%)	P Value for interaction
	No. of events/total no. (%)			
All patients	100/181 (55)	65/89 (73)		
Sex				0.97
Male	63/114 (55)	43/59 (73)		
Female	37/67 (55)	22/30 (73)		
Age				0.009
≥70 yr	52/86 (60)	23/38 (61)		
<70 yr	48/95 (51)	42/51 (82)		
MR				
Functional	26/48 (54)	12/24 (50)		0.02
Degenerative	74/133 (56)	53/65 (82)		
LVEF				0.06
<60%	35/68 (51)	15/28 (54)		
≥60%	64/111 (58)	50/61 (82)		

Figure 8.2 Subgroup analyses for the primary endpoint at 12 months. Shown are the difference in rates of the primary efficacy endpoint (freedom from death, from mitral valve surgery, and from grade 3+ or 4+ mitral regurgitation; MR) between patients in the percutaneous-repair group and those in the surgery group for all randomized patients and those in four post hoc subgroups. In the subgroup for the comparison of the left ventricular ejection fraction (LVEF), data were missing for two patients, including one patient who had MR of more than grade 2+. The horizontal lines indicate 95% confidence intervals. *Source:* From Ref. (6).

EVEREST II High-Risk Registry

Patients enrolled in the EVEREST I registry and EVEREST II randomized trial were considered acceptable candidates for mitral valve surgery. The purpose of the EVEREST II HRR was to evaluate the MitraClip® device in patients with elevated surgical risk (8). Seventy-eight patients with moderate to severe MR and an estimated surgical mortality risk of ≥12% (measured with Society of Thoracic Surgery calculator or based on assessment by a surgeon) were enrolled. Prespecified criteria qualifying a patient as high risk included age >75, LVEF <35%, prior chest surgery, and creatinine >2.5 mg/dL. The echocardiogram screening process and qualifying anatomic criteria were identical to EVEREST I and EVEREST II. Thirty-six patients who did not meet the anatomic screening criteria, based on transthoracic or transesophageal echo assessment, were used as a matched control group.

The HRR patients were clearly the sickest of the EVEREST series. The majority of patients were elderly (>75 years) men with congestive heart failure and coronary artery disease. A substantial number of patients in the high-risk group had previous cardiac surgery (62%), previous myocardial infarction (56%), COPD (35%), and moderate to severe renal disease (23%). The majority of the patients in the HRR had functional MR (59%); a contrast to the EVEREST I and EVEREST II randomized trials, where approximately 20% of MR was functional and the remainder degenerative.

Successful device placement occurred in 96% of patients. The majority of patients had a reduction in MR at discharge (83%), with 71.8% achieving a reduction in MR ≤2+. Overall 30-day mortality in the HRR group and control groups were similar, (7.7% and 8.3% respectively) and significantly lower

than predicted surgical mortality of 18.2% for open heart MV surgery in this patient cohort (p = 0.006). Survival was improved in the HRR group compared with the control group at one year (76.4% vs. 55.3%, p = 0.047).

At 30 days, 6 months, and 12 months, patients with MR 2+ or less were 72.9%, 73.3%, and 77.8% respectively, which represented a statistically significant change from baseline. Annual hospitalizations for heart failure in the HRR were decreased as a result of MitraClip® therapy by 45% from baseline. Significant improvements were seen in LV dimensions, NYHA class, and quality-of-life scores at 30 days and one year. These beneficial effects were present in both the functional MR and degenerative MR groups.

REALISM

The REALISM Continued-Access Registry was created when the EVEREST II trial completed enrollment in September 2008. The aim of REALISM is to continue to offer MitraClip® therapy to select patients with moderate to severe MR. REALISM is a prospective, multi-center, continued access registry of the EVEREST II study. Patients are currently being enrolled at 38 centers in the United States. Patients are assigned to either a high-risk arm or non-high-risk arm. Clinical, laboratory, and echocardiographic follow-up data are collected at 30 days, 6 months, and 12 months. Quality-of-life and functional capacity following MitraClip® therapy is one of the emphasized endpoints of the study. To date, the registry has primarily enrolled elderly patients with functional MR who are at high risk for mitral valve surgery. This pattern of patient selection is consistent with the subgroup analysis in EVEREST II, and also with the utilization of MitraClip® in the European experience since it became commercially available in 2008 (9).

UNDERSTANDING THE TRIALS

EVEREST I, EVEREST II randomized trial, and the EVEREST II HRR provided valuable insight into the potential role of the MitraClip® device in the current era of MR therapy. Specific anatomic features were identified on echocardiography, which were found to be most predictive of device success with percutaneous therapy. A direct comparison with the surgical "gold standard" was made, which validated the MitraClip® therapy in carefully selected cases. Finally, specific patient populations emerged who may benefit most from this novel device.

Case Selection

It became clear from the EVEREST trials that a careful evaluation of mitral valve anatomy is critical for optimal patient selection. It is crucial that the operator understand the anatomy of the mitral valve leaflets and the location of the mitral regurgitant jet origin prior to the procedure to ensure that clip implantation is feasible. For patients with functional MR, key inclusion criteria in the EVEREST trials included a coaptation length of ≥2 mm and a coaptation depth of ≤11 mm. For patients with leaflet flail, a flail gap of <10 mm and a flail width of <15 mm were required. In all patients, the origin of the MR jet was within the central two-thirds of the line of coaptation in the short axis color Doppler examination. Patients with mitral stenosis or diminished mitral orifice area (MV orifice area <4 cm^2) were excluded, as were those with significant calcification within the target zone.

The detailed anatomic information required for selecting candidates for the MitraClip® device are obtained from a quality transthoracic echocardiogram. Extensive interrogation of the mitral valve should be performed in multiple views, particularly in the parasternal short axis. If a more detailed examination of the mitral valve is needed, transesophageal echocardiography should be performed to complement TTE findings. Echocardiography technicians and interpreting physicians should undergo training regarding proper interrogation of the mitral valve and specific features which are relevant for patient selection for the MitraClip® device.

MitraClip® Vs. Surgical Repair/Replacement

EVEREST II was the first randomized trial to compare a catheter-based MR therapy with surgical intervention. This landmark study demonstrated that despite the more profound reduction in MR severity in the surgical group, patients who underwent percutaneous repair had significantly reduced LV end diastolic dimensions, improved NYHA grade, and improved quality of life compared with baseline and benefited from the superior safety profile of the catheter-based approach.

Several potential explanations exist for why MitraClip® recipients derived significant clinical benefit in EVEREST II despite lesser reductions in MR grade compared with surgery. The absolute degree of MR reduction may be less important than reducing the regurgitation below a critical threshold where ventricular remodeling and symptom improvement occur. The MitraClip® is apparently effective in reducing the

MR below this threshold, accounting for the clinical improvements despite higher degrees of residual MR compared with surgery.

Additionally, the echo estimates of post MitraClip® MR may have been inaccurate in EVEREST II. A double-orifice MR jet can have a significant effect on echo assessment of MR grade. In vitro models have demonstrated that the same volume of MR through a double orifice can appear to have a much greater MR area than the same volume through a single orifice, even when the area of the single- and double-orifice valves are equal (10). Thus, the severity of post MitraClip® MR in EVEREST II may have been overestimated.

EVEREST II demonstrated that there is a substantial difference in safety outcomes between MitraClip® therapy and surgery. The safety endpoint was driven by an over threefold increase in blood transfusion >2 units in the surgical arm. There is a demonstrated mortality penalty associated with blood transfusions after open heart operations. Patients who receive transfusions after cardiac surgery have a higher mortality rate beyond five years postoperatively compared with patients who do not receive transfusions (11). The risks are correlated with the number of units of blood transfused, and persist after propensity adjustment with a relative risk of >1.7 (12–17). Thus, it is clear from the cardiac surgical literature that transfusions are not benign. The increased incidence of both blood loss requiring transfusion and prolonged mechanical ventilation in the surgical group underscores decreased patient tolerance of an open thoracotomy versus a venous puncture.

Patient Population

Data from the EVEREST trials, along with published European experiences with the device, have provided insight into patient populations who may benefit most from the MitraClip® device. Subgroup analysis of EVEREST II showed the best outcomes in patients older than 75 years, with functional rather than degenerative MR, and with LVEF <60% (Fig. 8.2). In anatomically appropriate patients with functional MR and at high risk for surgical intervention, MitraClip® therapy may be the most reasonable first option.

The high-risk patient population included in EVEREST HRR represents a group, which has never been treated with surgery in the past and has been excluded from surgical registries. These generally older, poorly functioning patients have poor prognosis and limited therapeutic options. In addition, the majority of the patients in the EVEREST HRR had functional MR. The favorable effect of MitraClip® therapy on the LV dimensions, clinical heart failure symptoms, and quality-of-life parameters in these patients is striking. The results of the HRR are largely consistent with the European experience for patient selection since commercialization of the device there in 2008, where a large proportion of patients who are undergoing the MitraClip® procedure have functional MR, are at a high risk for surgery, and have derived significant anatomical and functional benefits from this technology (9).

LIMITATIONS OF THE EVEREST TRIALS AND THE MITRACLIP® DEVICE

Although the EVEREST trials were robust and well designed, with a inclusion of a randomized controlled trial and a core echocardiography laboratory allowing for standardization of echocardiogram interpretation, several limitations of the trials should be appreciated. The specific challenges of the MitraClip® device and implantation procedure must also be acknowleged.

EVEREST II, despite its randomized controlled design, was not blinded. Thus, a certain amount of expectation bias may have occurred during the follow-up evaluation. More patients who were randomized to surgery discontinued participation in the study protocol, which decreased the available long-term data in the surgical group.

Reported follow-up of the EVEREST trials did not extend past three years, which makes long-term durability of the device difficult to assess. The long-term durability of MR reduction is unknown. The surgical experience with isolated edge-to-edge repair has shown durable results to 12 years (18).

The majority of patients selected for participation in the EVEREST trials had degenerative mitral regurgitation. However, one of the main conclusions of the randomized trial and HRR was that the therapy appeared to be most beneficial in patients with functional mitral regurgitation. Additional trials which include patients with functional MR, along with review of the emerging European experience will clarify the role of the MitraClip® in various types of mitral valve and regurgitant jet anatomy.

A large proportion of the patients studied in the EVEREST trials, with the exception of the EVEREST HRR, were acceptable candidates for mitral valve surgery. However, it appears from the extensive European experience that patients who may benefit most from the favorable safety profile of the MitraClip® procedure are at high risk for surgery due to age and multiple comorbidities. Although percutaneous repair does not appear to provide as robust an echocardiographic result as open surgical procedures, the HRR showed that its clinical benefit is clearly better than medical therapy in the high-risk population. More investigation must be conducted in higher-risk populations to solidify this point.

Despite its obvious potential, there are several recognized limitations to the MitraClip® device and procedure. The device requires introduction of a 24 Fr guide catheter into the femoral vein, which has the potential to cause vascular damage and injury of the intra-atrial septum. Despite this, blood transfusions continue to be far more prevalent in the surgical arm of the randomized trial. The septum heals in the vast majority of patients and ASD has not been a significant problem in the trial experience to date.

Delivery of the implantable clip is technically demanding, and requires training and acceptance of a large learning curve. This was evident in the feasibility registry, where procedure times in the first third of the cohort were an hour longer than the final third of the cohort, even when performed by interventionalists with extensive experience in catheter-based procedures. New sites that have started using this device commercially in Europe have benefitted from the prior experience, and the learning curve has been shortened with the accumulation of shared knowledge. In the United States, familiarity with the device is also increasing, and device success rates have continued to improve from 90% in the early experience to 98% in the most recent continued access registries.

There is some concern that the chance for surgical repair may be lost after placement of a MitraClip®. Patients have undergone successful repair as long as five years after placement of a clip. In some cases repair may not be possible after a MitraClip® procedure. It appears that many of the valve replacements after prior MitraClip® implantation have been in patients at higher risk for failed repair, such as those with anterior or bileaflet prolapse, or with calcified mitral annulus. It is important that a surgeon who intends to remove a MitraClip® understands how to unlock the device, to avoid damage to the leaflets (19).

The MitraClip® device is not applicable to all subsets of patients with MR, particularly those with rheumatic disease, annular calcification involving the grasping area of the leaflets, or ruptured papillary muscles. Patients must meet specific anatomic criteria to be considered for the device, and many potential candidates are turned down due to inappropriate mitral valve anatomy. Additionally, concerns have been raised by the surgical community that percutaneous edge-to-edge repair alone, despite its demonstrated ability to improve LV dimensions, may not be sufficient to fully prevent annular dilatation in functional MR. As is the case for surgical annuloplasty for functional MR, the primary problem for many patients is LV dysfunction, which is not remedied by conventional mitral repair.

Percutaneous annuloplasty devices which address progressive annular dilatation are in phase I trials, and may eventually be used alone, or in combination with the MitraClip® to address annular dilation. As more novel percutaneous therapies become available, a wider range of patients will be considered candidates for catheter-based MR therapy.

CONCLUSIONS

The U.S. EVEREST trial experience, in combination with the commercial use of the MitraClip® device in Europe has enabled over 3000 patients to benefit from this novel therapy. It is clear from the EVEREST trial experience that the MitraClip® offers significant clinical and quality-of-life benefit to patients, with an excellent safety profile compared with surgical intervention. The patient population who benefits most from this therapy appears to be older, at a high risk or inoperable patients with functional or degenerative MR, who otherwise have limited or no therapeutic options. Additional experience with the device in the United States will continue to clarify the ideal candidates and clinical settings for MitraClip® therapy.

DISCLOSURES

Dr Feldman is a consultant for and receives research grants from Abbott, Boston Scientific, and Edwards Lifesciences. Dr Perlowski has nothing to disclose.

REFERENCES

1. Bonow RO, Carabello BA, Chatterjee K, et al. Focused update incorporated into the ACC/AHA 2006 guidelines for the management of patients with valvular heart disease: a report of the American college of cardiology/American heart association task force on practice guidelines (writing committee to develop guidelines for the management of patients with valvular heart disease. J Am Coll Cardiol 2008; 52: e1–142.

2. St. Goar FG, Fann JI, Komtebedde J, et al. Endovascular edge-to-edge mitral valve repair: acute results in a porcine model. Circulation 2003; 108: 1990–3.

3. Fann J, St. Goar F, Komtebedde J, et al. Off pump edge-to-edge mitral valve technique using a mechanical clip in a chronic model. Circulation 2003; 108: IV–493.

4. Fann JI, St. Goar FG, Komtebedde J, et al. Beating heart catheter-based edge-to-edge mitral valve procedure in a porcine model: efficacy and healing response. Circulation 2004; 110: 988–93.

5. Feldman T, Wasserman HS, Herrmann HC, et al. Percutaneous mitral valve repair using the edge-to-edge technique: six-month results of the everest phase i clinical trial. J Am Coll Cardiol 2005; 46: 2134–40.

6. Feldman T, Foster E, Glower DG, et al. Percutaneous repair or surgery for mitral regurgitation. N Engl J Med 2011; 364: 1395–406.

7. Mauri L, Garg P, Massaro JM, et al. The EVEREST II Trial: design and rationale for a randomized study of the evalve mitraclip® system compared with mitral valve surgery for mitral regurgitation. Am Heart J 2010; 160: 23–9.

8. Whitlow PL, Feldman T, Pederson W, et al. The EVEREST II high risk study: acute and 12 month results with catheter based mitral leaflet repair. J Am Coll Cordiol 2012; 59: 130–9.

9. Franzen O, Baldus S, Rudolph V, et al. Acute outcomes of mitraclip® therapy for mitral regurgitation in high-surgical-risk patients: emphasis on adverse valve morphology and severe left ventricular dysfunction. Eur Heart J 2010; 31: 1373–81.

10. Lin BA, Forouhar AS, Pahlevan NM, et al. Color Doppler jet area overestimates regurgitant Volume when multiple jets are present. J Am Soc Echocardiogr 2010; 23: 993–1000.

11. Murphy GJ, Reeves BC, Rogers CA, et al. Increased mortality, post-operative morbidity, and cost after red blood cell transfusion in patients having cardiac surgery. Circulation 2007; 116: 2544–52.

12. Engoren MC, Habib RH, Zacharias A, et al. Effect of blood transfusion on long-term survival after cardiac operation. Ann Thorac Surg 2002; 74: 1180–6.

13. Koch CG, Li L, Duncan AI, et al. Morbidity and mortality risk associated with red blood cell and blood-component transfusion in isolated coronary artery bypass grafting. Crit Care Med 2006; 34: 1608–16.

14. Koch CG, Li L, Duncan AI, et al. Transfusion in coronary artery bypass grafting is associated with reduced long-term survival. Ann Thorac Surg 2006; 81: 1650–7.

15. Kuduvalli M, Oo AY, Newall N, et al. Effect of peri-operative red blood cell transfusion on 30-day and 1-year mortality following coronary artery bypass surgery. Eur J Cardiothorac Surg 2005; 27: 592–8.

16. Scott BH, Seifert FC, Grimson R. Blood transfusion is associated with increased resource utilisation, morbidity and mortality in cardiac surgery. Ann Card Anaesth 2008; 11: 15–19.

17. Surgenor SD, DeFoe GR, Fillinger MP, et al. Intraoperative red blood cell transfusion during coronary artery bypass graft surgery increases the risk of postoperative low-output heart failure. Circulation 2006; 114: I43–8.

18. Maisano F, Vigano G, Blasio A, et al. Surgical isolated edge-to-edge mitral repair without annuloplasty: clinical proof of principle for an endovascular approach. Eurointervention 2006; 2: 181–6.

19. Argenziano M, Skipper HD, Letsou GV, et al. Surgical revision after percutaneous mitral repair with the MitraClip® device. Ann Thorac Surg 2010; 89: 72–80.

9   Outcomes for functional mitral regurgitation
James Hermiller, Douglas Segar, David Heimansohn, and Nauman Siddiqi

INTRODUCTION

Left ventricular (LV) dysfunction is frequently complicated by functional mitral regurgitation (FMR) in patients with ischemic heart disease and idiopathic dilated cardiomyopathy. FMR often results in further progression of LV systolic dysfunction, adverse LV remodeling, and worsening heart failure (1). Although surgical results in FMR are not as effective as surgical results in degenerative mitral regurgitation (MR), surgical treatment is selectively used to lessen the degree of MR. The most frequently employed surgical method used to treat FMR is undersized ring annuloplasty; however, significant MR recurs in up to a third of patients (2–4). Furthermore, unlike surgery for degenerative MR, surgical repair in FMR has not enhanced survival.

Besides ring annuloplasty, chordal-sparing valve replacement and other reconstructive procedures, including the "edge-to-edge" technique, have also been used to treat FMR (3,5,6). Edge-to-edge repair using a surgical approach to create a double orifice was first performed by Alfieri in 1991 (Fig. 9.1) (7). Durable results in surgically treated patients without annuloplasty have subsequently been described in a selected group of patients for as long as 12 years after initial repair (6). Previous studies with the edge-to-edge repair for ischemic FMR have also been reported (8). When edge-to-edge is used as a first choice repair method in properly selected FMR patients, results are improved compared with the use of edge-to-edge as a bail-out for a repair when other surgical techniques have failed. (6,8–10). Based on the concept of the "edge-to-edge" surgical repair, the MitraClip® device (Abbott Vascular, San Jose, California, USA) employs a percutaneously delivered clip rather than suture to secure and repair the mitral valve (MV) (11) and is delivered using femoral vein and transseptal access to the MV. In the randomized Endovascular Valve Edge-to-edge REpair STudy (EVEREST) II trial, compared with surgical repair, the MitraClip® was safer, although not as effective at reducing MR. However, MitraClip® did demonstrate equivalent improvements in functional class, quality of life at one year and LV remodeling (12). A post hoc analysis of the EVEREST II randomized data was performed examining the impact of MR etiology and other higher risk predictors including LV ejection fraction (EF) and age above 70. This analysis found that the primary endpoint of the study was not different between surgery and MitraClip® in those with functional MR, reduced LV function, and age over 70 (12). This chapter focuses on the results of the MitraClip® in FMR patients.

DEVICE AND TECHNIQUE DESCRIPTION

The MitraClip® device and percutaneous mitral repair system have been described previously (11–15). The MitraClip® implant is approximately 4 mm wide and 12 mm long (Fig. 9.1). Anterior and posterior mitral leaflet tissue is independently secured between two components of the clip creating permanent coaptation of a portion of the leaflets, simulating the Alfieri edge-to-edge suture repair (Fig. 9.2). The clip is delivered using a coaxial guide and delivery catheter system. The procedure is performed under general anesthesia using fluoroscopy and transesophageal, and on occasion transthoracic, echocardiographic guidance (15). Figure 9.3 demonstrates a typical case of severe FMR treated with a single mitral clip.

Functional MR patients were selected for therapy if they met basic criteria for intervention from the 1998/2006 American College of Cardiology/American Heart Association Joint Task Force recommendations regarding therapy for valvular heart disease (16). Functional MR was defined as MR occurring without demonstrated echocardiographic structural valve defects. Patients with moderate-to-severe (3+) or severe (4+) functional MR who were symptomatic with an EF $\geq 25\%$, or if asymptomatic with a compromised LV function [EF <60% or left ventricular end-systolic dimension (LVESD) >40 mm] were candidates (Table 9.1). All baseline and follow-up echocardiograms were assessed by an independent core laboratory (UCSF, San Francisco, California, USA). MR was graded according to the criteria of the American Society of Echocardiography guidelines (17) using strict definitions for multiple quantitative (regurgitant volume, regurgitant fraction, vena contracta width, and regurgitant orifice area) and qualitative criteria (color flow Doppler and pulmonary venous flow) for MR severity assessment (18). Key anatomic inclusion criteria included a regurgitant jet origin associated with the A2-P2 scallop segments of the mitral valve, and an available coaptation depth of at least 2 mm. Although during the randomized portion of the study, a coaptation depth of not more than 11 mm was necessary, coaptation depth greater than 11 mm is no longer an exclusion, a criterion particularly relevant to FMR, where leaflet tethering leads to a increased coaptation depth (Fig. 9.3).

RESULTS OF MITRACLIP® USE IN FMR

Early Experience: Roll-in EVEREST I and II Patients

The initial data suggesting that the MitraClip® effectively treats functional MR was derived from roll-in patients from the EVEREST I and II studies (19). There were 23 patients with functional MR who underwent percutaneous mitral repair with the MitraClip® device. Median age was 75 years (74% were older than 65 years), 87% had a history of congestive heart failure, and 83% were New York Heart Association (NYHA) functional class III or IV. Ten patients (43%) had one or more prior median sternotomies. In this very early

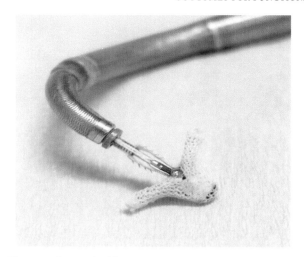

Figure 9.1 Photograph of the MitraClip® device and delivery catheter. The clip is opened with two arms extended to allow for grasping of the mitral leaflets.

experience, overall acute procedural success (APS), defined as placement of one or more clips resulting in discharge MR severity less than or equal to moderate (2+) as determined by the core echocardiographic lab, was achieved in 19/23 (83%) of patients. Of the patients with APS, 53% were discharged with 1+ or less. There were no in-hospital or 30-day deaths. Eighty-three percent of the 23 patients remained surgery free after a median follow-up of 369 days (range, 27–1077 days). Four of the 23 patients (17%) had MV surgery after an unsuccessful clip procedure, one of which occurred during the initial hospitalization. The remaining three patients underwent MV surgery as planned for recurrent MR post-clip implant. Clinical improvement occurred in 75% of patients who achieved APS. Mean NYHA functional class decreased significantly from 2.8 ± 0.5 at baseline to 1.8 ± 1.1 at 12 months (p = 0.0087). One patient (8%) had worsened symptoms at 12 months associated with chest pain requiring cardiac catheterization with angioplasty and stenting. This patient's MR was assessed as mild (1+) at 12 months. Improvements in symptoms were supported by objective measures of reverse left ventricular remodeling at 12 months. Patients with matched data at baseline and 12 months experienced a statistically significant decrease in LV dimensions and volumes, including: left ventricular end-diastolic dimension (LVEDD), LVESD, and LV end-systolic volume (LVEDV) (p <0.05) along with a non–statistically significant decrease in LVESV (p = 0.012). EF remained stable in this population from baseline to 12 months. In terms of durability, Kaplan–Meier (K-M) freedom from death was 89% at 12 months and 2 years. K-M freedom from surgery was 95% at 12 months and 2 years. Freedom from surgery, or reoperation, is the commonly reported endpoint after isolated MV repair surgery and also reflects the clinical durability of the device (Fig. 9.4).

FMR Patients: EVEREST I, II, and High-Risk Registry: 2-Year Follow-Up

A subsequent analysis examined 122 patients with FMR consecutively treated within the EVEREST I and II studies, including the high registry, who underwent percutaneous mitral repair with the MitraClip® device and who had the two-year follow-up (Table 9.2) (20) outlines the enrollment details in these patients. The median age of this group was 71.1 years, 55% were male, 57% had a prior myocardial infarction, 55% had prior sternotomy, 50% had a history of atrial fibrillation, 14% had severe renal dysfunction, and 31% had significant COPD. Nearly 80% had NYHA functional class III or IV symptoms. Moderately severe (3+) or severe (4+) MR was present in 95% and the overall mean EF was 48.2% + 10%.

A high percentage (97%) of patients had successful placement of at least one MitraClip®; in 3/122 no clip was placed. A single clip was placed in 2/3 and one clip in the others. APS was achieved in 94/122 (Fig. 9.5). Mean procedural time was 188 + 69 min. Thirty-day major complication rate was 8.2% excluding transfusion and 21.3% when a 2-unit or more transfusion is included (Table 9.3). Ninety six percent were discharged to home without home health care. Four patients died within the 30 days of procedure. In one patient myocardial infarction on the day of procedure occurred, and the patient died the following day. In the second patient, acute pulmonary edema and hemodynamic instability occurred two days post procedure, and he died on day 4. In the third patient, retroperitoneal bleed during procedure, led to a multiorgan failure, stroke, and death on day 11. The fourth patient died of refractory CHF on day 19.

Two-year follow-up data were available in high percentage of patients as outlined in the table. Over 90% were free of MV surgery at two years (Fig. 9.6). Survival at one and two years was 84% and 71%, respectively. Functional class was substantially improved with favorable results noted at one year becoming stable at two years. MR was reduced with over 80% of patients at two years having less than 3+ MR (Fig. 9.7). The results at one year were durable through two years. Favorable LV remodeling at one year was maintained at two years with significant reductions in LV end-systolic and end-diastolic dimensions/volume compared with baseline (Fig. 9.8). Quality-of-life metrics significantly improved as well.

These data suggested that the MitraClip® procedure provided significant clinical benefits in FMR patients, including symptomatic improvement as well as favorable LV remodeling. These results were durable through two years, as indicated by a sustained reduction of MR grade and LV size, improved NYHA functional class, and very low need for MV surgery in one to two years.

High-Risk Functional Mitral Regurgitation: EVEREST II

The role of the MitraClip® has been increasingly focused on patients at high risk for surgical treatment, and given that the majority of patients treated in the commercial setting have

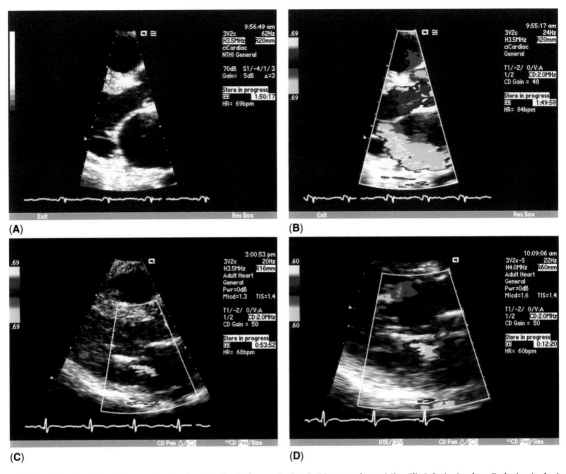

Figure 9.2 Transthoracic echocardiograms showing functional mitral regurgitation (MR) pre- and post-MitraClip® device implant. Each view is obtained at the same time of the cardiac cycle during late systole with the similar machine settings. (A) The incompetent valve appears normal without color flow Doppler. (B) Color flow Doppler shows severe baseline functional MR. (C) Thirty days post MitraClip® implant shows mild central MR by color flow Doppler. Arrow indicates the MitraClip® device. (D) Two years post MitraClip® implant shows ongoing reduction of the MR by color flow Doppler.

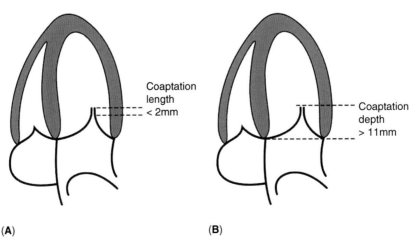

Figure 9.3 Illustrations of key anatomic exclusion criteria. (A) Patients were excluded if the coaptation length is less than 2 mm. (B) In EVEREST I and the randomized portion of EVEREST II, patients were excluded if the coaptation depth was greater than 11 mm. Subsequently, in this case it was not an exclusion.

FMR and are at high surgical risk, the outcomes in this subgroup are particularly relevant(21). Most recently, high–surgical risk patients with FMR were studied. These patients were enrolled in the EVEREST II High-Risk Registry and the ongoing continued-access REALISM studies. Patient enrollment details are shown in Figure 9.9. One-year follow-up is available for this group. Table 9.4 outlines the high-risk demographics of this group in comparison with The Society of Thoracic Surgeons (STS) database for MV repair and replacement. Much like the results from earlier analyses, outcomes in this cohort were favorable with low 30-day major adverse cardiac events rates for these high-risk patients (Table 9.5). Mitral grade of 2+ or less was noted in nearly 90% of patients at one-year follow-up (Fig. 9.10). Reductions in the severity of MR were coupled with significant improvements in indices of left ventricular remodeling, LV end diastolic volume and dimension both significantly declining. Particularly important in this group was the substantial improvement in functional class and quality-of-life indices

Table 9.1 Inclusion Criteria for EVEREST Studies

1. Candidate for mitral valve repair or replacement surgery
2. Moderate to severe (3+) or severe (4+) chronic mitral valve regurgitation, and:
   Symptomatic with LVEF >25% and LVESD ≤ 55 mm or,
   Asymptomatic with one or more of the following:
   i. LVEF >25–60%
   ii. LVESD ≥ 40 mm to 55 mm (60 mm EVEREST High-Risk Ongoing Access) Registry and Realism
   iii. New onset of atrial fibrillation
   iv. Pulmonary hypertension defined as pulmonary artery systolic pressure >50 mmHg at rest, or >60 mmHg with exercise.

Abbreviations: LVEF, left ventricular ejection fraction; LVESD, left ventricular end-systolic dimension.

(Fig. 9.10). Furthermore, hospitalization rates were significantly reduced by MitraClip® therapy (Fig. 9.11).

DISCUSSION
These results, derived from the EVEREST studies of functional MR, demonstrate that percutaneous MV repair using the Mitra-Clip® device can be successfully accomplished with low morbidity and mortality and with acute MR reduction to less than moderate (2+) in the majority of patients. A substantial proportion of patients remain free from need for MV surgery or recurrent MR greater than moderate at one-year follow-up. Furthermore, MitraClip® treatment in these patients improves functional class, quality-of-life metrics, the frequency of hospitalization for CHF, and ventricular remodeling. The favorable one-year results remained durable to two years.

Surgical Treatment of Functional Mitral Regurgitation
The best surgical approach for the treatment of FMR remains controversial. While FMR has been associated with decreased survival no clear survival benefit has been demonstrated for patients undergoing surgery for FMR, and the survival in patients undergoing surgical treatment of FMR has been reported to be lower than the survival in patients undergoing surgical treatment for degenerative MR (22–24). The double-orifice, or edge-to-edge, surgical MV repair technique involves using suture to create permanent coaptation of the MV scallops at the origin of MR. Excellent results utilizing the isolated edge-to-edge repair (no annuloplasty or leaflet resection) approach to repair the valve in selected patients with degenerative or functional MR have been reported with up to 12-year follow-up (10). Although ring annuloplasty alone in FMR patients results in excellent freedom from reoperation, early

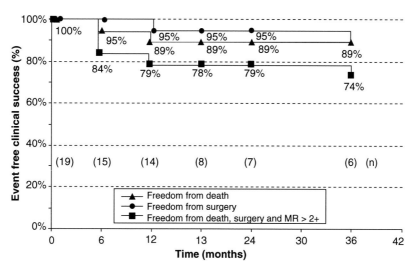

Figure 9.4 Kaplan–Meier curves for functional mitral regurgitation (MR) patients (n = 19) who achieved acute procedural success. The top curve is freedom from death, the middle curve is freedom from surgery, and the bottom curve represents a stringent reporting of survival by combining all key durability measures including freedom from death, freedom from surgery, and freedom from MR >2+. Time = months after clip implant.

reoccurrence of moderate to severe MR is frequent (25). McGee et al. reported a 28% MR (>2+) reoccurrence rate at 6 months. These results indicate alternative treatment options are needed for these patients.

The poor survival rates of FMR patients after surgery may be attributable to their underlying disease (26). Most often surgery for FMR is adjunctive to treatment for coronary artery disease. In the EVEREST studies, however, patients were excluded if they required surgery for any underlying cardiac disease other than FMR. The advent of percutaneous mitral repair creates the potential for performing staged percutaneous valve and coronary intervention.

Table 9.2 Functional MR Patients Treated with the MitraClip® Device in Clinical Studies Worldwide

EVEREST Clinical Trials	
EVEREST I	9
EVEREST II Roll-in	19
EVEREST II Randomized	48
EVEREST II High-Risk Registry[a]	46
REALISM	360
European Experience	
ACCESS-EU Registry	400
TOTAL FMR Patients	882

[a]High risk defined predicted surgical mortality ≥12% using Society of Thoracic Surgeons risk calculator or surgeon estimate (based on prespecified comorbidities).

Patient Selection for Treatment of Functional Mitral Regurgitation

Patient selection for these studies was strictly protocol based and employed anatomic descriptors and careful evaluation of the severity of MR. The prospective use of echocardiograms for these evaluations assured a patient population in need of therapy and well suited for the MitraClip® device. All patients were symptomatic or asymptomatic with LV dysfunction and importantly were carefully screened for moderate-to-severe or severe FMR (3+ or 4+). Surgical literature has reported on surgery of patients with moderate MR (2+), but this often includes patients undergoing surgery for coronary artery disease, who have adjunctive MV surgery. Eligibility for the EVEREST study required no other underlying cardiac disease requiring surgery; therefore, MR of at least moderate to severe (3+) was defined as an inclusion criterion. With a median age of 75 years, EVEREST patients were older than the first-time isolated MV repair or replacement patients reported in the 2002 STS database (median age of 59 and 64 years old, respectively) (27). Specific morphologic features of the valve leaflets and left ventricle size were required for treatment eligibility. The exclusion of patients with an EF less than 20% or an LVESD greater than 60 mm or coaptation overlap less than 2 mm excludes those patients with globally dilated hearts in whom annuloplasty or other surgical techniques are frequently reported to fail (16,28). The function of a significantly globally dilated LV may be primarily impacted by other underlying cardiac disease, and the relative importance of MR or coronary ischemia is unknown. Additionally, anatomic inclusion criteria are intended to assure sufficient

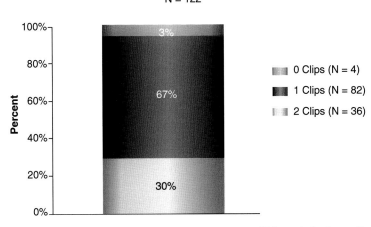

Figure 9.5 Clip implant rate in these 122 patients was 97%. Two-thirds required only one clip.

tissue availability for successful coaptation of the leaflets and reduction of MR with the MitraClip® device (3).

Mechanisms of Treatment

In surgical practice, undersized annuloplasty is currently performed in most of the operations for FMR. This technique is believed to assist with leaflet coaptation to create a competent valve and provide support for the annulus to prevent further dilation. In the case of the MitraClip® device, as in surgical edge-to-edge repair, the clip assists with coaptation of the leaflets to reduce MR. In addition, over time, a tissue bridge from the

anterior to posterior leaflet in the septolateral direction has been observed both in animals and humans (29,30). This healing response may support the repair and help prevent future annular dilatation (31). Whether the clip-initiated tissue bridge provides support for the percutaneous repair and helps prevent septolateral dilatation similar to the function of an undersized full annuloplasty ring remains to be seen and is pending additional long-term follow-up.

Preserving annular contractile function by avoiding annuloplasty may be an advantage of percutaneous mitral repair with the MitraClip® device, especially in patients with decreased LV and annular function. The Kaplan–Meier curves show (Figs. 9.7 and 9.8) failures primarily occurring within the first 6 months following the MitraClip® procedure, which is similar to the period or recurrent MR reported in the surgical literature (25). The rate of MR recurrence reported in this select patient group indicates that percutaneous mitral repair for FMR may offer an alternative treatment with similar rates of MR recurrence without the increased risk of mortality and morbidity associated with open heart surgery. The significant reduction in LV dimensions and volumes achieved by the percutaneous repair may contribute to the preservation of contractility and reduce the risk of annular dilatation.

Table 9.3 30-Day Major Adverse Events: EVEREST Functional MR Treated Patients

30-Day Major Adverse Events	Patients Experiencing Event (N = 122)
Death	4 (3.3%)
Major stroke	1 (0.8%)
Reoperation of mitral valve	0
Urgent/emergent cardiovascular surgery	2 (1.6%)
Myocardial infarction	2 (1.6%)
Renal failure	3 (2.5%)
Deep wound infection	0
Ventilation >48 hrs	2 (1.6%)
New-onset permanent atrial fibrillation	1 (0.8%)
Septicemia	0
GI complication requiring surgery	0
Transfusions ≥2 units	20 (16.4%)
Total	21.3%
Total excluding transfusions	8.2%

Procedural Outcomes

The MitraClip® device provides a therapy for reducing MR without requiring open chest heart surgery. Patients remained hemodynamically stable throughout the percutaneous procedure allowing operators to optimize results in a controlled environment. Complications to date in this population are primarily related either to cardiac catheterization in general or to the transseptal procedure. There have been no thromboembolic

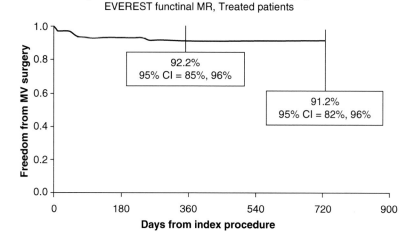

Kaplan-meier freedom from mitral-valve surgery
EVEREST functinal MR, Treated patients

92.2%
95% CI = 85%, 96%

91.2%
95% CI = 82%, 96%

At Risk:	0 Days	6m	1yr	1.5yr	2yr
Device N	122	102	95	87	71

Figure 9.6 Kaplan–Meier analysis of freedom from mitral valve surgery. Rate of mitral valve surgery is low in these patients with FMR undergoing MitraClip® treatment.

**Mitral regurgitation grade
baseline, 1 and 2 years (matched)**

EVEREST functional MR, Treated patients

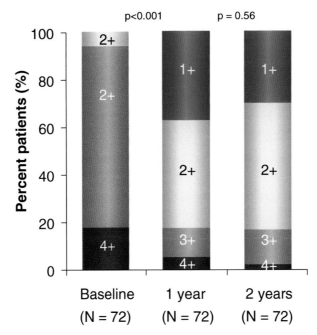

Figure 9.7 Baseline, 1 year, and 2 year matched residual mitral regurgitation.

**LV End diastolic and end systolic volumes baseline,
1 and 2 years (matched)**

EVEREST functional MR, Treated patients

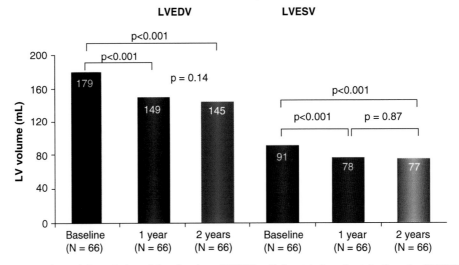

Figure 9.8 Baseline, 1 year, and 2 year left ventricular end diastolic volume (LVEDV) and left ventricular end systolic dimension (LVESD) at baseline, 1 year, and 2 year. Significant favorable LV remodeling was noted and was sustained.

Patient accountability

EVEREST high surgical risk cohort

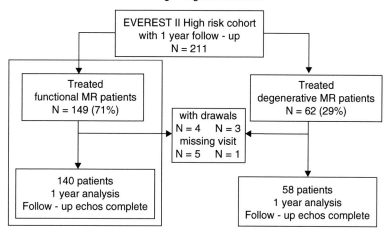

Figure 9.9 There are 211 patients from the EVEREST II high-risk cohort, of which 149 (71%) had functional mitral regurgitation.

Table 9.4 Baseline Demographics and Comorbidities: EVEREST II High–Surgical Risk Cohort Vs. Surgical Candidates

Demographics and Comorbidities	EVEREST II High–Surgical Risk Cohort	STS Data 2002–2006	
	FMR patients N = 149 (%)	Mitral valve replacement N = 21,229 (%)	Mitral valve repair N = 21,238 (%)
Age ≥75 years	45	21	14
Male	61	57	41
NYHA functional class III/IV	87	59	40
Prior Myocardial infarction	57	12	7
Prior cardiovascular surgery	63	28	9
Atrial fibrillation	62	27	13
Moderate to severe renal disease	32	10[a]	4[a]
Cerebrovascular disease	22	11	5
Diabetes	44	17	10

Abbreviations: EVEREST, Endovascular Valve Edge-to-edge REpair STudy; NYHA, New York Heart Association; STS, Society of Thoracic Surgeons; FMR, functional mitral regurgitation.

Table 9.5 30-Day Major Adverse Events: EVEREST II High–Surgical Risk Cohort

30-day events	EVEREST II High–Surgical Risk Cohort # Patients
	FMR patients N = 149
Death	7 (4.7%)
Myocardial infarction	3 (2.0%)
Reoperation for failed surgical MV repair or replacement	0
Non-elective cardiovascular surgery for adverse events	1 (0.7%)
Stroke	4 (2.7%)
Renal failure	3 (2.0%)
Deep wound infection	0
Ventilation >48 hrs	3 (2.0%)
GI complications requiring surgery	0
New-onset permanent atrial fibrillation	1 (0.7%)
Septicemia	1 (0.7%)
Transfusions ≥2 units	21 (14.1%)
Total	31 (20.8%)

Note: Total number of patients may not equal the sum of patients in each row since one patient may experience multiple events. *Abbreviations*: FMR, functional mitral regurgitation; MV, mitral valve.

events reported and the hospital stay has been considerably shorter than for MV surgery. The vast majority of patients treated were discharged home with self-care.

Durability and Left Ventricular Remodeling

Neither the 1998, nor the updated 2006 ACC/AHA Guidelines for the Management of Patients with Valvular Heart Disease recommend surgery for moderate (2+) MR (16,32). The EVEREST protocol eligibility criteria and MR reduction goal were defined to be consistent with these guidelines. Although the 12-month MR effectiveness endpoint of the trial defined success as MR severity of moderate (2+); however, the clinical procedural goal is to reduce MR to mild or less with optimal placement of the MitraClip® device. Overall approximately 80% of patients with FMR treated with the MitraClip® achieve APS with a reduction in MR to 2+ or less. Among patients successfully treated initially in these FMR cohorts, MR at one year was

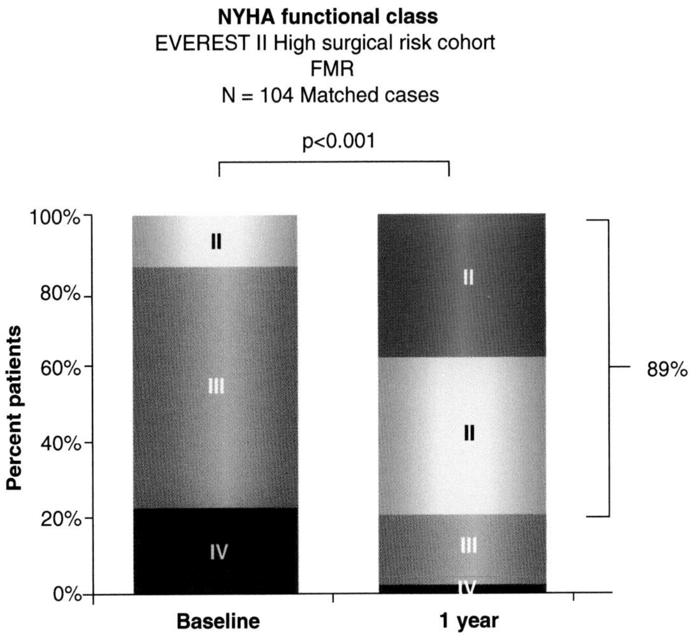

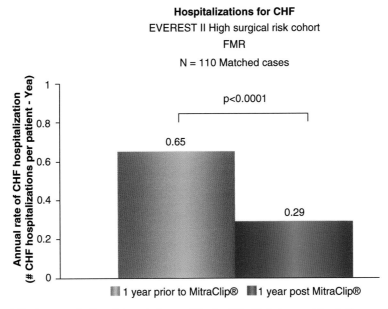

Figure 9.10 Functional class was substantially improved in this high-risk surgical cohort with FMR treated with the MitraClip®.

Figure 9.11 Hospitalizations were significantly lower in the year following MitraClip® placement than in the year prior to treatment.

1+ in a third of patients, 2+ in a half of patients, and the remainder had 3+ MR. These 12-month results remained stable to two-year follow-up.

In patients with severe heart failure or dilated cardiomyopathy, reverse LV remodeling is associated with improved LV function and favorable one-year survival after cardiac resynchronization (33). Yu et al. indicate significant reverse LV remodeling with a >9.5% reduction in LVESV is a predictor for lower long-term mortality and decreased heart failure events. In the current study, the APS patients with matched data at baseline and 12 months and 2-year matched echos experienced LV favorable reverse remodeling with reductions in LVESV, LVEDV, left ventricular end-diastolic dimension, and LVESD. Importantly, the improvements in LV dimensions and volumes provide objective evidence of reverse LV remodeling in a population, where MR severity of 3+ or greater was reduced to 2+ or less. These data support the definition of 2+ MR as a successful outcome when treating patients with 3+ or greater MR severity.

Conclusions

The best treatment of FMR is a subject of ongoing debate. A survival benefit has not been demonstrated with surgical treatment in patients who have compromised cardiac function. The MitraClip® is a percutaneous therapy, which reduces MR while avoiding concomitant injury to the heart, and appears to provide a viable solution for the treatment of FMR. Although MitraClip® was initially thought to be best suited for the treatment of degenerative MR, its use in treating FMR appears promising with low complication rates in these high-risk patients and good acute success, significant reverse remodeling, and encouraging two-year durability. Treatment of FMR in a setting that avoids the physiologic stress that occurs with surgical correction of MR may provide an important treatment alternative for some patients, particularly those at high risk for surgery. These results provide initial data suggesting the Mitra-Clip® device may be a new method for treatment of FMR.

REFERENCES

1. Yiu SF, Enriquez-Sarano M, Tribouilloy C, Seward JB, Tajik AJ. Determinants of the degree of functional mitral regurgitation in patients with systolic left ventricular dysfunction. a quantitative clinical study. Circulation 2000; 102: 1400–06.
2. Tahta SA, Oury JH, Maxwell JM, Hiro SP, Duran CM. Outcome after mitral valve repair for functional ischemic mitral regurgitation. J Heart Valve Dis 2002; 11: 11–19.
3. Calafiore AM, Gallina S, Di Mauro M, et al. Mitral valve procedure in dilated cardiomyopathy: repair or replacement. Ann Thorac Surg 2001; 71: 1146–52.
4. Hung J, Handschumacher MD, Rudski L, et al. Persistence of ischemic mitral regurgitation despite annular ring reduction: mechanistic insights from 3D echocardiography. Circulation 1999; 100: I–73.
5. Miller DC. Ischemic mitral regurgitation redux –to repair or to replace? J Thorac Cardiovasc Surg 2001; 122: 1059–62.
6. Maisano F, Vigano G, Blasio A, et al. Surgical isolated edge-to-edge mitral valve repair without annuloplasty: clinical proof of the principle for an endovascular approach. Euro Interv 2006; 2: 181–6.
7. Alfieri O, Maisano F, De Bonis M, et al. The double-orifice technique in mitral valve repair: a simple solution for complex problems. J Thorac Cardiovasc Surg 2001; 122: 674–81.
8. Umana JP, Salehizadeh BS, DeRose JJ, et al. "Bow-tie" mitral valve repair: an adjuvant technique for ischemic mitral regurgitation. Ann Thorac Surg 1998; 66: 1640–6.
9. Kinnaird TD, Munt BI, Ignaszewski AP, Abel JG, Thompson CR. Edge-to-edge repair for functional mitral regurgitation: an echocardiographic study of the hemodynamic consequences. J Heart Valve Dis 2003; 12: 280–6.
10. Bhudia SK, McCarthy PM, Smedira NG, et al. Edge-to-edge (alfieri) mitral repair: results in diverse clinical settings. Ann Thorac Surg 2004; 77: 1598–606.
11. Feldman T, Wasserman HS, Herrmann HC, et al. Percutaneous mitral valve repair using the edge-to-edge technique: six-month results of the EVEREST phase 1 clinical trial. J Am Coll Cardiol 2005; 46: 2134–40.
12. Feldman T. EVEREST II trial NEJM.
13. Herrmann HC, Rohatgi S, Wasserman HS, et al. Mitral valve hemodynamic effects of percutaneous edge-to-edge repair with the mitraclip® device for mitral regurgitation. Catheter Cardiovasc Interv 2006; 68: 821–8.
14. Feldman T, Leon MB. Prospects for percutaneous valve therapies. Circulation 2007; 116: 2866–77.
15. Silvestry FE, Rodriguez LL, Herrmann HC, et al. Echocardiographic guidance and assessment of percutaneous repair for mitral regurgitation with the evalve mitraclip®: lessons learned from EVEREST I. J Am Soc Echocardio 2007; 20: 1131–40.
16. Bonow RO, Carabello BA, Chaterjee K, et al. ACC/AHA 2006 guidelines for the management of patients with valvular heart disease: a report of the american college of cardiology/american heart association task force on practice guidelines. Circulation 2006; 114: 450–7.
17. Zoghbi WA, Sarano ME, Foster E, et al. Recommendations for the evaluation of the severity of native valvular regurgitation with two-dimensional and doppler echocardiography. J Am Soc Echocardiogr 2003; 16: 777–802.
18. Foster E, Wasserman HS, Gray W, et al. Quantitative assessment of severity of mitral regurgitation by serial echocardiography in a multi-center clinical trial of percutaneous mitral valve repair. Am J Cardiol 2008; 100: 1577–83.
19. Hermiller JB. ACC Late Breaking Clinical Trial 2007.
20. Hermiller JB. Transcather Valve Therapy (TVT) 2011.
21. Hermiller JB. TCT 2011.
22. Bursi F, Enriquez-Sarano M, Jacobsen SJ, Roger VL. Mitral regurgitation after myocardial infarction: a review. Am J Med 2006; 119: 103–12.
23. Gillinov AM, Blackstone EH, Rajeswaran J, et al. Ischemic versus degenerative mitral regurgitation: does etiology affect survival? Ann Thorac Surg 2005; 80: 811–19.
24. Wu AH, Aaronson KD, Bolling SF, et al. Impact of mitral valve annuloplasty on mortality risk in patients with mitral regurgitation and left ventricular systolic dysfunction. J Am Coll Cardiol 2005; 45: 381–7.
25. McGee EC, Gillinov AM, Blackstone EH, et al. Recurrent mitral regurgitation after annuloplasty for functional ischemic mitral regurgitation. J Thorac Cardiovasc Surg 2004; 128: 916–24.
26. Mihaljevic T, Lam BK, Rajeswaran J, et al. Impact of mitral valve annuloplasty combined with revascularization in patients with functional ischemic mitral regurgitation. J Am Coll Cardiol 2007; 49: 2191–201.
27. STS U.S. Cardiac surgery database. mitral valve repair and replacement patients. incidence of complications summary. 2003. www.sts.org.
28. Wisenbaugh T, Skudicky D, Sareli P. Prediction of outcome after valve replacement for rheumatic mitral regurgitation in the era of chordal preservation. Circulation 1994; 89: 191–7.
29. Fann JI, St Goar FG, Komtebedde J, et al. Beating heart catheter-based edge-to-edge mitral valve procedure in a porcine model: efficacy and healing response. Circulation 2004; 110: 988–93.
30. Privitera S, Butany J, Cusimano RJ, et al. Alfieri mitral valve repair: clinical outcome and pathology. Circulation 2002; 106: e173–4.

31. De Bonis M, Lapenna E, La Canna G, et al. Mitral valve repair for functional mitral regurgitation in end-stage dilated cardiomyopathy. Circulation 2005; 112(Suppl I): I-402–8.

32. Bonow RO, Carabello BA, de Leon AC Jr, et al. Guidelines for the management of patients with valvular heart disease: executive summary. a report of the american college of cardiology/american heart association task force on practice guidelines (committee on management of patients with valvular heart disease). Circulation 1998; 98: 1949–84.

33. Yu CK, Bleeker GB, Fung JWH, et al. Left ventricular reverse remodeling but not clinical improvement predicts long-term survival after cardiac resynchronization therapy. Circulation 2005; 112: 1580–6.

10   The role of percutaneous mitral repair for high-risk patients
Willis Wu and Patrick Whitlow

INTRODUCTION

For patients with severe mitral regurgitation (MR) who are at low risk for operative morbidity and mortality, surgical repair is the standard of care to achieve optimal long-term results and reduce mortality. If performed by experienced surgeons at high-volume centers, surgical mitral valve repair can be performed with negligible risk of mortality and low rates of complications (1). Unfortunately, because of advanced age, reduced left ventricular (LV) function, and/or other significant comorbid conditions, a significant number of patients are at prohibitively increased risk for adverse events following surgery and are not offered surgical management (2). The MitraClip® is a device that is delivered via a percutaneous approach; it reduces MR by clipping together the free edges of the anterior and posterior mitral leaflets, thereby reducing the regurgitant orifice area. Recently, the MitraClip® device has been shown to provide an alternative treatment to conventional surgery for patients with severe MR who were candidates for mitral valve repair or replacement (3). Because the percutaneous technique of the MitraClip® implantation is less invasive than the open heart or robotic-assisted surgical repair of the mitral valve, it has emerged as an option for those patients at high risk for perioperative mortality or morbidity. Recent studies have demonstrated echocardiographic, hemodynamic, and symptomatic benefits of MitraClip® implantation in this high-risk surgical population.

DEFINITION OF HIGH-RISK PATIENTS

There is no standard or universally-accepted criterion that defines a high-risk surgical candidate. However, there are certain patient characteristics and comorbid conditions that can be incorporated into risk assessment tools to help estimate perioperative risk. Although risk scores, such as the logistic European System for Cardiac Operative Risk Evaluation (EuroSCORE) (4) and the Society of Thoracic Surgeons (STS) (5) risk score, are not all-encompassing and are not able to account for all factors, they do provide an approximation of risk that is useful for determining whether or not to operate on a patient.

The EuroSCORE incorporates patient-related factors (age, sex, previous cardiac surgery, serum creatinine level, presence of chronic pulmonary disease, extra cardiac arteriopathy, neurologic dysfunction affecting ambulation, or critical preoperative state), cardiac-related factors (presence of unstable angina, LV dysfunction, myocardial infarction within 90 days, and pulmonary hypertension), and operation-related factors (other than isolated coronary bypass grafting, surgery on the thoracic aorta, or presence of post-infarct septal rupture).

The STS risk model takes into account other elements such as demographic information (ethnicity), patient characteristics (height, weight, presence of diabetes, hypertension, peripheral or cerebrovascular disease, use of immunosuppressive medications) cardiac status (need for resuscitation, intra-aortic balloon pump or inotropes, presence of heart failure, arrhythmias, and shock), and severity of coronary and valvular disease.

An STS risk score of ≥12% and/or a logistic EuroSCORE ≥ 20% have been used as criteria to define these patients in the clinical trials that have evaluated the role of MitraClip® therapy in high-risk surgical patients (6–10). In certain cases, however, accurate estimation of perioperative risk cannot be made by using risk assessment tools alone. Certain diagnoses or clinical findings are not captured by the risk calculators but confer significantly increased risk at the time of surgery. Such clinical risk factors include the presence of a porcelain aorta, mobile ascending aorta atheroma, history of mediastinal radiation, and hepatic cirrhosis (10).

The clinical trials that have evaluated the utility of the MitraClip® in high-risk surgical patients, though limited in number, have been successful in enrolling patients with elevated risk. In these studies, the mean logistic EuroSCOREs ranged from 27% to 41% and the mean STS scores varied between 10% and 24% (6–13). However, it is important to note that the patient populations in the MitraClip® trials involving high-risk patients differed significantly between the European and U.S. experiences. Specifically, the European trials enrolled a large proportion of patients with dilated cardiomyopathies, evidenced by low ejection fraction and elevated LV dimensions and volumes, whereas the trials that enrolled patients from the United States evaluated patients without severe LV dilatation.

The EVEREST II High-Risk study (HRS) (10) was an arm of the original EVEREST II clinical trial that was specifically designed to enroll patients with elevated surgical risk. This study included patients with an estimated mortality of at least 12% based on the STS calculator or surgeon estimation. The EVEREST II Real World Expanded Multicenter Study of the MitraClip® System (REALISM) is a prospective, continued access registry that is designed to evaluate outcomes with "real-world" use of the MitraClip®. Patients from the REALISM study who satisfied the high-risk criteria as defined in the HRS study have been pooled together with the patients from the HRS study and are collectively referred to as the EVEREST II high-risk surgical cohort. This cohort consists of a total of 211 patients: 78 patients from the HRS study and 133 of the original 294 patients from the REALISM high-risk study who were available for follow-up of at least one year. Combining the two groups was feasible because the procedure, the definition

Table 10.1 High-Risk Surgical Cohort and EVEREST II RCT Non-High-Risk Baseline Demographics and Comorbidities

Demographics and Comorbid Conditions	High-Risk Cohort N = 211	Concurrent Control (N = 36)	EVEREST II RCT Non–High Risk	
			Device (N = 178)	Control (N = 80)
Age (yrs)	76 ±10	77 ±13	67 ±13	65 ±13
≥75 yrs, (%)	57	64	29	24
Predicted mortalitya (%)	15.0	16.4	4.6	3.9
Prior cardiac surgery (%)	58	50	23	16%
History myocardial infarction (%)	49	36	22	22
Prior stroke (%)	14	14	2	3
COPD/chronic lung disease (%)	30	31	15	14
Moderate-to-severe renal failure (%)	31	31	3	3
History atrial fibrillation (%)	64	53	33	39
Diabetes mellitus (%)	40	42	8	9
Mean ejection fraction (%)	49	55	60	61
LV ESD (mm)	4.2	3.8	3.7	3.4
NYHA class III or IV (%)	86	84	50	50
Etiology – functional MR, (%)	71	64	27	23

aBased on a Society of Thoracic Surgery score of ≥12% or an assigned mortality rate of 12% for prespecified comorbid conditions.
Abbreviations: COPD, chronic obstructive pulmonary disease; LVESD, left ventricular end-systolic diameter; MR, mitral regurgitation; NYHA, New York Heart Association; RCT, randomized controlled trial.

of high surgical risk, the eligibility criteria, and the definitions for major adverse events were identical across both trials. In addition, all echocardiograms were core-lab reviewed, and 28 of 37 institutions and investigators were shared amongst the two trials. While results from the EVEREST II HRS have been published in a peer-reviewed journal, data from the pooled high-risk surgical cohort have been presented at an international meeting but have yet to be published.

Overall, the estimated preoperative risk of mortality of the high-risk surgical cohort was 15%. This elevated risk was mostly a reflection of the significant degree of comorbidities associated with the patients. This combined high-risk surgical cohort was comprised of a population that was at a significantly increased risk than those of the randomized EVEREST II study (Table 10.1). In contrast to the HRS group, only about 30% of patients in the EVEREST II study were more than 75 years; 22% had had a previous myocardial infarction; 15% had chronic pulmonary disease, and 21% had prior coronary artery bypass grafting. Although a significant proportion of patients had a history of congestive heart failure, only a 52% of the EVEREST II randomized patient population was classified as New York Heart Association (NYHA) class III or IV (3). In contrast, 86% of the patients in the high-risk surgical cohort were classified as NYHA functional class III or IV.

Despite the significant differences in comorbidities between the high-risk cohort and the EVEREST II randomized trial, an important commonality between the two studies is that they enrolled patients with LV dysfunction without severe LV dilatation. The mean ejection fraction in the high-risk cohort was 49%, which in the setting of severe MR and reduced afterload,

signified the presence of LV dysfunction. Despite the systolic dysfunction, however, the patients in the high-risk surgical cohort did not have severely dilated hearts, evidenced by a mean LV end-systolic diameter (LVESD) of 42 mm. In fact, both the HRS study and the REALISM high-risk study specifically excluded those with an LVESD >60 mm. Similarly, the EVEREST II trial only enrolled patients with an LVESD between 40 and 55 mm.

CLINICAL RESULTS OF HIGH RISK FOR SURGERY TRIALS IN THE UNITED STATES
Feasibility
The EVEREST II HRS study and the REALISM high-risk trial demonstrated the feasibility of implanting the MitraClip® in a high-risk population. Patients were considered eligible for the trial if they had symptomatic, significant (3 to 4+) MR, whether it be functional or degenerative in etiology. The trials required that the primary regurgitant jet originate from leaflet malcoaptation at the A2-P2 region. Patients were excluded if they had evidence of an acute myocardial infarction in the two weeks prior, an LV ejection fraction ≤20%, and/or severe LV dilatation with an end-systolic diameter >60 mm, or prior mitral leaflet surgery. In addition, patients were prohibited from enrolling if there was echocardiographic evidence of an intracardiac mass, thrombus, or vegetation, or if the leaflet anatomy precluded implantation or proper positioning of the MitraClip®. Specifically, the criteria used for determination of unsuitability for clip implantation included an elevated risk of post-procedural mitral stenosis (mitral valve area <4 cm²), and factors that would predispose to clip failure (flail gap ≥10 mm, flail width ≥ 15 mm, and coaptation length <2 mm).

Though data on feasibility of MitraClip® implantation in the REALISM high-risk study are not available, procedural success rates for the EVEREST II HRS trial have been reported. Specifically, 75 of the 78 patients (96%) had one or two MitraClips® successfully implanted. Of the three procedures that were failures, one was due to an inability to adequately reduce the degree of MR. Another procedure was stopped due to a transseptal complication. The third procedure was aborted because an exclusion criterion was encountered when an intracardiac thrombus was diagnosed on transesophageal echo after induction of general anesthesia but prior to the beginning of the actual procedure. Of the patients with successful MitraClip® implantation, 62 (79.5%) immediately achieved at least a one-grade reduction in MR and 56 (71.8%) demonstrated a reduction of regurgitation to ≤2+ (10).

Major Adverse Events

Eleven of the 211 patients in the high-risk cohort died within 30 days, giving an observed periprocedural mortality rate of 5.2%. This rate was significantly less than the predicted perioperative mortality of 15% that was based on the STS risk calculator or prespecified comorbidities. This mortality rate was also less than that of a retrospectively assigned comparator group, which was slightly higher at 8.3% (estimated perioperative mortality of this group was 16.4%). However, the 5.2% mortality rate was higher than that of patients in the randomized EVEREST II trial, likely reflecting the elevated baseline risk of

the patients in the high-risk cohort versus those in the randomized study. In the randomized trial, 1.1% of those who had received the MitraClip® device and 2.5% of those in the control group had died within 30 days. Kaplan–Meier curves illustrating freedom from all-cause mortality at one- or two-year follow-up in the high-risk cohort and the high-risk comparator group are shown in Figure 10.1. Data were only available for the comparator group through one year, but the separation of the curves favoring the patients who underwent MitraClip® implantation began within the first few months. However, overall survival was still better in the device and control groups of the randomized EVEREST II trial than in the high-risk cohort, again emphasizing the difference in comorbid conditions and overall health between the groups.

Overall, 42 of the 211 patients (19.9%) in the high-risk cohort experienced a major adverse event within 30 days of the procedure. However, excluding the 20 patients (13.7%) who received ≥2 units of blood transfusions, the most frequent adverse event, this number was reduced to 20 patients (9.5%). Stroke occurred in six patients (2.8%), and four (1.9%) developed renal failure. Other notable major adverse events occurred infrequently (Table 10.2).

Importantly, no patients required reoperation of the mitral valve during the 30-day follow-up period and only one patient (0.5%) required urgent or emergent cardiovascular surgery. Even at the one and two-year intervals, ≥98% of patients in the high-surgical risk cohort did not require mitral valve surgery based on Kaplan–Meier curve estimates.

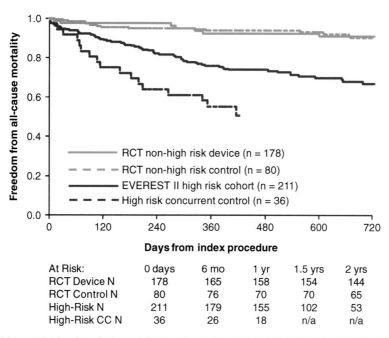

At Risk:	0 days	6 mo	1 yr	1.5 yrs	2 yrs
RCT Device N	178	165	158	154	144
RCT Control N	80	76	70	70	65
High-Risk N	211	179	155	102	53
High-Risk CC N	36	26	18	n/a	n/a

Figure 10.1 EVEREST II high surgical risk and non-high surgical risk randomized controlled trial (RCT) Kaplan–Meier freedom from all-cause mortality.

Efficacy

MitraClip® implantation was associated with a reduction in echocardiographic grade of MR, and the result was durable even up to two years after the procedure. A large majority of patients in the high-risk cohort had 3+ to 4+ MR by echocardiography at baseline, but this was reduced to ≤2+ MR at the one and two-year follow-up (Fig. 10.2). For the 123 patients that were available for follow-up for one year, the decrease in MR severity by echo was statistically significant. Similarly,

Table 10.2 EVEREST II High Surgical Risk 30-Day Major Adverse Events

30-Day Major Adverse Events	High-Risk Cohort N = 211, % Patients (N)
Death	5.2 (11)
Stroke	2.8 (6)
Reoperation of mitral valve	0
Urgent/Emergent Cardiovascular surgery	0.5 (1)
Myocardial infarction	1.4 (3)
Renal failure	1.9 (4)
Deep wound infection	0
Ventilation >48 hrs	1.9 (4)
New-onset permanent atrial fibrillation	0
Septicemia	0.5 (1)
GI complication requiring surgery	0.5 (1)
Transfusions ≥2 units	13.7 (29)
Total	19.9 (42)
Total excluding transfusions	9.5 (20)

for the 42 patients available for follow-up for two years, there was a statistically significant difference in the percentage of patients with ≤2+ regurgitation as compared with baseline.

Patients who underwent MitraClip® placement also had hemodynamic improvement, evidenced by a decrease in LV volumes. Overall in the high-risk cohort, the LV end-diastolic volume decreased from a mean of 163 mL at baseline to 141 mL at one year. There was further reduction at two years to 136 mL. Likewise, there was a decrement in LV end-systolic volume from 86 mL at baseline to 77 mL at one year, and then 71 mL at the two-year mark. For those patients who had only one year of follow-up, the decreases in both LV end-systolic and end-diastolic volumes were both statistically significant. For those patients who were available for two-year follow-up, the changes in LV volumes were statistically significant between baseline and two years, but not between years 1 and 2 (Fig. 10.3).

Possibly related to the improved hemodynamics from reduced LV volumes, patients who underwent MitraClip® device treatment had symptomatic benefit in heart failure as well (Fig. 10.4). At baseline, most of the patients in high-risk cohort were classified as NYHA class III or IV. At the one- and two-year intervals, this proportion had changed such that most patients were class I or II. This was true for those patients available for one- or two-year follow-up. This improvement in heart failure symptoms likely contributed to the observed 47% reduction in heart failure hospitalizations after the procedure was performed (Fig. 10.5).

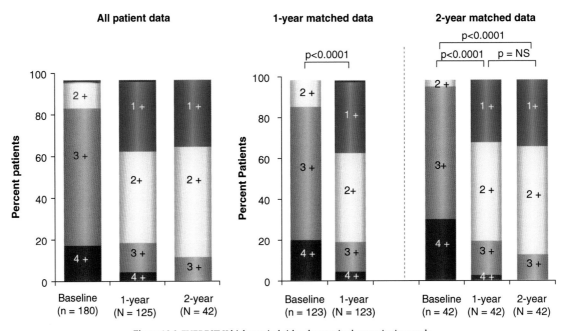

Figure 10.2 EVEREST II high surgical risk cohort: mitral regurgitation grade.

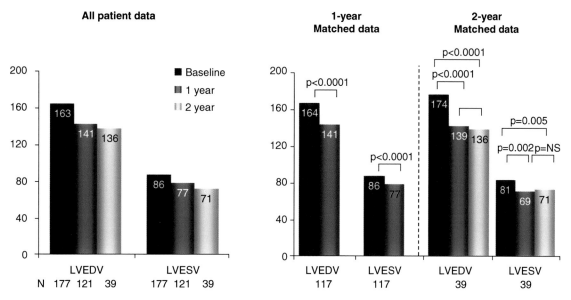

Figure 10.3 EVEREST II high surgical risk cohort: left ventricular end-diastolic and -systolic volumes (LVEDV and LVESV).

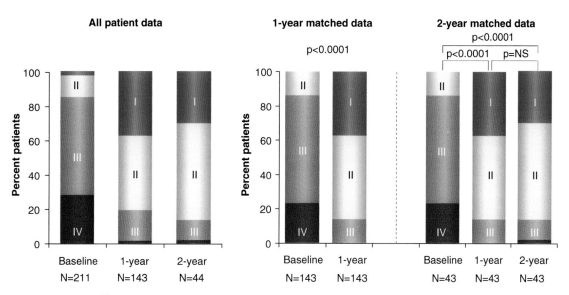

Figure 10.4 EVEREST II high surgical risk cohort: New York Heart Association functional class.

Etiology of Mitral Regurgitation: Functional Vs. Degenerative

In the EVEREST II trial, functional mitral regurgitation (FMR) comprised only 27% of the study population compared with 73% with degenerative valvular disease (degenerative MR) (3). In contrast, 71% of the combined high-risk surgical cohort had FMR as the etiology of their valvular disease and still demonstrated benefit. Likewise, in the EVEREST II HRS study specifically, 59% of patients had functional regurgitation while 41% had degenerative leaflets. It did not appear that the etiology of the regurgitation significantly influenced outcome, as 79% or the patients with functional regurgitation and 75% of patients with degenerative disease had ≤2+ insufficiency on echo. In addition, an equivalent percentage of patients from both groups (74% functional and 75% degenerative) were NYHA class I or II a year following the procedure. Eighty percent of those with FMR and 89% with degenerative MR had improvement in NYHA class by ≥1 grade that was sustained at one year. Mortality data were also similar between the

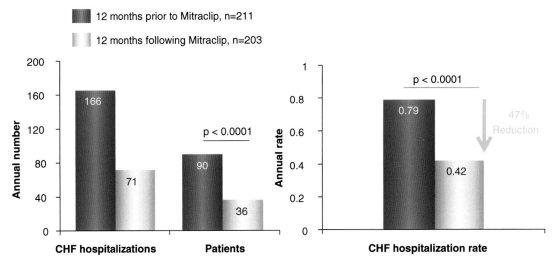

Figure 10.5 EVEREST II high surgical risk cohort: hospitalization for congestive heart failure.

two groups, as death occurred in 26% of patients with FMR compared with 22% in patients with degenerative mitral disease (10).

CLINICAL RESULTS FROM EUROPEAN CENTERS

The present design of the MitraClip® was meant to coapt the P2 and A2 mitral leaflet segments in ventricles with an end-systolic diameter of <60 mm. Patients with MR from advanced systolic heart failure and dilated ventricles pose a challenge to MitraClip® placement because the length of the device may not be able to span the annular diameter, thus leading to incomplete or ineffective clipping of the mitral leaflets. Furthermore, functional MR that results from ventricular dilatation is a fundamentally different disease process than MR stemming from degenerative mitral leaflets and the two have different natural histories with regards to progression of LV dilation. Theoretically, patients with degenerative MR will have a slowing of ventricular dilation once the MR is reduced. Conversely, those with a cardiomyopathy and a primary defect with the myocardium may not exhibit a similar cessation of ventricular enlargement. The utility of the MitraClip® in patients with severe ventricular dilation has been examined predominantly outside of the United States. However, recent European studies have explored the beneficial use of the MitraClip® in patients with primary cardiomyopathy and dilated ventricles with varying success (13).

Feasibility

The feasibility of MitraClip® implantation in a high-risk population is excellent despite the severity of systolic dysfunction and LV dilatation in these patients. In some reports, the device can be delivered successfully in >90% of cases (6–13).

Efficacy

In the cases of successful MitraClip® device implantation in patients with severely dilated LV dimensions, early evidence suggests echocardiographic and clinical benefit similar to that seen in patients with mildly dilated LV dimensions. For example, in the study performed by Treede et al., 186 out of 202 patients (92%) were able to achieve ≤2+ MR after Mitra-Clip® implantation, an even greater number than that seen in the HRS trial (11). In this trial, there was a drop in MR by 1 grade in 30% of patients, by 2 grades in 52%, and by 3 grades in 13%.

The benefits of the MitraClip® were not limited to echocardiographic parameters, as device implantation also resulted in clinical improvement in heart failure as well. Franzen et al. noted that the MitraClip® was able to decrease NYHA class by 1 grade in 30 out of 49 patients (61%) at the time of discharge and a decrease in NYHA class by 2 grades in 14 of 49 patients (29%) (7). In the study by Rudolph et al., nearly 70% of the 81 patients who survived for one year after the procedure had class I or II symptomatology, whereas all of them were class III or IV at baseline (12). Associated with the change in symptom severity was a parallel increase in six-minute walk distances (8,13), but there were also inconsistent results with regards to improvement in NT-ProBNP levels(6,8,9,13) or quality of life as assessed by questionnaires (6,12,13).

The degree to which MitraClip® therapy can reverse the negative remodeling of the heart is not entirely clear. In the study by Rudolph et al., the LV end-diastolic volume decreased from 221 mL to 183 mL while the LV end-systolic volume decreased from 125 mL to 102 mL at one-year follow up (12). Even when the left ventricular end-diastolic diameter (LVEDD) was as high as 64 mm, the MitraClip® was able to reduce this to 62 mm at the 6-month follow-up, which was statistically significant (9). In contrast, other trials have not documented any statistically significant changes in LVEDD, LV end-diastolic volume, or LV end-systolic volume at one month (6,8) or LVEDD at 12 months (11).

Acute and Long-Term Major Adverse Events

Despite enrolling patients with significantly elevated risk of surgical death and dilated left ventricles, there is some evidence to suggest that the MitraClip® procedure can be performed with low mortality and morbidity. Three studies did not record a single mortality during the index hospitalization (6–8). Three other studies reported in-hospital death rates of less than 7% (9,12,13) older age and NYHA functional class IV appeared to be risk factors for early death in at least one of these studies. In this same study, NYHA functional class IV also appeared to be associated with poorer survival six months post procedure as well (13).

Rates of other adverse events after catheter-based mitral valve repair with the MitraClip® were relatively low, but tended to be either procedure-related or cardiac in etiology. Franzen et al. (13) do raise the possibility of creating significant mitral stenosis in their study because of the discovery of a mean gradient across the valve of ≥5 mmHg in 4 out of 19 patients who were available for follow-up measurements at six months. Though this event occurred in a small proportion of patients, there may have been an association with the number of clips required during the procedure, as three out of the four patients with the elevated gradient had two clips deployed. Despite the clinical and echocardiographic benefit demonstrated after MitraClip® placement for dilated cardiomyopathy, many patients still required hospitalization after their initial procedure. Franzen et al. witnessed a 58% re-hospitalization rate within six months in patients who were initially treated successfully with the MitraClip® (13). Twenty-seven percent of patients in the study by Rudolph et al. were admitted again within the follow-up period due to cardiac decompensation (12).

CONCLUSION

Surgical mitral valve repair can be performed safely with a risk of mortality of approximately 1% in patients who are otherwise healthy or have few comorbid conditions (1). However, in patients with elevated surgical risk, operative repair may not be an option because of prohibitive risk. Given the less-invasive percutaneous approach of the mitral clip and the encouraging data available, there appears to be an emerging role for the MitraClip® in treating patients with severe MR and high surgical risk.

MitraClip® trials in the United States have primarily studied patients with either degenerative or ischemic FMR with normal-to-moderate LV systolic impairment but without severe LV dilatation. MR from a primary cardiomyopathy is mechanistically different than the MR studied in the EVEREST and REALISM trials. Patients with dilated cardiomyopathy have a primary disease of the LV muscle leading to dilation of the ventricular cavity and secondary MR. Similarly, patients with ischemic FMR have both mitral valve dysfunction from tethering of one or both leaflets and LV dysfunction from ischemia or infarction. Patients with degenerative disease have primary mitral regurgitation and secondary LV dysfunction. Conceptually, the MitraClip® halts progression of LV dilation by correcting the volume overload caused by degenerated or tethered regurgitant leaflets. On the other hand, in patients with a cardiomyopathic process it is unlikely that simply joining the mitral leaflets without treating the underlying primary myocardial disease will prevent further LV enlargement. Therefore, it will not be surprising if long-term outcomes from mitral valve clipping vary somewhat depending on the degree and possible progression of ventricular dysfunction.

Studies such as the HRS trial and the REALISM high-risk study have shown high rates of successful MitraClip® deployment, and have shown a reduction in echocardiographic assessment of mitral insufficiency. The reduction in regurgitation severity leads to a reduction in intracardiac volume, which translates clinically to an improvement in NYHA functional class and heart failure hospitalizations. In patients without severe dilation of the left ventricle, the MitraClip® can be performed with low complication rates with an uncommon need for future reintervention. Future randomized trials are needed to assess the durability of benefits beyond one or two years in high-risk surgical patients, both in terms of clinical symptoms and potential remodeling. Small nonrandomized trials also suggest a low periprocedural complication rate and significant reduction in MR grade along with clinical improvement in selected patients with dilated cardiomyopathy and severe MR. Further study in this group with dilated hearts is needed to define the role of mitral valve clip placement for this indication.

REFERENCES

1. David TE, Ivanov J, Armstrong S, Rakowski H. Late outcomes of mitral valve repair for floppy valves: implications for asymptomatic patients. J Thorac Cardiovasc Surg 2003; 125: 1143–52.
2. Mirabel M, Iung B, Baron G, et al. What are the characteristics of patients with severe, symptomatic, mitral regurgitation who are denied surgery? Eur Heart J 2007; 28: 1358–65.
3. Feldman T, Foster E, Glower DD, et al. Percutaneous repair or surgery for mitral regurgitation. N Engl J Med 2011; 364: 1395–406.
4. European System for Cardiac Operative Risk Evaluation. http://www.euroscore.org.
5. The Society of Thoracic Surgeons Risk Calculator. http://www.sts.org/sections/stsnationaldatabase/riskcalculator.
6. Van den Branden BJ, Post MC, Swaans MJ, et al. Percutaneous mitral valve repair using the edge-to-edge technique in a high-risk population. Neth Heart J 2010; 18: 437–43.
7. Franzen O, Baldus S, Rudolph V, et al. Acute outcomes of mitra-clip® therapy for mitral regurgitation in high-surgical-risk patients: emphasis on adverse valve morphology and severe left ventricular dysfunction. Eur Heart J 2010; 31: 1373–81.
8. Pleger ST, Mereles D, Schulz-Schönhagen M, et al. Acute safety and 30-day outcome after percutaneous edge-to-edge repair of mitral regurgitation in very high-risk patients. Am J Cardiol 2011; 108: 1478–82.
9. Van den Branden BJ, Swaans MJ, Post MC et al. Percutaneous edge-to-edge mitral valve repair in high-surgical-risk patients do we hit the target? JACC Cardiovasc Interv 2012; 5: 105–11.

10. Whitlow PL, Feldman T, Pedersen WR et al. Acute and 12-month results with catheter-based mitral valve leaflet repair the EVEREST II (endovascular valve edge-to-edge repair) high risk study. J Am Coll Cardiol 2012; 59: 130–9.

11. Treede H, Schirmer J, Rudolph V, et al. A heart team's perspective on interventional mitral valve repair: percutaneous clip implantation as an important adjunct to a surgical mitral valve program for treatment of high-risk patients. 2012; J Thorac Cardiovasc Surg 143: 78–84.

12. Rudolph V, Knap M, Franzen O, et al. Echocardiographic and clinical outcomes of mitraclip® therapy in patients not amenable to surgery. J Am Coll Cardiol 2011; 58: 2190–5.

13. Franzen O, van der Heyden J, Baldus S, et al. Mitraclip® therapy in patients with end-stage systolic heart failure. Eur J Heart Fail 2011; 13: 569–76.

11 Echocardiographic evaluation for mitral regurgitation grading and patient selection

Ehrin J. Armstrong and Elyse Foster

INTRODUCTION

Echocardiography is the cornerstone of patient selection for percutaneous edge-to-edge repair of mitral regurgitation (MR). The accurate assignment of MR severity is critical to the appropriate triage of patients for intervention, and echocardiography has become the primary tool for grading MR severity. However, echocardiographic findings must be viewed in the context of the overall clinical picture, including symptoms, the patient's hemodynamics at the time of the study, and current medical treatment. Two-dimensional transthoracic echocardiography with Doppler provides crucial information about both qualitative and quantitative grading of MR, although it remains incumbent upon the expert echocardiographer to assign an integrated score of MR severity. Both transthoracic and transesophageal echocardiograms are essential for identifying the mechanism of MR and anatomic suitability for percutaneous implantation of a MitraClip® device. In the asymptomatic patient, echocardiographically-determined evaluation of left ventricular size and function also provide the critical thresholds for intervention according to current guidelines.

This chapter discusses the echocardiographic grading of MR severity in the context of consideration for percutaneous edge-to-edge repair of MR. The next chapter extends the clinical discussion of patient selection by addressing the anatomic suitability for MitraClip® implantation and the clinical limitations of patient selection.

GRADING OF MITRAL REGURGITATION SEVERITY

Defining the severity of MR has significant subtleties and variations. Within a given patient, dynamic changes in loading conditions (e.g., elevated left atrial pressure or hypertension) may alter the apparent severity of MR. Between patients, the anatomic heterogeneity of MR and the spatial relationship of the regurgitant jet to the left atrial wall (e.g., central vs. eccentric) may also alter the apparent severity of MR. For these reasons, rigorous and reproducible methodologies for standardization of MR are paramount to successful clinical trial application.

The EVEREST (Endovascular Valve Edge-to-edge REpair STudy) studies were the first clinical trials to utilize a core echocardiography laboratory that employed strict guideline-based qualitative and quantitative assessment of MR. In order to ensure adequate image acquisition, detailed imaging protocols were provided to each site and training sessions were conducted (1).

Detailed attention to echocardiographic image acquisition allowed measurement of overall MR severity grade in 98.4% of the EVEREST I trial patients (2). The importance of this approach cannot be overemphasized, as prior trials had significant discordance in actual severity as measured by performing institutions and the core laboratory, or lacked a definitive protocol for reporting MR severity (3). Translating the detailed and stringent approach used in a clinical trial to practice is akin to the clinical application of core laboratory criteria for determination of stenosis severity in trials of new coronary stents. However, as percutaneous repair methods gain approval and are used more widely, it is imperative that MR severity is accurately assessed to assure that this unique technology is appropriately utilized.

The protocol employed for assessment of MR severity in the EVEREST trials was based on the American Society of Echocardiography guidelines for grading of MR severity (Table 11.1) (4). In the core laboratory, two qualitative and four quantitative measurements were used to determine a composite MR grade. The composite grade is an important overall assessment of MR severity that takes into the account the limitations of each individual measurement of MR severity. In clinical practice, additional criteria can be integrated into the overall assessment. These include the peak mitral E-wave velocity, pulmonary artery systolic pressure, and the density of the MR continuous wave jet.

Qualitative Measurements

Color Doppler flow (CDF) and pulmonary vein flow patterns are the two major qualitative characteristics used to judge the severity of MR. While each of these characteristics is important for initial identification of MR, they also have significant limitations (Table 11.2).

Color Doppler Flow Jet Area

CDF is often the first criterion used when screening for severity of MR (Fig. 11.1). The visual correlation between regurgitant flow and color Doppler signal makes CDF an attractive method for semiquantitative grading of MR severity (5). CDF can also provide important anatomic information regarding the cause of MR, including the area of flow convergence, the origin of the regurgitant jet, and the orientation of the jet within the left atrium. Characteristics of CDF consistent with more severe MR include an eccentric jet demonstrating wall impingement, or a large central jet with an area >40% of the left atrial area and a Doppler signal extending into one or more pulmonary veins (6).

Table 11.1 Quantitative Measurements of Mitral Regurgitation Severity

Variable	Mild (1+)	Moderate (2+)	Moderate to Severe (3+)	Severe (4+)
CDF	• Small • Central • (<4 cm² or <10% of LA area)	• Moderate • Central • (4–6 cm² or 10–30% of LA area)	• Large • Central • (>6 < 8 cm² or >30% <40% of LA area) or Eccentric to 1st PV	• Large • Central • (>8 cm² or >40% of LA area) or eccentric to 2nd PV
PV flow	Systolic dominant	Diastolic dominant	All diastolic	Systolic reversal
RV (mL)	<30	30–44	45–59	≥60
RF (%)	<30	30–39	40–49	≥50
EROA, cm²	<0.20	0.20–0.29	0.30–0.39	≥0.40
Vena contracta width (cm)	<0.30	0.30–0.70	0.30–0.70	≥0.70

Abbreviations: CDF, color Doppler flow; EROA, effective regurgitant orifice area ; LA, left atrial; MR, mitral regurgitation; PV, pulmonary vein; RF, regurgitant fraction; RV, regurgitant volume.

Table 11.2 Advantages and Disadvantages of Criteria for Mitral Regurgitation

Method	Advantages	Disadvantages
CDF	Provides anatomic information about MR etiology	May underestimate severity of MR with eccentric jet
PV flow	Systolic flow reversal specific for severe MR	Less useful if a patient has atrial fibrillation
RV	Can be applied to a double-orifice valve	Requires accurate volumetric assessment of left ventricle
RF	Normalizes regurgitation to filling volumes	Requires accurate volumetric assessment of left ventricle
EROA	Correlated with long-term outcomes in degenerative MR	Assumes a hemispheric flow convergence. May underestimate severity of functional MR.
Vena contracta	Validated with other measures of MR severity. Relatively easy to image	Discriminates between severe and mild, but less sensitive in moderate MR. Cannot be applied to a double-orifice valve

Abbreviations: CDF, color Doppler flow; EROA, effective regurgitant orifice area; MR, mitral regurgitation; PV, pulmonary vein; RF, regurgitant fraction; RV, regurgitant volume.

CDF has important limitations that limit its utility as the sole criterion for MR grading. Doppler area has a poor correlation with quantitative measurements of MR severity, and the Doppler flow depends on hemodynamics, the Nyquist limit, and the imaging sector (7). Additionally, an eccentric jet of MR will appear less severe by CDF than a central jet of similar severity, because the eccentric jet is constrained by the adjacent wall and not able to entrain as much blood (8). This results in a 30–40% decrease in apparent jet area by CDF for the same regurgitant fraction (RF) (9). Quantitative measurements of MR severity are therefore preferable when the MR jet is eccentric (10).

Pulmonary Vein Flow

Pulsed wave Doppler can be used to identify the inflow patterns of the pulmonary vein on TTE and TEE. Pulmonary vein inflow to the left atrium occurs predominately during ventricular systole. With increasing severity of MR, there is blunting of the inflow pattern and an eventual systolic flow reversal (Fig. 11.2) (11).

Numerous hemodynamic disturbances can affect pulmonary vein inflow patterns, thereby limiting the specificity and utility of this measurement among patients with MR (12). A significant percentage of patients with severe MR will develop atrial fibrillation prior to definitive therapy. In the setting of atrial fibrillation, pulmonary vein inflow patterns are informative only if the pattern is systolic dominant (consistent with 1+ MR) or a systolic flow reversal (consistent with 4+ MR). In the echocardiographic substudy of the EVEREST I trial, pulmonary vein flow was the most difficult parameter to assess, due to contamination by the MR jet or coexistent atrial fibrillation (2).

Quantitative Characteristics

While qualitative characteristics are important screening tools for identifying the severity of MR, quantitative techniques have improved reproducibility and correlation with patient outcomes. In the echocardiographic substudy of the EVEREST I trial, there was excellent inter-observer correlation of all quantitative characteristics, with correlation coefficients ≥0.80 for all parameters and inter-observer agreement in regurgitation severity among 84% of cases (2).

Although they are more time intensive to calculate, quantitative measurements of MR also provide an important tool for longitudinal assessment of MR severity. RF and regurgitant volume are especially important tools in the setting of MitraClip® device implantation, where creation of a double-orifice valve may alter the CDF characteristics and result in overestimation of MR severity (13).

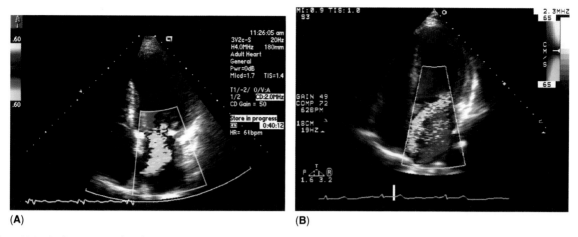

(A)   **(B)**

Figure 11.1 Mitral regurgitation by color Doppler flow. Color Doppler flow (CDF) can be used to semi-quantitatively assess severity of MR. (A) A central jet of MR with a color Doppler area >40% is consistent with severe MR. (B) In eccentric MR, the CDF area may underestimate the severity of MR when compared with quantitative methods.

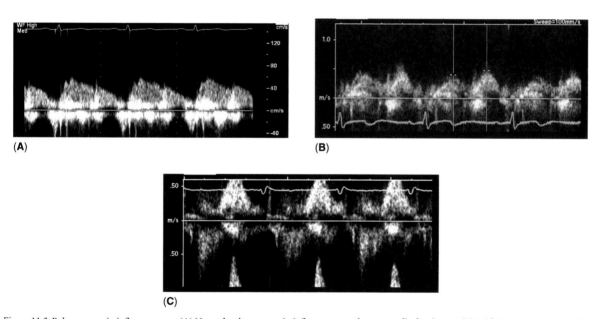

Figure 11.2 Pulmonary vein inflow patterns. (A) Normal pulmonary vein inflow patterns show a systolic dominance. (B) With increasing severity of MR, the systolic inflow pattern in blunted. (C) In severe MR, there is systolic flow reversal of the pulmonary vein inflow pattern.

Regurgitant Volume

Regurgitant volume can be calculated using a variety of methods. Prior to development of Doppler echocardiography, regurgitant volume was often calculated based on invasive left ventricular cineangiography. Echocardiographic measurements of regurgitant volume are based on relative flow through the mitral valve and aortic valve: the difference between diastolic flow through the mitral valve and systolic flow through the aortic valve is equivalent to the regurgitant volume. Although simple in concept, this approach can have significant error when measuring mitral annulus area, especially in the setting of mitral annular calcification and when there is more than trivial aortic regurgitation. Regurgitant volume can also be derived from the proximal isovelocity surface area (PISA) methods used to calculate the effective regurgitant orifice area (EROA; see below), by multiplying EROA by the velocity time integral of the MR jet.

Another echocardiographic technique for measuring regurgitant volume is based on volumetric measurements of the left ventricle and flow through the left ventricular outflow tract (LVOT) (10,14). Regurgitant volume is calculated using the following relationships between forward stroke volume and total stroke volume (Fig. 11.3):

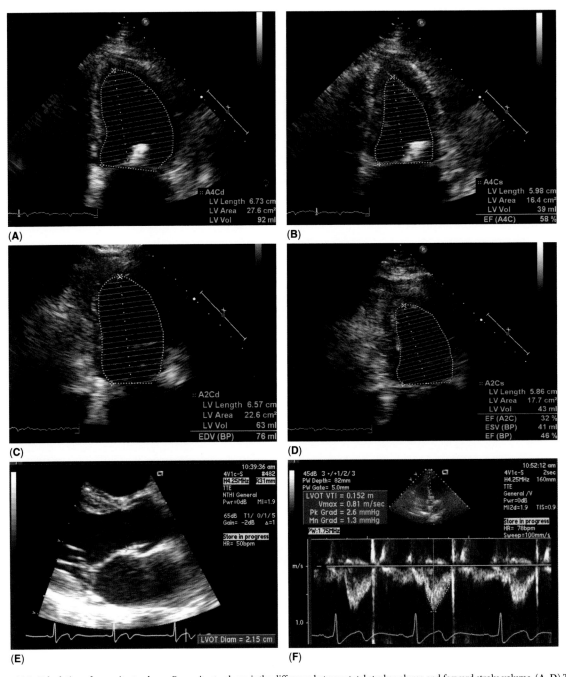

Figure 11.3 Calculation of regurgitant volume. Regurgitant volume is the difference between total stroke volume and forward stroke volume. (A–D) Total stroke volume is calculated using the volumetric measurements of left ventricular end diastolic and left ventricular end systolic volumes. (E–F) Forward stroke volume is obtained by multiplying the left ventricular outflow tract (LVOT) cross-sectional area by the velocity time integral of the LVOT.

$$\text{Forward stroke volume (FSV)} = \text{VTI}_{\text{LVOT}} \times \text{Area}_{\text{LVOT}} \quad (11.1)$$

$$\text{Total stroke volume (TSV)} = \text{LVEDV} - \text{LVESV} \quad (11.2)$$

$$\text{Regurgitant volume (RV)} = \text{TSV} - \text{FSV} \quad (11.3)$$

where VTI_{LVOT} is the velocity time integral of the LVOT, $\text{Area}_{\text{LVOT}}$ is the cross-sectional area of the LVOT, LVEDV is the left

ventricular end diastolic volume, and LVESV is the left ventricular end systolic volume. This approach has the advantage that LVOT measurements are widely reproducible. Additionally, these measurements are independent of mitral valve intervention and can therefore be used during screening of MR severity and also to track MR reduction over time after Mitra-Clip® implantation. The major limitation of this approach is

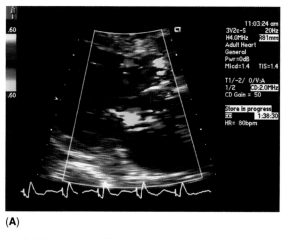 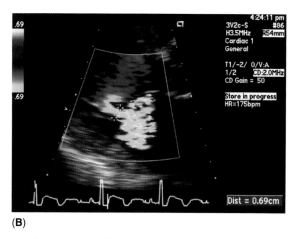

(A) **(B)**

Figure 11.4 Vena contracta. The vena contracta is the narrowest portion of the regurgitant jet. (A) In mild MR, the vena contracta is <0.3 cm. (B) In severe MR, the vena contracta exceeds 0.7 cm.

possible poor endocardial definition leading to errors in the measurement of left ventricular volumes. However, careful attention to echocardiographic technique and use of left-sided echocardiographic contrast agents can improve volumetric measurements (15). This method also remains valid in the presence of significant aortic insufficiency and mitral inflow obstruction.

A regurgitant volume ≥60 mL/beat is consistent with severe MR (16). Among patients with functional MR, a lower threshold of 30 mL/beat may be associated with subsequent adverse outcomes (17). This lower cutoff may reflect in part the hemodynamic impact of a smaller regurgitant volume in the face of a compromised left ventricle.

Regurgitant Fraction
RF is related to the regurgitant volume:

$$\text{Regurgitant Fraction} = \frac{\text{Regurgitant Volume}}{(\text{LVEDV}-\text{LVESV})} \quad (11.4)$$

An advantage of using RF over regurgitant volume is that RF may better reflect the hemodynamic effects of MR for a given left ventricular size. Similar to regurgitant volume, RF has been validated with left ventricular cineangiography and scintigraphy (18). Because it is based on the same volumetric and cross-sectional measurements as regurgitant volume, RF is subject to the same potential measurement errors.

Vena Contracta
The vena contracta is the narrowest width of CDF from the origin of the regurgitant jet (Fig. 11.4). It is slightly smaller than the actual width of regurgitant flow, due to boundary effects (19). Because the vena contracta is narrow, it is important to optimize visualization by zooming the field of view, thereby minimizing the measurement error. The vena contracta is also best measured in a modified parasternal long axis view, in order to maximize axial resolution. Because the

regurgitant flow is parallel to the probe in the apical two-chamber view, measurement in this window will result in overestimation of vena contracta width. With careful imaging, the vena contracta is useful for both central and eccentric jets (20).

Vena contracta width has been extensively validated against other measurements of MR severity (20–22). A vena contracta width of <0.3 cm is consistent with mild MR, while a width of 0.6–0.8 cm can be used as a cutoff for severe MR. Because of the overlap in MR severity with intermediate values of the vena contracta, other methods should also be employed to confirm MR severity. Because vena contracta width has not been previously applied to a double-orifice valve, vena contracta measurements were performed as part of the initial evaluation of MR severity in the EVEREST trials, but not in the follow-up assessment of MR.

Effective Regurgitant Orifice Area
Measurement of EROA is based on the principle of flow convergence (23,24). As a jet of blood approaches an orifice, the flow converges in hemispheric shells of increasing velocity and decreasing surface area: the PISA. Flow through the orifice can then be calculated as the product of PISA × the aliasing velocity (Fig. 11.5):

$$\text{Flow} = 2\pi r^2 \times V_a \quad (11.5)$$

where r is equal to the radius of the isovelocity hemispheric shell and V_a is equal to the aliasing velocity based on the Nyquist limit. Because

$$\text{Flow} = \text{EROA} \times \text{peak velocity} \quad (11.6)$$

EROA can then be calculated as

$$\text{EROA} = 2\pi r^2 \times V_a/V_{peak} \quad (11.7)$$

where V_{peak} is equal to the peak flow velocity of the mitral regurgitant jet, as determined by continuous wave (CW) Doppler. Imaging of the PISA and calculation of EROA is best performed in the apical four-chamber view, with the Nyquist limit adjusted to a value that achieves the most hemispheric-appearing PISA.

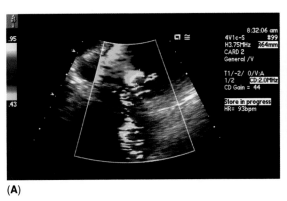
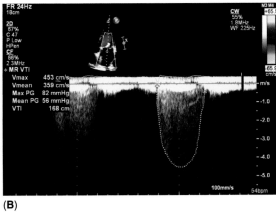

(A)   **(B)**

Figure 11.5 Calculation of effective regurgitant orifice. (A) By lowering the Nyquist limit in the apical four-chamber view, a hemispheric area of proximal isovelocity surface area can be visualized. The radius of this convergence is then measured. (B) Continuous wave Doppler of the mitral regurgitant jet is used to measure the peak regurgitation velocity.

Because the EROA is inversely related to regurgitant jet velocity, the CW Doppler measurement must also be optimized; a smaller CW velocity measurement will result in overestimation of EROA (25). As with vena contracta measurements, EROA was used for baseline measurement of MR severity in the EVEREST trials, but not for follow-up measurement of MR after MitraClip® implantation because this measure of MR severity has not been validated for double-orifice valves (2).

EROA has been studied in numerous clinical situations. Among a population of asymptomatic patients with degenerative MR, an EROA ≥40 mm² was independently associated with both overall and cardiac mortality, independent of other measurements of MR severity. The increased predictive value of EROA may reflect indirect measurement of both kinetic energy (regurgitation) and potential energy (increased left atrial pressure) with EROA. In functional MR, the regurgitant orifice is often elongated, and EROA may underestimate the severity of the MR. Consistent with this, an EROA of 20 mm² has been found to predict heart failure and adverse outcomes among patients with functional MR (17,26). Alternative methods including hemiellipsoid area calculations may correct for the underestimation of hemispherical EROA measurements among patients with functional MR, but such methods require prospective validation (27).

Composite Score

No single measurement of MR severity can capture the anatomic and hemodynamic complexity of MR. Each parameter has important technical limitations. For this reason, it is important to take all the above measurements into consideration, but to then assign an overall MR severity score ranging to from 1+ (mild) to 4+ (severe). This composite score can then be used to track changes in disease severity over time and after therapeutic intervention.

In the EVEREST trials, patients with a score of 3+ or 4+ on three or more parameters met inclusion criteria for moderately severe or severe MR. This formalized and stepwise approach to the grading of MR severity ensured that all patients enrolled met strict criteria for moderately severe or severe MR.

CONCLUSIONS

Quantitative measurements of MR severity add significantly to the discriminatory power of echocardiography to classify MR. Once MR is confirmed as moderately severe (3+) or severe (4+), important anatomic characteristics must also be taken into consideration to determine suitability for percutaneous edge-to-edge repair. While many of these criteria can be screened with TTE, TEE is also important at this stage to identify subtle anatomic findings that may further refine the mechanism and pathology of the MR. These anatomic characteristics are discussed in detail in the next chapter.

REFERENCES

1. Gottdiener JS, Bednarz J, Devereux R, et al. American society of echocardiography recommendations for use of echocardiography in clinical trials. J Am Soc Echocardiogr 2004; 17: 1086–119.
2. Foster E, Wasserman HS, Gray W, et al. Quantitative assessment of severity of mitral regurgitation by serial echocardiography in a multicenter clinical trial of percutaneous mitral valve repair. Am J Cardiol 2007; 100: 1577–83.
3. Acker MA, Bolling S, Shemin R, et al. Mitral valve surgery in heart failure: insights from the acorn clinical trial. J Thorac Cardiovasc Surg 2006; 132: 568–77; 577 e1–4.
4. Zoghbi WA, Enriquez-Sarano M, Foster E, et al. Recommendations for evaluation of the severity of native valvular regurgitation with two-dimensional and Doppler echocardiography. J Am Soc Echocardiogr 2003; 16: 777–802.
5. Miyatake K, Izumi S, Okamoto M, et al. Semiquantitative grading of severity of mitral regurgitation by real-time two-dimensional Doppler flow imaging technique. J Am Coll Cardiol 1986; 7: 82–8.
6. Spain MG, Smith MD, Grayburn PA, Harlamert EA, DeMaria AN. Quantitative assessment of mitral regurgitation by Doppler flow imaging: angiographic and hemodynamic correlations. J Am Coll Cardiol 1989; 13: 585–90.

7. Sahn DJ. Instrumentation and physical factors related to visualization of stenotic and regurgitant jets by Doppler color flow mapping. J Am Coll Cardiol 1988; 12: 1354–65.

8. Cape EG, Yoganathan AP, Weyman AE, Levine RA. Adjacent solid boundaries alter the size of regurgitant jets on Doppler color flow maps. J Am Coll Cardiol 1991; 17: 1094–102.

9. Chen CG, Thomas JD, Anconina J, et al. Impact of impinging wall jet on color Doppler quantification of mitral regurgitation. Circulation 1991; 84: 712–20.

10. Enriquez-Sarano M, Bailey KR, Seward JB, et al. Quantitative Doppler assessment of valvular regurgitation. Circulation 1993; 87: 841–8.

11. Seiler C, Aeschbacher BC, Meier B. Quantitation of mitral regurgitation using the systolic/diastolic pulmonary venous flow velocity ratio. J Am Coll Cardiol 1998; 31: 1383–90.

12. Pu M, Griffin BP, Vandervoort PM, et al. The value of assessing pulmonary venous flow velocity for predicting severity of mitral regurgitation: a quantitative assessment integrating left ventricular function. J Am Soc Echocardiogr 1999; 12: 736–43.

13. Lin BA, Forouhar AS, Pahlevan NM, et al. Color Doppler jet area overestimates regurgitant volume when multiple jets are present. J Am Soc Echocardiogr 2010; 23: 993–1000.

14. Rokey R, Sterling LL, Zoghbi WA, et al. Determination of regurgitant fraction in isolated mitral or aortic regurgitation by pulsed Doppler two-dimensional echocardiography. J Am Coll Cardiol 1986; 7: 1273–8.

15. Hundley WG, Kizilbash AM, Afridi I, et al. Administration of an intravenous perfluorocarbon contrast agent improves echocardiographic determination of left ventricular volumes and ejection fraction: comparison with cine magnetic resonance imaging. J Am Coll Cardiol 1998; 32: 1426–32.

16. Dujardin KS, Enriquez-Sarano M, Bailey KR, et al. Grading of mitral regurgitation by quantitative Doppler echocardiography: calibration by left ventricular angiography in routine clinical practice. Circulation 1997; 96: 3409–15.

17. Grigioni F, Enriquez-Sarano M, Zehr KJ, Bailey KR, Tajik AJ. Ischemic mitral regurgitation: long-term outcome and prognostic implications with quantitative Doppler assessment. Circulation 2001; 103: 1759–64.

18. Blumlein S, Bouchard A, Schiller NB, et al. Quantitation of mitral regurgitation by Doppler echocardiography. Circulation 1986; 74: 306–14.

19. Roberts BJ, Grayburn PA. Color flow imaging of the vena contracta in mitral regurgitation: technical considerations. J Am Soc Echocardiogr 2003; 16: 1002–6.

20. Hall SA, Brickner ME, Willett DL, et al. Assessment of mitral regurgitation severity by Doppler color flow mapping of the vena contracta. Circulation 1997; 95: 636–42.

21. Fehske W, Omran H, Manz M, et al. Color-coded Doppler imaging of the vena contracta as a basis for quantification of pure mitral regurgitation. Am J Cardiol 1994; 73: 268–74.

22. Mele D, Vandervoort P, Palacios I, et al. proximal jet size by Doppler color flow mapping predicts severity of mitral regurgitation. clinical studies. Circulation 1995; 91: 746–54.

23. Vandervoort PM, Rivera JM, Mele D, et al. Application of color Doppler flow mapping to calculate effective regurgitant orifice area. An in vitro study and initial clinical observations. Circulation 1993; 88: 1150–6.

24. Enriquez-Sarano M, Seward JB, Bailey KR, Tajik AJ. Effective regurgitant orifice area: a noninvasive Doppler development of an old hemodynamic concept. J Am Coll Cardiol 1994; 23: 443–51.

25. Enriquez-Sarano M, Miller FA Jr, Hayes SN, et al. Effective mitral regurgitant orifice area: clinical use and pitfalls of the proximal isovelocity surface area method. J Am Coll Cardiol 1995; 25: 703–9.

26. Grigioni F, Detaint D, Avierinos JF, et al. Contribution of ischemic mitral regurgitation to congestive heart failure after myocardial infarction. J Am Coll Cardiol 2005; 45: 260–7.

27. Matsumura Y, Fukuda S, Tran H, et al. Geometry of the proximal isovelocity surface area in mitral regurgitation by 3-dimensional color Doppler echocardiography: difference between functional mitral regurgitation and prolapse regurgitation. Am Heart J 2008; 155: 231–8.

12 Understanding the limits of patient selection for edge-to-edge repair
Ehrin J. Armstrong and Jason H. Rogers

INTRODUCTION

Development of percutaneous edge-to-edge repair has expanded the treatment options for severe mitral regurgitation (MR). Concomitant with development of this technique, there has been a newfound interest in understanding the anatomic heterogeneity of MR and the complex interplay among leaflets, annulus, and the chordal apparatus (1). Unlike aortic stenosis, where the majority of cases in the elderly are due to calcific senile degeneration of the valve, MR can occur due to primary defects in the leaflets (leading to prolapse), the chordal structures (leading to more severe prolapse and flail leaflets), or the left ventricle (leading to functional MR [FMR]) (2). Further complicating this categorization, clinically severe MR may result from a number of regurgitant jet sizes and locations. For these reasons, no single technique can successfully repair all anatomic subtypes of MR. When screening a patient for percutaneous edge-to-edge repair, it is therefore crucial to have an understanding of measurements of MR severity, as well as the anatomic inclusion and exclusion criteria that make this approach feasible (3–5).

This chapter discusses the major anatomic inclusion and exclusion criteria for MitraClip® device implantation among patients with severe MR (Table 12.1). The complete list of inclusion and exclusion criteria for the Endovascular Valve Edge-to-edge REpair STudy (EVEREST) studies, including other clinical criteria, have previously been published (6). The discussion is focused on the rationale for these criteria and the echocardiographic criteria for these measurements. We also briefly discuss the application of MitraClip® device implantation to high-risk subgroups.

ECHOCARDIOGRAPHIC SCREENING FOR ANATOMIC SUITABILITY

Jet Origin

A central jet of MR originating from the A2–P2 interface is a primary inclusion criterion for MitraClip® device implantation. A central jet allows creation of a symmetric double-orifice valve while avoiding the chordae. Screening for a central jet can be performed primarily with transthoracic echocardiography, although transesophageal echocardiography (TEE) may be necessary to confirm an A2–P2 origin of the jet (Fig. 12.1). Although commissural jets can technically be closed with the MitraClip® device, it is more difficult to maneuver the device within the left ventricle, and there is theoretically a greater risk of entangling the MitraClip® device arms within the chordae.

Because the goal of MitraClip® implantation is to create a competent double-orifice valve, the presence of multiple significant jets is also a relative exclusion criterion for MitraClip® implantation; patients with multiple jets of MR were excluded from the EVEREST randomized trial, but were included in the high-risk registry. The rationale for this criterion is that two devices need to be placed in anatomically distinct areas of the valve to effect adequate reduction of MR. This could result in the formation of a triple-orifice valve and a higher transmitral gradient.

Mitral Valve Area

Because a double-orifice valve impairs central leaflet excursion, edge-to-edge repair reduces the mitral valve area and may increase transvalvular gradients. In the initial descriptions of the Alfieri technique, the valve area was measured directly at the conclusion of the surgery using Hegar dilators; a valve area >2.5 cm^2 was considered adequate and unlikely to cause iatrogenic stenosis (7). Among patients with FMR undergoing surgical edge-to-edge repair, echocardiographic study of the mitral valve showed that mean mitral valve area after surgery was 3.8 cm^2 by planimetry and 2.0 cm^2 by pressure half-time. Almost all patients have a mean mitral valve gradient <5 mm Hg after surgical edge-to-edge repair (8). In a population of patients including the Alfieri technique for both myxomatous and FMR, the mean gradient was 3.7 mm Hg and did not increase over time (9). In almost all of these patients, surgical edge-to-edge repair was accompanied by concomitant annuloplasty.

Based on the results of surgical studies with the Alfieri technique, patients enrolled in the EVEREST studies were required to have a baseline mitral valve area of ≥4.0 cm^2 (Fig. 12.2). In an echocardiographic substudy of 24 patients from the EVEREST I study, the mean mitral valve gradient increased from a mean of 1.79 to 3.31 mm Hg after device deployment. Valve area decreased slightly when measured both by pressure half-time or planimetry, but not when calculated by direct invasive measurement (10). During a 12-month follow up, there was a small increase in peak mitral valve gradient, but the mean gradient did not change significantly.

Most of the patients in the initial echocardiographic substudy had a degenerative etiology of MR, and only three of the patients had two MitraClip® devices implanted. A follow-up study included 96 patients from the EVEREST I registry and EVEREST II roll-in; 22 (23%) of the patients had FMR, and 30 (31%) of patients had two MitraClip® devices implanted (11). Patients with FMR had slightly lower baseline and post-procedure mitral valve areas than those with degenerative MR, but these results were not significant. Patients with two MitraClips® implanted had slightly smaller post-procedure valve areas as assessed by pressure half-time, but the measurements were not significantly different by planimetry or invasive assessment. On average, the mitral valve area decreased by 40% after MitraClip® implantation.

Table 12.1 Major Anatomic Inclusion and Exclusion Criteria for MitraClip® Device Deployment

Inclusion Criteria	
Jet origin	Primary regurgitant origin from a malcoaptation of A2–P2 interface

Exclusion Criteria	
Mitral valve orifice area	Mitral valve area <4.0 cm²
Flail width	Flail width of ≥15 mm
Flail gap	Flail gap of ≥10 mm
Coaptation depth[a]	Coaptation depth >11 mm
Coaptation length	Coaptation length <2 mm
Adverse leaflet anatomy	
Leaflet calcification	Calcification in the grasping area of A2 and P2
Cleft	Presence of any cleft in the valve
Severe bileaflet flail	Bileaflet flail or severe bileaflet prolapse
Chordal support	Lack of both primary and secondary chordal support

[a]Coaptation depth applied as an exclusion criterion for the EVEREST II randomized trial, but not for the High-Risk Registry. All other criteria applied to both the randomized trial and High-Risk Registry.

Based on these results, MitraClip® implantation results in a small but significant decrease in mitral valve area and concomitant increase in mitral valve gradient. When using inclusion criteria that include a valve area of ≥4.0 cm², the risk of iatrogenic mitral stenosis is small.

Coaptation Depth

Left ventricular remodeling and geometric distortion alter the balance between leaflet closure and tethering among patients with FMR (12). The extent of this tethering can be assessed by the measurement of the coaptation depth, defined as the distance from the mitral valve annulus to the point of leaflet coaptation at end systole (Fig. 12.3). The magnitude of the coaptation depth may integrate many measurements of MR severity: coaptation depth increases with increased sphericity and annulus size, and varies inversely with ejection fraction (13).

Initial surgical reports suggested that a preoperative coaptation depth >10 mm was an independent predictor of MR recurrence after annuloplasty (13). For this reason, most surgeons recommend mitral valve replacement for patients with a

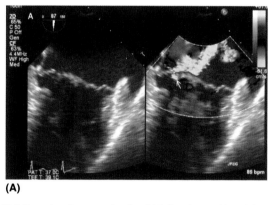
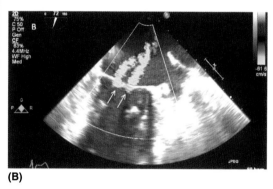

(A)   **(B)**

Figure 12.1 Examples of noncentral and multiple Jets. A central jet origin at the A2–P2 interface ensures deliverability of the MitraClip® device and minimizes the likelihood of device entanglement in the chordae. (A) A noncentral (medial jet in this example) origin of the mitral regurgitation (MR) is a relative contraindication to device placement. (B) Multiple jets (arrows) of MR may not be ideally addressed with percutaneous edge-to-edge repair.

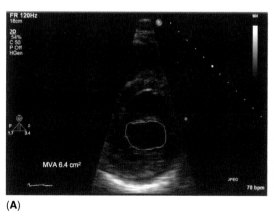
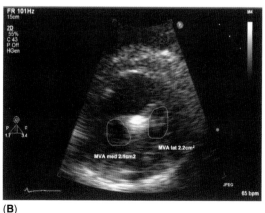

(A)   **(B)**

Figure 12.2 Mitral valve area. Creation of a double-orifice mitral valve may slightly decrease the mitral valve area. The mitral valve areas can be measured on transthoracic echocardiogram using planimetry of the short-axis view. A pre-procedure area of 4.0 cm² or more reduces the likelihood of clinically significant mitral stenosis after MitraClip® implantation.

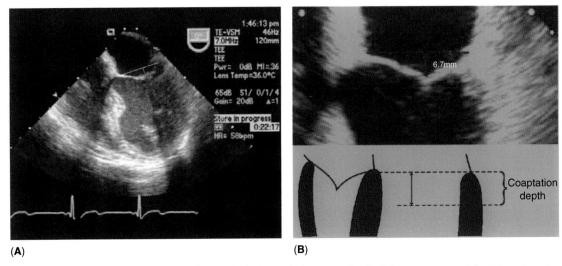

Figure 12.3 Coaptation depth. Among patients with functional mitral regurgitation, coaptation depth is a measurement of the distance from the mitral annular plan to the leaflet tips in systole. (**A**) Coaptation depth is measured in the four-chamber view on transesophageal echocardiography. (**B**) A magnified view shows the measurement of coaptation depth.

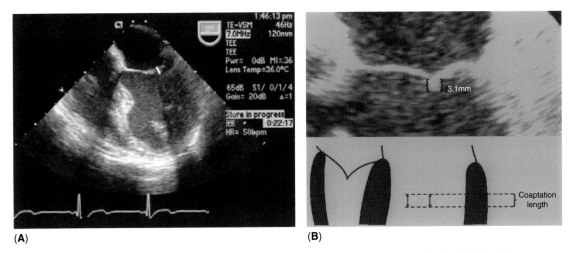

Figure 12.4 Coaptation length. Coaptation length is the length of leaflet apposition at the grasping area. A coaptation length of 2 mm is necessary to ensure adequate tissue for overlap for the MitraClip® device. This measurement is also made in the four-chamber magnified view.

coaptation depth exceeding 10 mm. Using this strategy, Calafiore et al. reported excellent long-term outcomes for surgical treatment of FMR (14). Consistent with this approach, a postoperative coaptation depth ≥5 mm also predicts long-term recurrence of MR (15). Interestingly, surgical edge-to-edge repair combined with an undersized annuloplasty has been reported as an effective treatment for patients with FMR and a coaptation depth >10 mm (16).

Because a goal of the EVEREST II randomized trial was to achieve mitral valve repair whenever surgically possible, a coaptation depth ≥11 mm was an exclusion criterion for inclusion in the trial. In the EVEREST II High-Risk Registry, coaptation depth was not part of the exclusion criteria, since patients were considered high risk for surgery. Although studies specifically examining the efficacy of MitraClip® implantation among subjects with coaptation depths ≥10 mm are not available, the surgical literature supporting edge-to-edge repair among patients with increased coaptation depth suggests that these patients may also benefit from MitraClip® implantation (16).

Coaptation Length

Coaptation length, defined as the length of the A2–P2 interface on 2D echocardiography, was required to be 2 mm or more for inclusion in the EVEREST studies (Fig. 12.4). The rationale for this measurement was that there must be an adequate plane of tissue overlap to allow edge-to-edge approximation with implantation of the MitraClip® device. In practice, most patients with MR possess adequate coaptation length to undergo MitraClip® implantation. A major group of patients who may be excluded based on this measurement are those with severe annular dilation and resultant failure of central coaptation. Because the mechanism of MR in these cases may result primarily from annular dilation, patients with this anatomic subset of MR also may benefit primarily from annuloplasty.

Flail Gap

Among patients with degenerative MR, the presence of a flail leaflet results in greater separation of the opposing leaflets during systole. A greater distance between apposing edges of the leaflets may make it difficult to adequately grasp both leaflets with the MitraClip® device. The flail gap, a measurement of this leaflet separation, is illustrated in Figure 12.5. On echocardiography, the flail gap is defined as the greatest distance between the ventricular side of the flail leaflet and the atrial side of the opposing leaflet. This gap should be measured in two orthogonal views if possible, with the measurement aligned perpendicular to the plane of the mitral valve annulus. In the EVEREST protocol, these distances were measured on TEE, using both four-chamber and left ventricular outflow tract views. In all clinical trials of the MitraClip® device including the High-Risk Registry, a flail gap of 10 of more millimeters was an exclusion criterion.

Flail Width

While flail gap is a measure of the vertical separation of the mitral leaflets, flail width assesses the length of leaflet along the coaptation line that has flail segments. The rationale for this measurement is patients with a wide flail width may not have adequate reduction of MR after MitraClip® implantation, due to the wide segment of regurgitation. The flail width is measured in the transthoracic echocardiogram short-axis view (Fig. 12.6). In the EVEREST studies, a flail width of 15 mm or more was an exclusion criterion for MitraClip® device implantation.

Other Important Anatomic Features

Mitral Annular and Leaflet Calcification

Extensive mitral annular calcification (MAC) may result in the disruption of annular integrity and success of surgical annuloplasty (17). As a result, patients with extensive MAC and MR are more likely to undergo mitral valve replacement rather than surgical repair. In order to maximize the chance for mitral valve repair among patients randomized to surgery, extensive MAC was an exclusion criterion for enrollment in the EVEREST studies. Because the MitraClip® device functions by grasping leaflet tissue at the A2–P2 interface, any significant disturbance of the tissue at the grasping

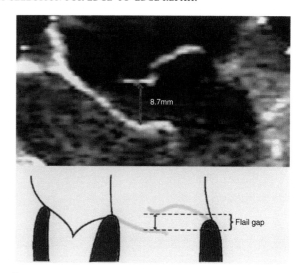

Figure 12.5 Flail gap. Flail gap is defined as the maximal separation between the ventricular side of the prolapsing leaflet and the atrial side of the more apposed leaflet. This measurement should be made with the flail gap aligned perpendicular to the annulus. A flail gap of 10 mm or less ensures that the arms of the MitraClip® device will be able to grasp both leaflets.

region may impact successful deployment of the device. Additionally, the presence of significant calcium or leaflet thickening may make the leaflets less pliable, thereby reducing the ability of the leaflets to coapt tightly after edge-to-edge repair. Any significant calcification of the leaflet at the grasping region is therefore a relative contraindication for MitraClip® device deployment (Fig. 12.7).

Short Posterior Leaflet

Progressive left ventricular dysfunction and remodeling leads to alterations in the geometry of the chordal apparatus among patients with FMR. The posterior leaflet is most often the more severely tethered of the two leaflets, due to inferoposterior remodeling of the left ventricle. The extent of the posterior leaflet restriction may impact the feasibility of MitraClip® device deployment. In the EVEREST studies, the posterior leaflet was required to have a sufficient mobility to make leaflet grasping feasible. Figure 12.8 shows two examples of patients with FMR and a short posterior leaflet.

Severe Bileaflet Prolapse or Multiple Ruptured Chordae

Because the goal of percutaneous edge-to-edge repair is to create a stable double-orifice valve, an intact mitral apparatus is necessary. A number of patients with a bileaflet prolapse and/or ruptured chordae were treated successfully with MitraClip® device implantation in the EVEREST studies. However, patients with a severe bileaflet prolapse or multiple ruptured chordae were excluded from MitraClip® implantation, because they lacked adequate mid-leaflet or basal-leaflet chordal support. Such patients likely require either mitral valve replacement or

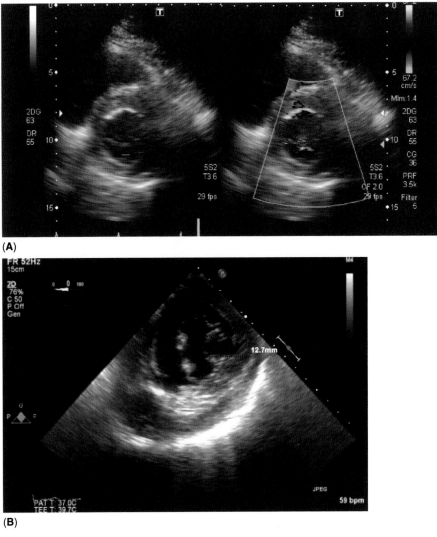

(A)

(B)

Figure 12.6 Flail width. Among patients with degenerative MR, flail width is the horizontal length of flail along the zone of leaflet apposition. If the flail width is 15 mm or more, the MitraClip® device may not effect adequate reduction in MR. (A) Flail width is best assessed using the transthoracic short-axis view, with and without Doppler. (B) In this example, the flail width is 12.7 mm.

complex reconstruction including the use of neochordae to buttress the valve apparatus.

Atrial Septal Defect
In the EVEREST trials, a pre-existing atrial septal defect (ASD) or symptomatic patent foramen ovale (PFO) was considered an exclusion criterion for percutaneous leaflet repair. An asymptomatic PFO was not considered an exclusion criterion.

Although the MitraClip® procedure is still feasible in subjects with pre-existing ASD or PFO, the rationale for this exclusion is that the 22 French transseptal sheath necessary for delivery of the MitraClip® device creates an iatrogenic ASD, which could additionally compromise the inter-atrial septum

in cases of a pre-existing ASD. The MitraClip® procedure requires a transseptal puncture superior and posterior in the fossa ovalis. This location may not always coincide with the location of a congenital PFO or ASD, and will therefore generate a second septal defect. If the location of the congenital PFO or ASD is in the proper location for the MitraClip® guide, it may be reasonable to perform the procedure at the operator's discretion. In rare cases, the creation of an iASD may also result in right to left shunting and significant hypoxia, thereby necessitating the device closure of the inter-atrial septum. Although iatrogenic ASDs (iASD) may be relatively common after transseptal puncture, most close spontaneously over time (18). In an analysis of iASD among patients undergoing

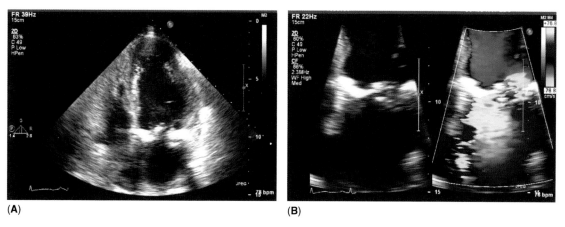

(A) **(B)**

Figure 12.7 Mitral annular and leaflet calcification. Extensive mitral annular or leaflet calcification may make surgical repair technically impossible, thereby necessitating valve replacement. (A) In this example, there is extensive calcification of the mitral annulus with encroachment on the leaflets. (B) Calcification of the leaflets, especially at the central grasping area near the A2–P2 interface, will impair the ability of the MitraClip® device to grasp each leaflet and also limits the ability of the leaflets to achieve an adequate degree of coaptation to reduce MR.

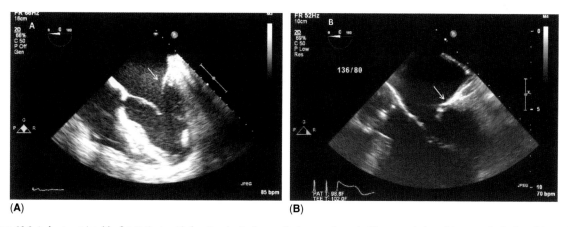

(A) **(B)**

Figure 12.8 A short restricted leaflet. Patients with functional mitral regurgitation may have significant restriction of the posterior leaflet. If the mobile segment of the leaflet is too short, the MitraClip® device may not be able to adequately grasp and coapt the leaflets. Panel A shows a short (<10 mm in length) P2 scallop in the four-chamber view. Panel B shows another patient with a short P2 scallop (arrow) in the magnified four-chamber view.

MitraClip® implantation, significant residual MR was a predictor of persistent iASD during a 12 month follow-up (19).

LEFT VENTRICULAR CRITERIA FOR PERCUTANEOUS MITRAL LEAFLET REPAIR

Although some investigators have reported good immediate surgical outcomes for MR among patients with severely depressed EF and severe MR, it is uncertain whether surgical repair of MR is beneficial among patients with severe left ventricular dysfunction (20,21). For this reason, EVEREST randomized trial inclusion criteria included a left ventricular ejection fraction >25% and left ventricular end systolic diameter <55 mm. In the High-Risk Registry, patients were required to have a left ventricular ejection fraction >20% and left ventricular end systolic diameter <60 mm.

Prior to development of transcatheter therapies for mitral leaflet repair, one concern of mitral valve surgery was that a repair of MR could acutely increase afterload and decrease cardiac output. However, these observations were confounded by the invasive nature of surgery. In a recent study of 96 patients from the EVEREST studies who underwent hemodynamic measurements pre- and post-device deployment, cardiac output and forward stroke volume improved acutely, while left ventricular end-diastolic volumes decreased (22). These observations suggest that repair of MR results in left ventricular unloading and an improved cardiac output.

Because MitraClip® therapy is less invasive than surgery, these findings provide a rationale for considering MitraClip® implantation among patients with severe MR and depressed left ventricular systolic function. In a study of 50 consecutive patients with New York Heart Association class III or IV heart failure, ejection fraction of 25% or less and 3+ or greater MR, Franzen et al. reported an acute procedural success rate of 94%, and 92% of patients were discharged with 2+ or less MR (23). At six-month follow-up, patients had improved six-minute walk tests and also had evidence of decreased left ventricular volumes. Among 51 patients who had continued MR despite cardiac resynchronization therapy, MitraClip® implantation also decreased left ventricular volumes over a six-month follow-up (24). These initial promising case series will require further confirmation with a control group to determine the potential benefit of MitraClip® implantation among patients with MR, heart failure, and severely depressed ejection fractions.

EXPERIENCE WITH ADVERSE VALVE MORPHOLOGY

The above discussion has focused on characteristics of leaflet morphology that were carefully considered for clinical trial design to maximize the chances of mitral valve repair either percutaneously or by a surgical approach. As techniques and procedural skills develop, there will be increased experience with patients with otherwise adverse leaflet morphology. The greatest clinical experience with this has been in Europe, where MitraClip® implantation has been performed in some cases that would not have met inclusion criteria for the EVEREST studies (25–27). While these reports provide initial evidence that MitraClip® implantation can have wider applicability in a real-world setting, these studies were performed by highly experienced operators and did not report a control group.

CONCLUSIONS

MitraClip® device implantation for percutaneous repair of MR has wide applicability in many etiologies of MR. When selecting a patient for possible MitraClip® implantation, several anatomic characteristics of the MR jet and valve apparatus must be taken into account before proceeding with definitive therapy. Close collaboration between interventional cardiologists and imaging specialists is crucial to understanding the anatomy of the mitral valve, echocardiographic characteristics that are favorable for device implantation, and the limitations of device implantation. As increasing experience is gained with this technique, the limitations of patient selection will undergo continued refinement.

REFERENCES

1. Van Mieghem NM, Piazza N, Anderson RH, et al. Anatomy of the mitral valvular complex and its implications for transcatheter interventions for mitral regurgitation. J Am Coll Cardiol 2010; 56: 617–26.
2. Feldman T, Cilingiroglu M. Percutaneous leaflet repair and annuloplasty for mitral regurgitation. J Am Coll Cardiol 2011; 57: 529–37.
3. Feldman T, Glower D. Patient selection for percutaneous mitral valve repair: insight from early clinical trial applications. Natl Clin Pract Cardiovasc Med 2008; 5: 84–90.
4. Maisano F, La Canna G, Colombo A, Alfieri O. The evolution from surgery to percutaneous mitral valve interventions: the role of the edge-to-edge technique. J Am Coll Cardiol 2011; 58: 2174–82.
5. Grayburn PA, Roberts BJ, Aston S, et al. Mechanism and severity of mitral regurgitation by transesophageal echocardiography in patients referred for percutaneous valve repair. Am J Cardiol 2011; 108: 882–7.
6. Mauri L, Garg P, Massaro JM, et al. The EVEREST II trial: design and rationale for a randomized study of the evalve mitraclip® system compared with mitral valve surgery for mitral regurgitation. Am Heart J 2010; 160: 23–9.
7. Alfieri O, Maisano F, De Bonis M, et al. The double-orifice technique in mitral valve repair: a simple solution for complex problems. J Thorac Cardiovasc Surg 2001; 122: 674–81.
8. Kinnaird TD, Munt BI, Ignaszewski AP, Abel JG, Thompson RC. Edge-to-edge repair for functional mitral regurgitation: an echocardiographic study of the hemodynamic consequences. J Heart Valve Dis 2003; 12: 280–6.
9. Bhudia SK, McCarthy PM, Smedira NG, et al. Edge-to-edge (Alfieri) mitral repair: results in diverse clinical settings. Ann Thorac Surg 2004; 77: 1598–606.
10. Herrmann HC, Rohatgi S, Wasserman HS, et al. Mitral valve hemodynamic effects of percutaneous edge-to-edge repair with the mitraclip® device for mitral regurgitation. Catheter Cardiovasc Interv 2006; 68: 821–8.
11. Herrmann HC, Kar S, Siegel R, et al. Effect of percutaneous mitral repair with the mitraclip® device on mitral valve area and gradient. EuroIntervent 2009; 4: 437–42.
12. Agricola E, Oppizzi M, Pisani M, et al. Ischemic mitral regurgitation: mechanisms and echocardiographic classification. Eur J Echocardiogr 2008; 9: 207–21.
13. Calafiore AM, Gallina S, Di Mauro M, et al. Mitral valve procedure in dilated cardiomyopathy: repair or replacement? Ann Thorac Surg 2001; 71: 1146–52; discussion 1152–3.
14. Calafiore AM, Di Mauro M, Gallina S, et al. Mitral valve surgery for chronic ischemic mitral regurgitation. Ann Thorac Surg 2004; 77: 1989–97.
15. Onorati F, Rubino AS, Marturano D, et al. Midterm clinical and echocardiographic results and predictors of mitral regurgitation recurrence following restrictive annuloplasty for ischemic cardiomyopathy. J Thorac Cardiovasc Surg 2009; 138: 654–62.
16. De Bonis M, Lapenna E, La Canna G, et al. Mitral valve repair for functional mitral regurgitation in end-stage dilated cardiomyopathy: role of the "edge-to-edge" technique. Circulation 2005; 112: I402–8.
17. Sherlock KE, Muthuswamy G, Basu R, Mitchell IM. The Alfieri stitch: the advantages for mitral valve repair in difficult circumstances. J Card Surg 2011; 26: 475–7.
18. McGinty PM, Smith TW, Rogers JH. Transseptal left heart catheterization and the incidence of persistent iatrogenic atrial septal defects. J Interv Cardiol 2011; 24: 254–63.
19. Smith T, McGinty P, Bommer W, et al. Prevalence and echocardiographic features of iatrogenic atrial septal defect after percutaneous edge-to-edge mitraclip® repair. Catheter Cardiovasc Interv 2012, [epub ahead of print]. doi: 10.1002/ccd.24460.
20. Bolling SF, Pagani FD, Deeb GM, Bach DS. Intermediate-term outcome of mitral reconstruction in cardiomyopathy. J Thorac Cardiovasc Surg 1998; 115: 381–6; discussion 387–8.
21. Wu AH, Aaronson KD, Bolling SF, et al. Impact of mitral valve annuloplasty on mortality risk in patients with mitral regurgitation and left ventricular systolic dysfunction. J Am Coll Cardiol 2005; 45: 381–7.
22. Siegel RJ, Biner S, Rafique AM, et al. The acute hemodynamic effects of mitraclip® therapy. J Am Coll Cardiol 2011; 57: 1658–65.

23. Franzen O, van der Heyden J, Baldus S, et al. Mitraclip® therapy in patients with end-stage systolic heart failure. Eur J Heart Fail 2011; 13: 569–76.

24. Auricchio A, Schillinger W, Meyer S, et al. Correction of mitral regurgitation in nonresponders to cardiac resynchronization therapy by mitraclip® improves symptoms and promotes reverse remodeling. J Am Coll Cardiol 2011; 58: 2183–9.

25. Franzen O, Baldus S, Rudolph V, et al. Acute outcomes of mitraclip® therapy for mitral regurgitation in high-surgical-risk patients: emphasis on adverse valve morphology and severe left ventricular dysfunction. Eur Heart J 2010; 31: 1373–81.

26. Franzen O, Seiffert M, Baldus S, et al. Percutaneous mitral valve repair as a bail-out strategy for patients with severe mitral regurgitation after cardiac surgery. J Thorac Cardiovasc Surg 2011; 142: 227–30.

27. Tamburino C, Ussia GP, Maisano F, et al. Percutaneous mitral valve repair with the mitraclip® system: acute results from a real world setting. Eur Heart J 2010; 31: 1382–9.

13 The basic technique for the Evalve MitraClip® procedure
Gretchen Gary and Ted Feldman

The MitraClip® System consists of a Steerable Guide Catheter (Guide) and a Clip Delivery System (CDS), which includes the detachable MitraClip® Device (Clip). The Clip is a polyester-covered mechanical device with two arms that are opened and closed by control mechanisms on the Delivery Catheter Handle (Fig. 13.1). The two arms have an opened span of approximately 2 cm when the Clip is opened to grasping position, defined as a 120° angle between the inner edges of both arms of the Clip. On the inner portion of the Clip is a U-shaped "gripper" that matches up to each arm and helps stabilize the leaflets from the atrial aspect as they are captured. Leaflet tissue is secured between the arms and each side of the gripper, and the Clip is then closed and locked to effect and maintain coaptation of the two leaflets. The width of the covered Clip is 5 mm (Fig. 13.2A–D). The CDS is used to advance and manipulate the implantable MitraClip® Device for proper positioning and placement on the mitral valve leaflets.

The tip of the Guide Catheter is delivered to the left atrium (LA) using the transseptal approach over a guidewire and tapered dilator. The Guide Catheter is 24-French (F) proximally, and tapers to 22-F at the point where it crosses the atrial septum. A steering knob on the proximal end of the guide catheter marked as ± allows for flexion and movement of the distal tip (Fig. 13.3).

The procedure is performed under general anesthesia using fluoroscopy and primarily transesophageal echocardiographic (TEE) guidance. Procedural success is best achieved by utilizing a systematic approach to the procedural steps with the corresponding echo views. It is critical that the interventional operator and the echocardiographer have a common anatomically based "vocabulary" for the standard procedural TEE views, so that clear communication can be maintained during the procedure. Efficient use of each echo view will assist in eliminating unnecessary device and TEE maneuvers.

For vascular access, a 6-F arterial and an 8-F venous sheath are placed in the left femoral artery and femoral vein, respectively. A 14-F sheath is placed in the right femoral vein for transseptal access and guide catheter delivery. Using the left femoral access, a 7-F balloon-tipped pulmonary artery catheter and a 6-F pigtail left ventricular (LV) catheter are placed. Cardiac output and baseline pulmonary capillary wedge, LV and pulmonary artery pressures are measured. An ACT (Acitivated Clotting Time) of 250–300 seconds is maintained throughout the procedure, with ACT measurements obtained every half an hour.

PROCEDURAL TECHNIQUE
The MitraClip® repair procedure consists of four main steps:

1. Transseptal puncture and Steerable Guide Catheter insertion
2. Steering and positioning of the Guide Catheter and CDS
3. Leaflet grasping, leaflet insertion assessment, and Clip closure
4. MitraClip® deployment and system removal

Transseptal Puncture and Steerable Guide Catheter Insertion
Initially, an 8-F Mullins sheath and then, a transseptal needle are advanced into the right atrium. To assure successful and adequate grasping of the mitral leaflets, it is critical that the transseptal puncture be placed relatively "high" and relatively posterior in the fossa ovalis. This "high" puncture is necessary to create sufficient distance above the mitral leaflets (ideal height from the annulus should be 3.5–4 cm) thereby allowing for an adequate working space for delivery catheter manipulations, Clip opening, and Clip retraction during grasping. If the transseptal puncture is placed too "low" in the fossa, the MitraClip® Device may come to lie just above and too close to the mitral annular plane and subsequent orientation of the CDS to position the Clip appropriately and grasp the leaflets may not be possible because of inadequate space in the LA above the annular plane. The transseptal puncture should be optimally positioned more posterior from an anterior-posterior perspective in order to enable the Guide tip positioning near the line of leaflet coaptation.

Using the TEE short-axis view at the base of the heart, the potential puncture site position is evaluated prior to needle advancement. The "tenting" of the atrial septum can be seen as the transseptal needle is pushed against it. Additionally, using the long-axis four-chamber view, the appropriate height above the valve should be confirmed. Transseptal puncture should only be performed if such tenting is clearly seen in both of these echo views. The transseptal crossing should be visualized and carried out using the TEE short-axis view at the base (Fig. 13.4A–F).

After the appropriate transseptal puncture is achieved and LA–LV pressure is measured at baseline, IV Heparin is given (50–70 units/kg) to achieve ACT ≥250 sec. A 0.035 inch, 260 cm, extra-stiff, J-tipped Amplatzer™ guidewire is carefully placed ideally in the left superior pulmonary vein or alternatively looped in the LA (Fig. 13.5).

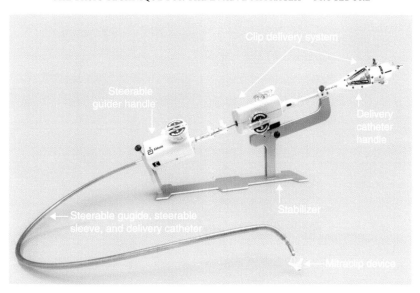

Figure 13.1 The MitraClip® System consists of a Steerable Guide Catheter (Guide) and a Clip Delivery System (CDS), which includes the detachable MitraClip® Device (Clip). The Clip is a Polyester-covered mechanical device with two arms that are opened and closed by control mechanisms on the Delivery Catheter Handle. The CDS is used to advance and manipulate the implantable MitraClip® Device for proper positioning and placement on the mitral valve leaflets.

After removal of the Mullin's sheath and dilator, the Steerable Guide Catheter and dilator assembly are advanced slowly toward the atrial septum over the 0.035 inch, 260 cm extra-stiff guidewire. The transseptal puncture site is slowly dilated to accommodate the 22-F distal end of the Guide Catheter by gentle pressure and forward movement of the dilator tip, which can be visualized by echo because of echogenic coils (Fig. 13.6A, B). Once the dilator tip is half to three-quarters across the septum, a few seconds' wait is often useful to allow the atrial septum to stretch. Advancement of the guide catheter tip across the septum is usually easier afterwards. It is very important not to place guide catheter tip too far into the LA, but rather to aim for a position of its tip about 1 or 2 cm across the atrial septum in the center of LA in the short-axis view at the base. (Fig. 13.7A, B)

Steering and Positioning of the Guide Catheter and CDS to the Mitral Line of Coaptation

Using the short and long-axis views of the LA by TEE, the orientation of the distal Guide curve plane relative to the mitral valve plane must be determined (perpendicular vs. parallel) (Fig. 13.8A–D). Ideally, the initial transseptal puncture site positions the guide catheter such that the clockwise rotation moves its tip posterior and cephalad. If the guide catheter tip is not in a favorable position, the Guide may be torqued or the tip deflected using the guide catheter ± steering knob.

It is critical to carefully de-air the guide catheter upon removal of the dilator and guidewire assembly once the guide catheter tip is 1–2 cm across the atrial septum and away from adjacent tissues. Aspirated blood from de-airing can be given back to the patient. Prior to insertion of the CDS, a slow

continuous heparinized saline flush through the CDS should be confirmed and must be maintained throughout the procedure. Proper insertion of the CDS into the Guide Catheter is assured when the longitudinal alignment marker on the CDS is aligned with the alignment marker on the proximal end of the Guide. The CDS is advanced through the Guide under fluoroscopic guidance until the tip of the Clip is even with the tip of the Guide. Under echocardiographic guidance the CDS is carefully advanced into the LA and the Guide iteratively retracted as needed to ensure that the tip of the Clip remains away from the left atrial wall while maintaining the Guide in the LA (Fig. 13.9A–C). Once the Clip and the CDS are safely outside the guide catheter tip and by verifying on fluoroscopy that the Guide radiopaque tip ring is between the radiopaque alignment markers of the CDS, the first positioning adjustments are made (Fig. 13.9D, E). Initial MitraClip® System positioning goals are to position the Clip centrally over the valve with respect to anterior-posterior and medial-lateral directions, align the Clip so that the DC shaft is perpendicular to the plane of the mitral valve, and positioning the distal tip of the Clip at least 1 cm above the leaflets (Fig. 13.10).

The Clip is directed medially toward the apex of the heart and thereby toward the mitral orifice typically by applying M knob to the CDS and modestly torquing the guide catheter clockwise (posterior) to avoid contacting either the posterior left atrial wall or the anteriorly located aortic root (Fig. 13.11A, B). The delivery catheter of the CDS tends to advance when deflection is applied to the steerable sleeve of the CDS thereby requiring periodic withdrawals of the delivery

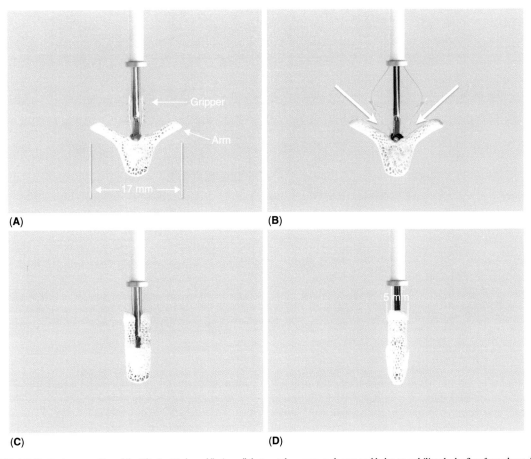

(A)   **(B)**

(C)   **(D)**

Figure 13.2 (**A**) On the inner portion of the Clip is a U-shaped "gripper" that matches up to each arm and helps to stabilize the leaflets from the atrial aspect as they are captured. The two arms have an opened span of approximately 2 cm when the Clip is opened to grasping position, defined as a 120° angle between the inner edges of both Clip arms. (**B**) Leaflet tissue is secured between the arms and each side of the gripper. (**C**) The Clip is closed and locked to effect and maintain coaptation of the two leaflets. (**D**) The width of the covered Clip is 5 mm.

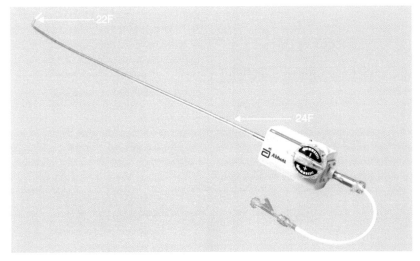

Figure 13.3 The Guide Catheter is 24-French (F) proximally, and tapers to 22-F at the point where it crosses the atrial septum. A steering knob on the proximal end of the guide catheter marked as ± allows for flexion and movement of the distal tip.

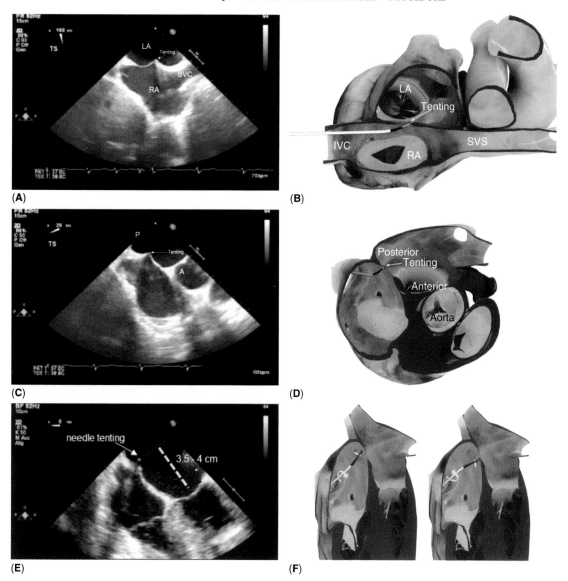

Figure 13.4 Using the TEE bicaval (**A, B**) and short-axis view at the base of the heart (**C, D**), the potential puncture site position is evaluated prior to needle advancement. Additionally, using the long-axis four-chamber view (**E, F**), the appropriate height of 3.5–4.0 cm above the valve should be confirmed. Clockwise rotation of the transseptal needle will move the tip posterior and increase the height above the mitral valve plane. Conversely, counterclockwise rotation will move the needle anterior and decrease the height above the valve. Transseptal puncture should only be performed if such tenting is clearly visualized on echo.

catheter handle (Fig. 13.12). Similarly, during Sleeve deflections it will be necessary to confirm that the Guide radiopaque tip ring is between the radiopaque alignment markers of the Sleeve prior to making maximum Sleeve deflections requiring occasional advancement of the CDS. The mid-esophageal two-chamber long-axis or "intercommissural" view allows for the evaluation of the Clip location medially and laterally along the line of mitral coaptation. The mid-esophageal long-axis LV outflow tract or "LVOT" view allows for assessment of Clip location anteriorly or posteriorly within the mitral orifice. The transgastric short-axis view or the 3D En Face view are the best views for evaluation of Clip arm orientation and supplement the intercommissural view for assessment of device position along the line of coaptation.

Fine adjustments in steering can be used incrementally to align the Clip and delivery catheter parallel with the long-axis of the heart and perpendicular to the mitral valve opening (Fig. 13.13A–C). Incremental medial steering changes of the

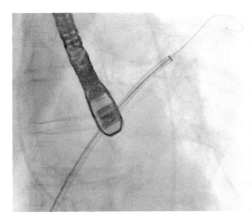

Figure 13.5 After the appropriate transseptal puncture is achieved, a 0.035 inch, 260 cm, extra-stiff, J-tipped Amplatzer™ guidewire is carefully placed ideally in the left superior pulmonary vein or alternatively looped in the left atrium.

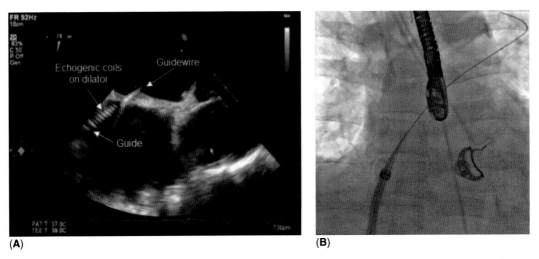

(A)   **(B)**

Figure 13.6 (A) Following removal of the Mullin's sheath and dilator, the Steerable Guide Catheter and dilator assembly are advanced slowly toward the atrial septum over the 0.035 inch, 260 cm extra-stiff guidewire. The transseptal puncture site is slowly dilated to accommodate the 22-F distal end of the Guide Catheter by gentle pressure and forward movement of the dilator tip, which can be visualized by echo because of echogenic coils. (B) Ideally, the tip of the guidewire should be in the left superior pulmonary vein.

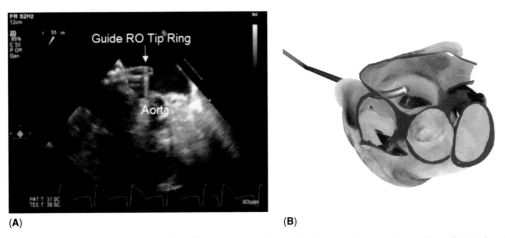

(A)   **(B)**

Figure 13.7 (A, B) It is very important not to place the guide catheter tip too far into the LA, but rather to aim for a position of its tip about 1 or 2 cm across the atrial septum in the center of LA in the short-axis view at the base.

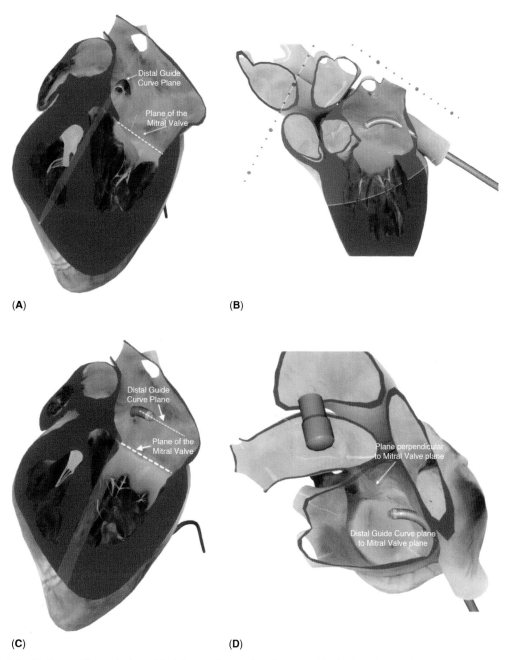

Figure 13.8 Using the short- and long-axis views of the left atrium by TEE, the orientation of the distal Guide curve plane relative to the mitral valve plane must be determined (perpendicular vs. parallel). The Guide curve plane is perpendicular to the mitral valve plane (A, B); the Guide curve plane is parallel to the mitral valve plane (C, D).

CDS in the intercommissural view by use of the M knob or modest advancement or withdrawal of guide catheter by sliding the stabilizer and the system together allow the Clip tip move to a position just over the middle scallop of the anterior (A2) and posterior (P2) leaflets of the mitral valve. Using the LVOT view, further fine steering movements in the anterior-posterior direction can be achieved by modest rotation of the guide catheter (counterclockwise for anterior, clockwise for posterior) or using the A/P knob to move the Clip to the appropriate position. These views must be checked several times to be certain that movement in one plane has not changed the position of the catheter in the orthogonal plane.

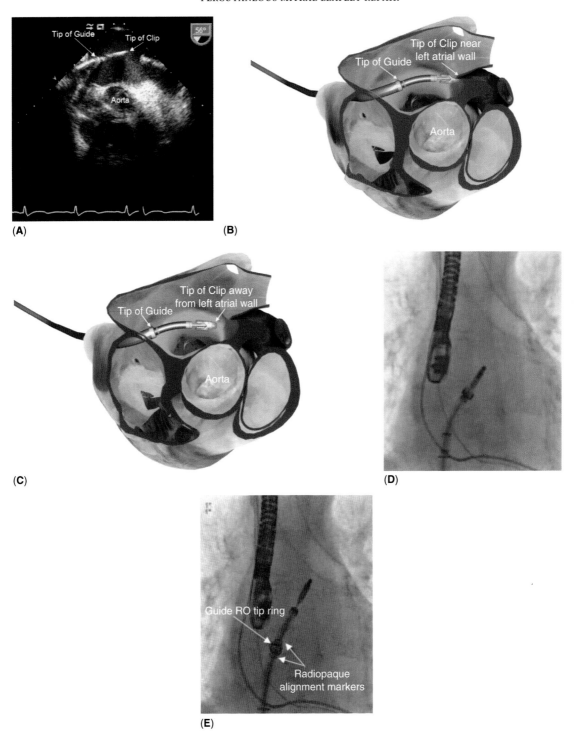

Figure 13.9 Under echocardiographic guidance the CDS is carefully advanced into the LA and the Guide iteratively retracted as needed to ensure that the tip of the Clip remains away from the left atrial wall while maintaining the Guide in the LA (**A, B, C**). The first positioning adjustments can be made once the Clip and the CDS are safely outside the guide catheter tip by verifying on fluoroscopy that the Guide radiopaque tip ring is between the radiopaque alignment markers of the CDS. In addition, during Sleeve deflections it will be necessary to confirm that the Guide radiopaque tip ring is between the radiopaque alignment markers of the Sleeve prior to making maximum Sleeve deflections requiring occasional advancement of the CDS (**D, E**).

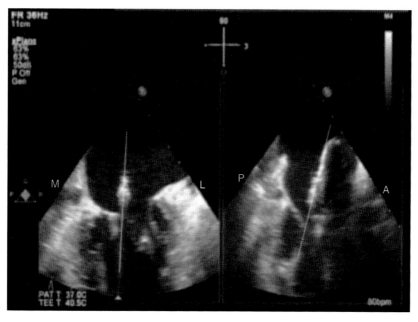

Figure 13.10 Initial MitraClip® System positioning goals are to position the Clip centrally over the valve with respect to anterior-posterior and medial-lateral directions and align the Clip so the DC shaft is perpendicular to the plane of the mitral valve.

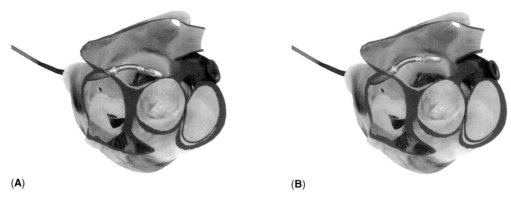

(A)   **(B)**

Figure 13.11 The Clip is directed medially toward the apex of the heart and thereby toward the mitral orifice typically by applying M knob to the CDS (**A**) and modestly torquing the guide catheter clockwise (posterior) to avoid contacting either the posterior left atrial wall or the anteriorly located aortic root (**B**).

The delivery catheter is then advanced 1–2 cm toward the mitral valve to assess the trajectory or path of the Clip. Once the Clip and delivery catheter are assessed to be parallel with the long axis of the heart and perpendicular to the mitral valve opening in both echo planes (LVOT and intercommissural views), color flow of the jet is evaluated. If the position of the Clip is correct, the Clip will split the MR jet in both views (Fig. 13.14). Both the guide catheter and the CDS can be advanced or pulled back slightly as one unit by pushing or pulling the stabilizing platform to help position the Clip over the origin of the MR jet without significantly changing the delivery catheter trajectory. While forward advancement moves the system laterally, its withdrawal moves it toward the medial commissure. Clockwise and counterclockwise guide catheter manipulation helps adjust the device position posteriorly and anteriorly without significantly affecting the delivery catheter trajectory.

The Clip arms are then opened to 180° in the LVOT view (Fig. 13.15A) and the grippers are fully raised using fluoroscopy (Fig. 13.15B). The transgastric short-axis view (if available, the 3D En Face view) is used while rotating the DC handle to align the Clip so that the Clip arms are oriented perpendicular to the line of coaptation. This step is critical

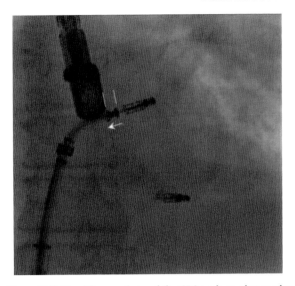

Figure 13.12 The delivery catheter of the CDS tends to advance when deflection is applied to the steerable sleeve of the CDS thereby requiring periodic withdrawal of the delivery catheter handle.

as significant deviation from a perpendicular alignment may result in an inadequate grasp of the mitral leaflets (Fig. 13.16). Multiple short to and fro translations are made with the delivery catheter handle during the rotation of the Clip in order to relieve the torque, which tends to be stored within the CDS.

Leaflet Grasping, Leaflet Insertion Assessment, and Clip Closure

After a perpendicular Clip arm alignment is achieved, the Clip is advanced into the LV so that the Clip arms are under the free edges of the mitral leaflets (Fig. 13.17). Free motion of the leaflet edges is important to note and the restriction of the leaflets by the Clip arms means the Clip is not far enough below the free edges to achieve a successful grasp. Generally, the most proximal portion of the gripper must be beneath the leaflets. Using LVOT and short-axis views (transgastric and/or 3D En Face), a final check of the perpendicular orientation is done with the Clip in the LV and the arms at 180° to be sure that no deviation of Clip arm orientation to the mitral leaflets has occurred during advancement into

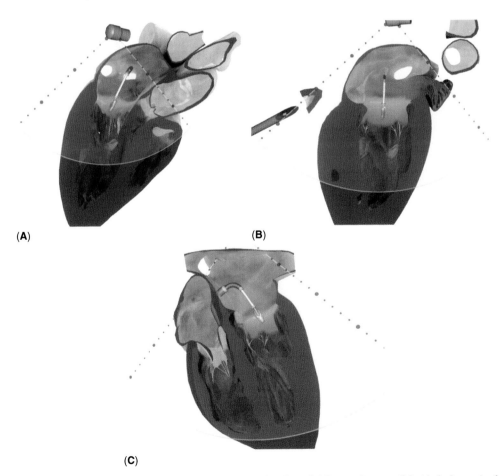

(A)

(B)

(C)

Figure 13.13 Fine adjustments in steering can be used incrementally to align the Clip and delivery catheter parallel with the long axis of the heart and perpendicular to the mitral valve opening in the left ventricular outflow tract (**A**), intercommissural (**B**), and four-chamber views (**C**).

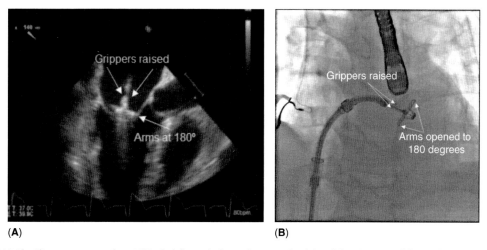

(A)   **(B)**

Figure 13.14 The Clip arms are opened to 180° in the left ventricular outflow tract view (**A**) and the grippers are fully raised using fluoroscopy (**B**).

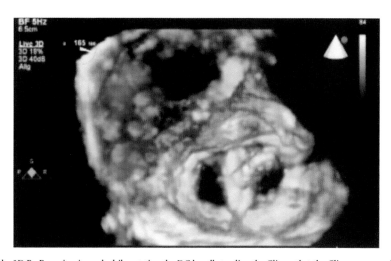

Figure 13.15 If available, the 3D En Face view is used while rotating the DC handle to align the Clip so that the Clip arms are oriented perpendicular to the line of coaptation. This step is critical as significant deviation from a perpendicular alignment may result in an inadequate grasp of the mitral leaflets.

the LV. The assessment of perpendicular orientation is greatly facilitated by the use of 3D echo, with the En Face or so-called "surgeons view" of the line of coaptation from the LA side. If there is deviation from the perpendicular or from coaxial delivery in the long axis of the LV, then the Clip arms can be everted and withdrawn into the LA, where readjustments in positioning can be performed and another passage to the LV can be made since the ability for substantial Clip arm orientation adjustment in the LV is very limited and not recommended.

The leaflets are grasped by retracting the delivery catheter handle while the Clip arms are open to approximately 120°. Mitral leaflet grasping during the pullback of the CDS is often best monitored in the LVOT view in order to observe the anterior and posterior leaflet capture within the open

Clip arms (Fig. 13.18A, B). In this view the open clip arms lay parallel to the mitral leaflets. Remarkably, the leaflets tend to fall into the Clip as the Clip is pulled back. Retraction should be done in a slow, smooth manner to capture the leaflet edges. If atrial fibrillation is present, or if the posterior leaflet is short in length, more than one attempt may be needed to capture the leaflets. When the leaflets are successfully immobilized by the open Clip, then the grippers are quickly lowered and the Clip is closed to about 60°. A successful grasp captures both mitral leaflets and produces a double-orifice mitral valve with reduction in MR. Careful interrogation in the LVOT, IC (Inter-Commissural), and short-axis views using a slow motion frame-by-frame analysis is very critical to make sure that both leaflets are captured by the Clip arms

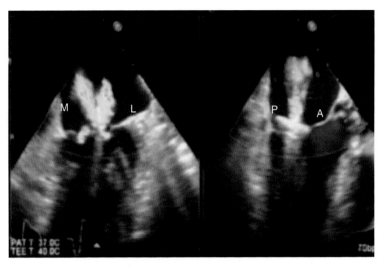

Figure 13.16 If the position of the Clip is correct, the Clip will split the MR jet in both the intercommissural and left ventricular outflow tract views.

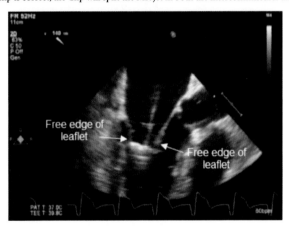

Figure 13.17 After perpendicular Clip arm alignment is achieved, the Clip is advanced into the LV so that the Clip arms are under the free edges of the mitral leaflets. Free motion of the leaflet edges is important to note and restriction of the leaflets by the Clip arms means the Clip is not far enough below the free edges to achieve a successful grasp.

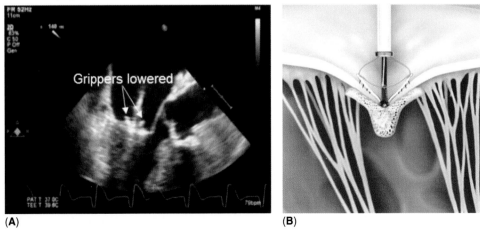

(A)   **(B)**

Figure 13.18 (A, B) Mitral leaflet grasping during a slow pullback of the CDS is often best monitored in the left ventricular outflow tract view in order to observe the anterior and posterior leaflet capture within the open Clip arms. The leaflets are successfully immobilized by the open Clip; then the grippers are quickly lowered.

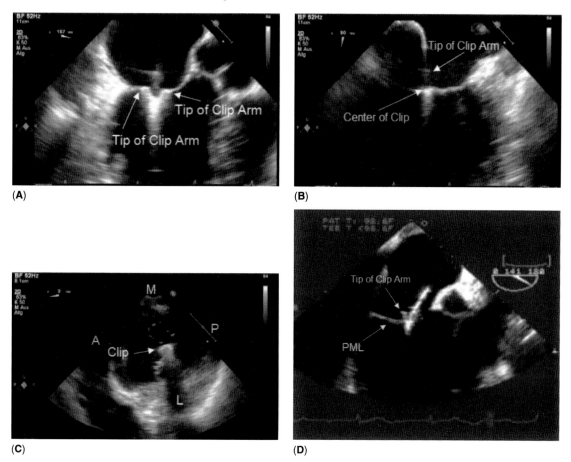

Figure 13.19 After the grippers are lowered, the Clip is closed to about 60°. Careful interrogation in the left ventricular outflow tract (A), intercommissural (B), and short-axis views (C) using slow motion frame-by-frame analysis is very critical to make sure that both leaflets are captured by the Clip arms. If the leaflet does not enter the clip between the arm and the gripper or if there is significant motion of the mitral leaflet just as it enters the Clip (Tip of Clip Arm), the resulting grasp is not adequate (D). Open the Clip and then repeat positioning and grasping steps.

(Fig. 13.19A–C). If there is significant motion of the mitral leaflet just as it enters the Clip, the resulting grasp may not be adequate for a long-term result (Fig. 13.19D). Open the Clip and then repeat positioning and grasping steps. If the leaflets are stable and immobile at the Clip entry point, an adequate grasp has been achieved (Fig. 13.20A). The presence of a stable double orifice should be confirmed in the short axis view (Fig. 13.20B). Assessment of the adequacy of leaflet insertion should be done before evaluating the reduction in the degree of MR. If both leaflets have not been adequately grasped, there is no point in evaluating the reduction in the degree of MR. Multiple TEE views with color and pulsed wave Doppler should be used to evaluate the reduction in the MR jet. Although the Clip has not been completely closed, a significant reduction in MR jet is expected. It is also important to remove the back tension from the delivery catheter by slightly advancing the CDS to allow proper assessment of the amount of residual MR. Once adequate leaflet insertion has been

confirmed at 60°, continue slowing closing the Clip just until the leaflets are coapted and MR is sufficiently reduced. Leaflet insertion assessment is repeated using LVOT, IC, and short axis views.

MitraClip® Deployment and System Removal

Prior to Clip release, the patient's systolic blood pressure should be raised using an alpha-agonist to the level of the baseline wakened state (or 10–20 mmHg higher) and the extent of the MR jet is reevaluated. A mean trans-mitral valve pressure gradient assessment should be performed using Doppler prior to proceeding to deployment. Once the desired endpoint in MR reduction is achieved, the function of the locking mechanism is confirmed by rotation of the Arm Positioner counterclockwise, toward the open direction, to confirm that the Clip remains closed and locked. After confirming the line moves freely, the lock control line is slowly removed by pulling the line coaxial to the lock lever. The Clip is

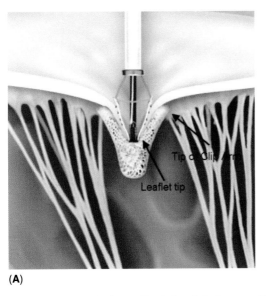
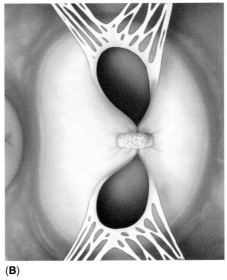

(A) **(B)**

Figure 13.20 (A) An adequate grasp has been achieved when the leaflets are stable and immobile at the Clip entry point (Tip of Clip Arm) and the leaflet tips are fully inserted to the base of the "V" between the gripper and the arms. (B) The presence of a stable double orifice should be confirmed in the short axis view.

released under fluoroscopic guidance and then the gripper line is pulled with the same slow technique as the lock line during which the operator can feel the line withdraw with each cardiac cycle. RAO (Right Anterior Oblique) caudal or LAO (Left Anterior Oblique) cranial views may be used for visualizing a side view of the Clip to confirm the degree of Clip closure prior to and after its deployment and also to ensure that a modest space is maintained between the delivery catheter tip and the implanted Clip during gripper line withdrawal (Fig. 13.21). After the Clip is free and both lines have been withdrawn, the CDS can be removed. It is critical that the tip of the CDS is carefully retracted back into the guide catheter to avoid damage to the LA (Fig. 13.22A, B). Careful and reverse steering to slowly straighten the guide curve with slow retraction of the CDS back into the guide catheter is performed using TEE. Once the CDS is retracted into the Guide, the guide catheter is withdrawn into the RA and removed from the insertion site using "figure of eight" subcutaneous sutures, which are removed after several hours, or sometimes the next morning. In about 40% of cases, a second Clip placement could be necessary for procedural success (≤2 + residual MR). If that is the case, a second CDS is advanced via the guiding catheter in the similar way as previously described with several important differences. During mitral valve crossing, the Clip arms are maintained in a more closed position to reduce interaction with the first Clip. TEE and fluoro are used to guide the second Clip either medial or lateral to the first, depending on where the residual MR jet is

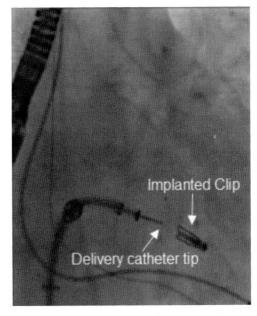

Figure 13.21 The Clip is released under fluoroscopic guidance and the gripper line is slowly removed. RAO caudal or left atriumO cranial views may be used to ensure that a modest space is maintained between the delivery catheter tip and the implanted Clip during gripper line withdrawal.

seen. Assessment of leaflet insertion may be more difficult due to acoustic shadowing of the TEE caused by the first Clip. Remaining steps are identical.

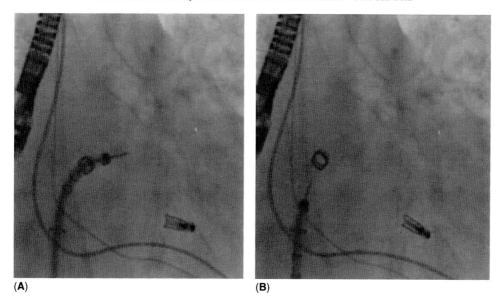

(A)　　　　　　　　　　　　　　　**(B)**

Figure 13.22 After the Clip is free and both the lock line and gripper line have been withdrawn, the CDS can be removed. It is critical that the tip of the CDS is carefully retracted back into the guide catheter to avoid damage to the left atrium (**A, B**). Careful and reverse steering to slowly straighten the guide curve with slow retraction of the CDS back into the guide catheter is performed using TEE.

SUMMARY

The MitraClip® procedure is novel and has a significant learning curve. In addition, the main procedure elements are well developed, and this chapter summarizes the four main steps: transseptal puncture and Steerable Guide Catheter insertion, steering and positioning of the Guide Catheter and CDS, leaflet grasping and leaflet insertion assessment, and MitraClip® deployment and system removal.

Saibal Kar and Wen-Loong Yeow

INTRODUCTION

MitraClip® therapy (Abbott Vascular, Santa Clara, California, USA) is the only percutaneous leaflet repair technology available for the treatment of selected patients with functional or degenerative mitral regurgitation (MR). Although the procedure is intuitive and methodical, there are tips and tricks at each step of the procedure which are necessary in different cardiac anatomies or during the treatment of different mitral valve pathologies.

Important aspects of the procedure to be discussed in this chapter include vascular access and hemostasis, transseptal puncture challenges, use of imaging during manipulation of the catheter, techniques in grasping leaflets, and MitraClip® procedure in special situations.

VASCULAR ACCESS AND HEMOSTASIS

In order to minimize vascular complications, and help early mobilization of patients, we advocate minimal access. A suitable size sheath should be placed in the internal jugular vein, for administration of fluid, medications by anesthesiologist, and a portal for performing the right heart study. A 4- or 5-French sheath is placed in the radial artery, for monitoring of arterial pressures and for a portal of introduction of catheters for the left heart study. The right femoral vein is used for introduction of the therapeutic catheter. In some instances after gaining access in the right femoral vein, two Perclose ProGlide sutures (Abbott Vascular) can (in an off-label fashion) be deployed at 60° to each other. At the end of the procedure the sutures are tightened to achieve hemostasis (Fig. 14.1). A figure-of-eight subcutaneous suture at the femoral venous puncture site can be used for additional hemostasis if necessary. We have found that the use of this vascular access regimen minimizes the bleeding complications, reduces the time of immobilization of the patient, and increases patient comfort.

TRANSSEPTAL ACCESS: ISSUES AND CHALLENGES

Access into the left atrium (LA) via a transseptal puncture is one of the most crucial steps of the MitraClip® procedure. The site of puncture is determined by the size of the LA, the level at which the leaflets coapt, as well as the working length of the delivery catheter beyond the guide catheter. The working length of the catheter is approximately 5 cm beyond the tip of the guide catheter. As a result, the distance between puncture site and the point of coaptation of leaflets should be 3.5–4 cm in order to allow enough length of clip delivery system above and below the valve. Puncturing the septum too close the plane of the mitral valve will not allow adequate steering of the delivery catheter above the valve, where as if

the puncture site is too far posterior from the plane of the valve, the clip delivery system will not be able to be advanced into the left ventricle.

In order to achieve an accurate puncture location, three transesophageal echocardiographic (TEE) views are used (1). The bicaval view helps in the inferior-superior orientation, and the short-axis view at the base of heart (45–50°) helps in the anterior-posterior orientation of the puncture. Movement of the transseptal needle clockwise allows the needle to be in a more posterior location, whereas advancing or retracting the needle allows the needle to position in the bicaval view. Finally the actual distance of the puncture site to the valve plane is determined in the mid-esophageal four-chamber view. In a patient with a flailed mitral valve leaflet, the plane of coaptation of the leaflets is at or above the plane of the annulus (Fig. 14.2). If this is the case it is important that the puncture site be posterior and superior in order to allow adequate distance from the puncture site to the leaflet plane. With functional MR with a large LA, the leaflet coaptation is often quite deep in the ventricle (Fig. 14.3). In this situation the puncture site needs to be more anterior and low on the fossa in order to achieve enough distance.

In addition to the above-mentioned situations, transseptal puncture may be challenging in instances where the right atrium is very large not allowing adequate tenting of the septum, or the area of interest might be too thick preventing the needle to enter the LA. There are some important techniques to overcome these challenges. In cases of large right atriums, or inadequate tenting of the septum, the curve of standard transseptal needle can be increased or a needle with a large pre-formed curve such as the BRK1 needle (St Jude Medical) can be used. In cases where the needle is not advancing through the septum, the style of the needle or the stiff end of an angioplasty wire can be advanced into the LA through the needle. Alternatively, transseptal puncture facilitated by radiofrequency energy can be performed in a thick unyielding septum. The source of radiofrequency energy is usually the standard surgical electrocautery device with the electrosurgical pen in direct contact with hub of the needle applied for a short period of time during the puncture. A similar technique can be done using the radiofrequency-powered transseptal needle (Baylis Medical Company, Inc.) (Fig. 14.4). This system consists of its proprietary needle and radiofrequency energy generator. These two techniques using radiofrequency energy allow accurate localization of a puncture without sliding on the septum as may occur using the standard transseptal techniques.

Rather than using a standard Mullins sheath we suggest the use of a SL1 transseptal sheath to enter into the LA. This sheath is

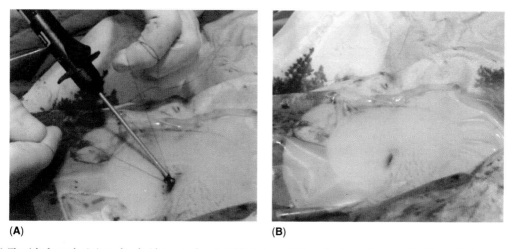

(A)　　　　　　　　　　　　**(B)**

Figure 14.1 The right femoral vein is preclosed with two Perclose ProGlide devices at 60° to each other and at the end is tightened in the same order as they were used, with good hemostasis.

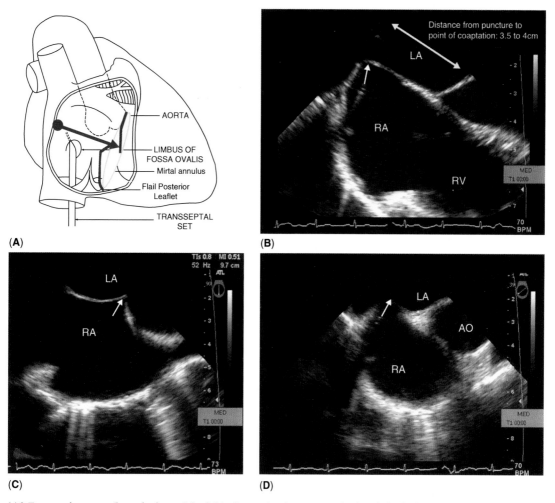

Figure 14.2 Transseptal puncture (base of red arrow) for flail leaflets needs to be very posterior (Panel A). The distance from transseptal puncture to the line of coaptation needs to be between 3.5 and 4 cm as seen in the 0° TEE (Panel B). In the bicaval view a superior position is required (Panel C) and the posterior position as seen in the short-axis view (Panel D). LA, Left atrium; RA, right atrium; AO, aortic valve; White arrow, tenting of the septum.

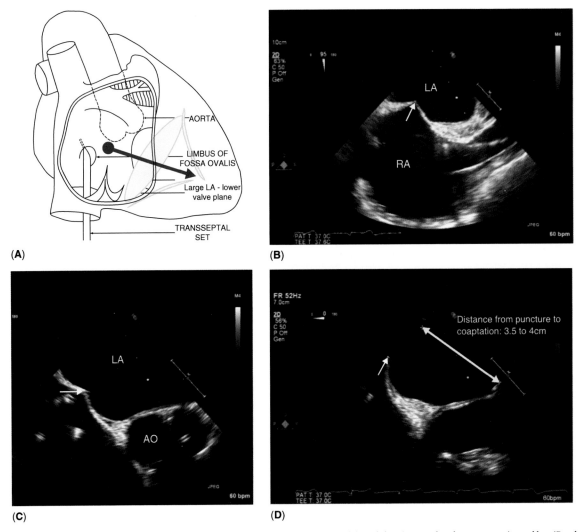

Figure 14.3 Transseptal puncture (base of red arrow) for functional mitral regurgitation with large left atrium needs to be more anterior and low (Panel A). In the bicaval view, a low puncture is required (Panel B) and a mid or anterior puncture in the short-axis view (Panel C). The same distance of 3.5-4 cm from the transseptal to line of coaptation is required (Panel D). LA, Left atrium; RA, right atrium; AO, aortic valve; White arrow, tenting of the septum.

easier to advance in the left pulmonary vein. Once the sheath is advanced in the pulmonary vein, intravenous heparin is administered, and repeated boluses of heparin can be given to maintain an activated clotting time greater than 250 seconds throughout the procedure. A J-tip, 0.035 inch, 260 cm long exchange length, super-stiff wire is then advanced through the transseptal sheath into the pulmonary vein. The sheath is then removed over the wire and the 22-F steerable guide catheter with the dilator is advanced into the LA via the femoral vein over this strong wire. Parking the super-stiff wire in the pulmonary vein provides a strong rail for a large bore sheath to be advanced in the LA.

The transseptal access into the LA is one of the most crucial steps of the procedure, and the above tips are vital to the success of the procedure. It is important to mention that constant visualization of the sheath in the LA using the TEE is a helpful step for the prevention of perforation of the LA free wall.

IMAGING TECHNIQUES

The MitraClip® procedure is performed under real-time echocardiographic and fluoroscopic guidance in a unique collaboration between the interventionalist and echocardiographer (1). Although the essential steps of the procedure are performed under guidance of real-time two-dimensional (2D) TEE, the availability of real-time 3D TEE has provided additional information in the understanding of the mitral valve pathology and the MitraClip® procedure. As 2D and 3D TEE are complementary imaging technologies, the combined

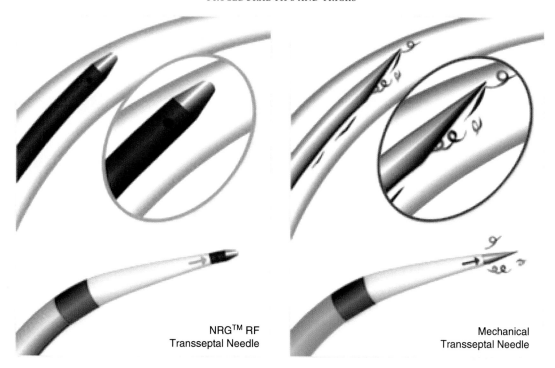

NRG™ RF
Transseptal Needle

Mechanical
Transseptal Needle

Figure 14.4 Radiofrequency Transseptal Needle (Baylis Medical, Mississauga, Ontario, Canada) uses radiofrequency energy to cross fibrotic or aneurysmal septa.

approach has greatly enhanced our interpretation of mitral valve anatomy and guidance of the percutaneous repair of the mitral valve (2,3). This unique procedure is primarily guided by real-time echocardiography, with a smaller but complementary role of fluoroscopy. We have found it very useful for both the echocardiographer and interventionalist to have simultaneous access to real-time TEE and fluoroscopic images. The interventionalist primarily uses the fluoro to visualize the components of the MitraClip® system, while the echocardiographer uses the fluoroscopic images to help quickly and accurately position the probe in line with the delivery catheter to allow optimal echocardiographic visualization of the MitraClip® system and valve (Fig. 14.5A). This dual imaging tool helps both key physicians in reducing the procedure time, improving the image guidance, and minimizing the movement of the probe and resultant trauma to the esophagus of the patient. The primary reliance on echo and minimal role of X-ray helps minimize the radiation exposure to the physicians and patients, and practically eliminates the need for contrast angiography and diminishes the risk of contrast-induced nephropathy.

Alignment of the clip orthogonal with the plane of the mitral valve annulus and the positioning of it just above the MR jet in a 3D space requires multiple imaging planes. Two orthogonal long-axis views are used to accomplish this: The mid-esophageal long-axis view, for anterior-posterior alignment and the mid-esophageal intercommissural view for medial-lateral positioning. The x-plane function of the 3D TEE probe of the Phillips i33 echocardiographic system allows two orthogonal planes to be displayed simultaneously on the screen (Fig. 14.6). This function greatly enhances our ability without moving the TEE probe to allow accurate and axial alignment of the clip, localize the transseptal puncture site as well help localize and quantify residual MR jets following a clip deployment.

The 3D TEE is valuable for determining the orientation of the clips arms perpendicular to the line of coaptation of the leaflets (Fig. 14.7). This modality also helps to confirm that the clip is directed over the appropriate segment of the mitral valve. This viewing modality avoids repetitive cross-checks and verification in multiple 2D planes.

Selective use of fluoroscopy during the procedure has important value. As mentioned earlier, it helps the interventionalist in visualizing the different components of the catheter system and aids in assessing the opening and closing angles of the clip. A magnified fluoroscopic view of the clip showing the closing angle of the clip should be recorded when the clip is locked and not deployed. While the clip is in its locked position, an attempt should be made to open it, and only if the clip does not open, and the efficacy of the lock confirmed, should be deployed. Fluoroscopy is also very helpful in guiding a second clip procedure. The first clip acts as a guide for the second clip. In a right

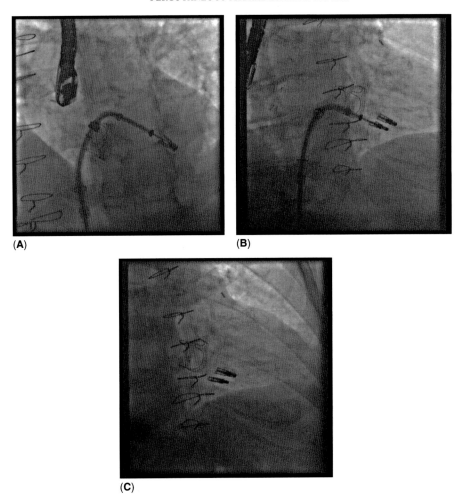

(A)   **(B)**

(C)

Figure 14.5 Fluoroscopic images allow greater visualization of the clip elements and assist in positioning the TEE probe (Panel A). While working in the right anterior oblique position, fluoroscopy assists in positioning the second clip (Panels B and C).

anterior oblique view the clip delivery system should be adjusted to be parallel and just medial or lateral to the first clip during deployment (Figs. 14.5B and 14.5C).

A judicious use of combined imaging modalities 2D and 3D TEE, and fluoroscopy is helpful in accomplishing the key steps of the procedure. The MitraClip® procedure is a unique structural heart disease procedure which emphasizes the importance of combined imaging modalities and a collaboration of the interventionalist and an imaging physician (1).

TECHNIQUES AND CHALLENGES
OF GRASPING OF LEAFLETS

Successful grasping of leaflets sometimes poses a challenge especially in some cases of significant flail segments or severe tethering of the mitral leaflets. The slow grasping technique has evolved as the preferred method to ensure a controlled adequate capture of both leaflets. The leaflets are grasped by slowly retracting the delivery catheter while the clip arms are open approximately 120°. The leaflets tend to fall into the clip as the clip is pulled back. When the leaflets are successfully immobilized by the open clip, the gripper is quickly lowered and the clip is closed. This technique allows the operator enough time to ensure adequate leaflet insertion without causing damage to the subvalvular apparatus.

As all patients undergoing the procedure are intubated and ventilated, certain ventilation maneuvers can facilitate MitraClip® placement (4). Respiratory movements are associated with side-to-side movement of the clip in relation to the mitral valve. In order to ensure that the leaflets are captured in the appropriate location it is important to make the final adjustment of the clip delivery system and grasping of the leaflets during temporary cessation of positive pressure ventilation. In some cases of functional MR with a dilated annulus, grasping is often challenging due to the poor coaptation of the leaflets. In such cases the anesthesiologist can perform a Valsalva maneuver which leads to a reduction of the preload, better leaflet coaptation, as

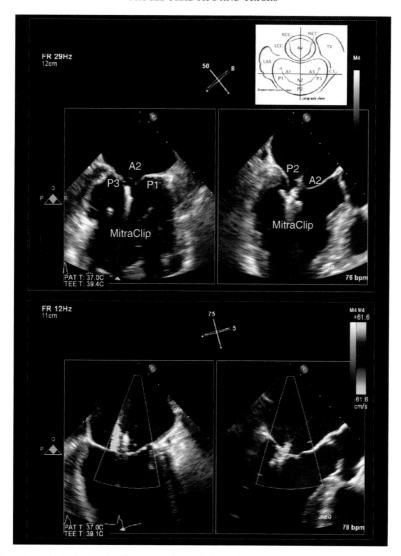

Figure 14.6 The X-plane function of the 3D TEE probe allows two orthogonal planes, the mid esophageal long-axis view and mid esophageal intercommissural view, to be displayed simultaneously on the screen. P1, P2, P3, medial, middle and lateral scallops of the posterior mitral leaflet: A2, middle segment of the anterior mitral leaflet

well as alteration of the relationship of the clip and the mitral valve. During the Valsalva maneuver the position of the clip delivery system is readjusted and the leaflets are grasped.

In spite of the above-mentioned strategies grasping of large flail segments or significantly tethered leaflets can be difficult. In such cases, a mandatory two-clip strategy can be used. The first clip is placed near the edge of the flail or tethered segment. This allows stabilization of the flail segment or improved coaptation of tethered leaflet, and then the second clip is deployed in the middle of the diseased segment. A two-clip strategy usually helps in better reduction of leakage, wider area of coaptation, and reduced stress on the leaflets and potentially a durable result. In a two-clip strategy it is important to make sure that the mitral valve orifice is large enough to accommodate two clips without causing significant mitral valve obstruction.

Finally, alteration of the heart rate with rapid pacing or transient adenosine-induced asystole have been used to aid grasping of leaflets in certain complex cases (5,6). In case of severe prolapse of the leaflet, rapid pacing at 180/min results in reduced amplitude of the mitral valve and safe and successful grasping of the leaflets. The use of this technique in functional MR with poor coaptation length has yet to be described. Creation of temporary atrioventricular block with adenosine is also helpful in difficult cases (6). A temporary pacing wire is required and a large dose of adenosine is injected via a central venous line by the anesthetist with mechanical ventilation on hold. The mitral leaflets should rest at the level of the annulus, buoyed up by the filled ventricle, and facilitate grasping.

As described in this section there are several ways to ensure successful grasping of leaflets. In a given patient one or more of

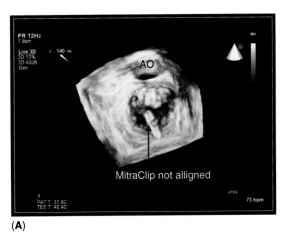
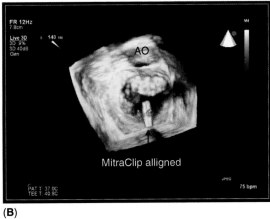

(A) **(B)**

Figure 14.7 The 3D TEE probe can accurately determine the orientation of the clips arms perpendicular to the line of coaptation of the leaflets. AO, aortic valve.

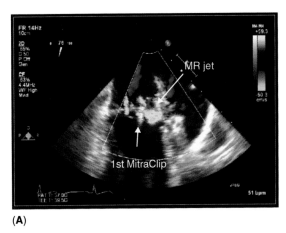
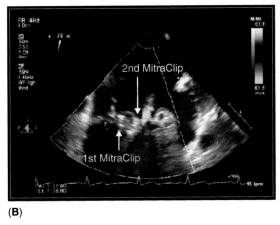

(A) **(B)**

Figure 14.8 Recurrent mitral regurgitation (MR) jet on the lateral side of the first clip (Panel A). Successful second clip procedure results in trivial MR (Panel B).

these techniques may have to be used to achieve a successful result. On the contrary in spite of all these tricks, adequate capture of leaflets may not be possible, emphasizing the importance of case selection as the most important determinant of success of the procedure.

MITRACLIP® IN SPECIAL SITUATIONS

Recurrent MR can occur in patients following an initial successful MitraClip® procedure due to either partial clip detachment or progression of mitral valve pathology. In case of the latter, provided the MR jet is close to the first clip, the second clip procedure can be performed. Unlike the situation with open surgery, a second elective clip procedure does not pose substantial additional risk to the patient (Fig. 14.8).

The MitraClip® procedure has been performed in selected patients with recurrent MR following surgical repair. Some patients with recurrent MR following successful ring placement

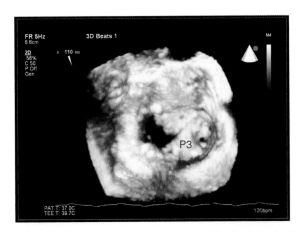

Figure 14.9 A 3D TEE view of the mitral valve following a single-clip procedure to close a P3 flail with the asymmetrical double orifice.

or due to recurrent flail segment following surgical placement of artificial chords can be treated with the MitraClip® procedure. The presence of a ring makes grasping of leaflets less of a challenge. In cases where the index surgery involved resection of a part of the leaflet, the MitraClip® procedure will be contraindicated.

The MitraClip® procedure can be performed in certain cases of degenerative mitral valve disease involving the medial or lateral segments of the mitral valve (Fig. 14.9). Such patients were excluded in the EVEREST trials since there is crowding of chords below the lateral and medial aspects of the mitral valve. In such cases the clip needs to be aligned just above the pathological segment, and the clip is then advanced just below the leaflets prior to grasping. A small number of patients with such a pathological condition have been treated in Europe and, on compassionate grounds, in the United States. The acute results are often dramatic.

CONCLUSION

The MitraClip® procedure is novel percutaneous treatment option for selected patients with functional or degenerative MR. There are several tips and tricks that can be used to acheive a successful result. The procedure requires multiple imaging modalities including 2D and 3D TEE and fluoroscopy. A close collaboration among the interventionalist, echocardiographer, and anesthesiologist is vital for the success of this procedure. Further modifications of the MitraClip® device will hopefully improve the primary success and durability of this procedure.

REFERENCES

1. Silvestry FE, Rodriguez LL, Herrmann HC, et al. Echocardiographic guidance and assessment of percutaneous repair for MR with the evalve mitraclip®: lessons learned from EVEREST I. J Am Soc Echocardiogr 2007; 20: 1131–40.
2. Biner S, Perk G, Kar S, et al. Utility of combined two-dimensional and three-dimensional transesophageal imaging for catheter-based mitral valve clip repair of MR. J Am Soc Echocardiogr 2011; 24: 611–17.
3. Altiok E, Becker M, Hamada S, et al. Optimized guidance of percutaneous edge-to edge repair of the mitral valve using real-time 3-D transesophageal echocardiography. Clin Res Cardiol 2011; 100: 675–81.
4. Mayr NP, Martin K, Hausleiter J, Brown A, Tassani P. Ventilation manoeuvres facilitate mitraclip® placement. Heart 2011; 97: 1717.
5. Paranskaya L, Turan I, Kische S, Nienaber C, Ince H. Rapid pacing facilitates grasping and mitraclip® implantation in severe mitral leaflet prolapse. Clin Res Cardiol 2012; 101: 69–71.
6. Borgia F, Di Mario C, Franzen O. Adenosine-induced asystole to facilitate mitraclip® placement in a patient with adverse mitral valve morphology. Heart 2011; 97: 864.

15 Training and simulation
Scott Lim

Percutaneous mitral leaflet repair using the MitraClip® system is unique in two aspects: for the skills required to perform the procedure and the degree of echocardiographic visualization required to accomplish the procedure. As such, there is a steep learning curve associated with this novel procedure (Figs. 15.1 and 15.2). However, the skills involved are unlike the traditional catheter-based procedures, and require familiarity with a large caliber mechanical system guided by transesophageal echocardiography that is specifically positioned relevant to the individual patient's mitral pathologic anatomy following transseptal puncture. Knowledge of mitral valve pathology and patience are also important for success. Therefore, the development of competence with the MitraClip® procedure appears to be independent of specialty discipline of the valve interventionalist (cardiovascular surgeon or interventional cardiologist), and therefore training for the procedure is of particular relevance (1). Following a training program, MitraClip® procedural results have been demonstrated to be similar between surgeon-treated and cardiology-treated patients, with low complications rates and similar improvements in mitral regurgitation reduction and functional class (2).

To address the training needs relevant to transcatheter valve procedures such as the MitraClip® therapy, there have been calls for professional societies to create standardized curriculum and performance evaluation metrics, as well as certification bodies (3,4). While research is underway to create this by the appropriate committees of these professional societies, no guidelines yet exist at the time of this writing. Therefore, when the need arose to develop the first center for MitraClip® procedural training, the multidisciplinary team at the University of Virginia Advanced Cardiac Valve Center created a de novo comprehensive training protocol incorporating didactic, simulator-based, and case-based training (Fig. 15.3). Inherent in this training protocol is the involvement of faculty from cardiac surgery, interventional cardiology, and imaging specialties as well as cardiac pathology. Also of importance is hands-on time with computer and physical simulator training and placing the MitraClip® on pathologic specimens.

An important part of training for the MitraClip® procedure is illustrating the importance of the multidisciplinary approach to both valve disease and transcatheter therapy of it. The optimal formation of the heart valve team should include experienced physicians from cardiac surgery, interventional cardiology, cardiac anesthesia, imaging specialist, and cardiac intensive care. While more than one of these roles may be owned by the same physician, the benefits of collaboration among many cannot be underemphasized. Additionally, for the MitraClip® procedure and entire valve program to be successful, inclusion of non-physician partners is important. In the MitraClip® training program at the University of Virginia, different didactic and hands-on sections are taught by faculty from these different disciplines, demonstrating in practice this concept.

In order to best understand the optimal role of the MitraClip® therapy in the armamentarium of therapies for mitral regurgitation, we have given training sections on surgical considerations for the different subtypes of mitral regurgitation pathologies, as well as our perspective on the results from the MitraClip® clinical trial data.

Given that the MitraClip® therapy is a unique and complicated mechanical device and delivery system, we feel it is important to understand the engineering and design, so as to better utilize its functionality as well as to be able to trouble shoot if problems arise (5). We have interspaced didactic lectures on the mechanics of the system with hands-on time on an actual MitraClip® system in a physical heart model, as well as an engineering video to better understand what is happening within the system's mechanical innards.

It is an old adage that "you can't fix what you can't see." This is apropos to the MitraClip® therapy, and therefore places imaging at the forefront of this therapy. At present time, that role of imaging has been done by the different modalities of echocardiography. We have therefore allocated a significant amount of training for the valve interventionalist on echocardiography, even to the point of stressing that prior to scrubbing in for the MitraClip® procedure, the valve interventionalist ought to place their hands on the transesophageal echocardiogram (TEE) probe, and understand the available views and pathology. This is particularly important if the procedure operator comes from an interventional cardiology or cardiac surgical background without extensive prior noninvasive imaging experience.

We start our imaging training section on understanding the role of the transthoracic echocardiogram in assessing the severity of mitral regurgitation, its effects on ventricular function and pulmonary hypertension, and the dynamic nature of functional mitral regurgitation. We then focus the training on the use of TEE to determine the mechanism of mitral regurgitation, and understand the types of pathologies that are suitable or should be excluded from the MitraClip® therapy. We also spend training time on clarifying the echocardiographic language used so that both imager and valve interventionalist can be clear in their communication. These didactic lectures on TEE are followed up by time using a TEE simulator designed for the MitraClip® (MitraClip® Virtual Procedure simulator program, Abbott Vascular; Fig. 15.4).

Since it is vitally important for all personnel involved in the MitraClip® procedure to understand the interactions between the MitraClip® device and different types of mitral anatomy, we

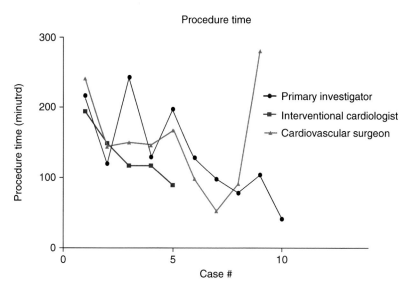

Figure 15.1 Graph demonstrates the fall in procedure time in consecutive cases performed either by an experienced MitraClip® primary investigator, interventional cardiologist MitraClip® trainee, or cardiovascular surgeon MitraClip® trainee. Data from cases performed at the University of Virginia using the MitraClip® system.

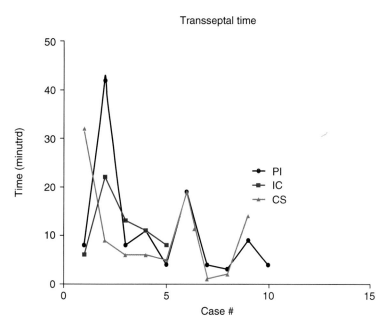

Figure 15.2 Graph demonstrates the fall in transseptal puncture time stratified by the performance of the transseptal either by the experienced MitraClip® primary investigator (PI), interventional cardiologist (IC) MitraClip® trainee, or cardiovascular surgeon (CS) MitraClip® trainee. Data from cases performed at the University of Virginia using the MitraClip® system at the University of Virginia.

then spend a significant amount of training time in the pathological suite. A cardiac pathologist illustrates to the trainees the issues of normal mitral valve anatomy, and gives the trainees opportunities to place the MitraClip® device on the leaflets in the appropriate position. This gives a sense of the three-dimensional (3D) relationship of the subvalve apparatus and the leaflets, and the pitfalls of manipulating a device in this space. We then demonstrate the same in different pathologic subsets, including degenerative and functional types, and how they interact with the MitraClip®. We also have selected some pathological examples that are not conducive to the MitraClip® therapy, such as rheumatic disease, commissural pathology, or congenital pathology.

Pre-procedural considerations are discussed, including anesthesia needs, issues related to the TEE and esophageal windows, device preparation, and antibiotic prophylaxis.

1. Introduction and History of the MitraClip procedure
2. Perspective on the clinical trial data
3. Advanced Cardiac Valve Center team approach
4. Surgical considerations for mitral regurgitation
   a. Degenerative
   b. Functional
5. MitraClip engineering and design
6. Echocardiography
   a. Mitral Regurgitation assessment
      i. TTE
         1. PISA/EROA method
         2. Importance of LA size
         3. Functional MR – dynamic nature
      ii. TEE
         1. Determine the mechanism
         2. Suitability/exclusions – emphasize short axis en face
7. Patient screening &selection
   a. Functional
   b. Degenerative
8. Mitral Valve Pathology – Hands-on in Pathology Suite
   a. Normal anatomy
   b. Degenerative disease
   c. Functional disease
9. Procedural considerations
   a. Pre procedure
   b. Intra procedure
      i. Communication
      ii. Transseptal puncture
      iii. Computer Simulator practice
      iv. TEE guidance of the MitraClip procedure
         1. 2D TEE
         2. 3D TEE
      v. *Physical Simulator practice*
      vi. Steering & Orientating
      vii. *Computer Simulator practice*
      viii. Grasping
      ix. *Physical Simulator practice*
      x. Deployment & System removal
      xi. 2nd Clip decision
   c. Post procedure
10. Complications
   a. Transseptal
   b. Chords
   c. Partial clip detachment
   d. Mitral stenosis
11. Live cases
   a. Pre-procedure case review
   b. Computer Simulator practice
   c. TEE in case assessment
   d. MitraClip procedure
   e. Post-procedure de-brief
   f. Computer Simulator practice

Figure 15.3 Demonstrates the curriculum used at the MitraClip® training program, University of Virginia.

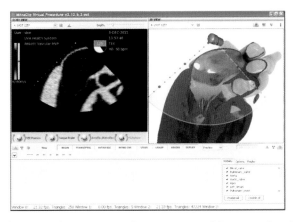

Figure 15.4 The computer simulation program used for transesophageal echocardiographic (TEE) training, Abbott Vascular.

Anesthetic considerations are discussed including effects of volume and systemic vascular resistance changes on mitral regurgitation, the need for indwelling monitoring lines, and a urinary catheter. The pre-procedure TEE issues relate to the experience and time available of the echocardiologist and sonography technician. We also discuss issues ranging from the mundane but important bite block to the more sophisticated 2D versus 3D imaging. Efficiency with the imaging for the procedure is also emphasized.

The importance of a good beginning to any endeavor cannot be underemphasized, and as such the transseptal puncture as it relates to the MitraClip® procedure is discussed in detail. While traditionally for left atrial diagnostic procedures as well as those directed at mitral stenosis, the transseptal puncture was performed using only fluoroscopic guidance. However, this technique is not adequate for the MitraClip® procedure. Utility of echocardiography for guidance of the transseptal puncture at the appropriate location for the mechanical system to work relative to the mitral pathology is demonstrated, as is an understanding of the relationship between the important anatomic structures involved (Fig. 15.5). As this schematic demonstrates, the standard transseptal puncture location through the center of the fossa ovalis brings the MitraClip® delivery system of the anterior leaflet near the aorta. Trainees need to understand that for the MitraClip® system to work optimally, a posterior transseptal direction is frequently needed. Three-dimensional echocardiographic images are used to teach the relationships between the atrial septum and the mitral valve particular to the MitraClip® device positioning (Fig. 15.6).

As illustrative as 3D echocardiographic images are for transseptal puncture, they also have certain limitations that the MitraClip® trainees need to understand, particularly in terms of physical and temporal resolution. Therefore, the training program then utilizes proscribed 2D TEE images (bicaval, short axis, and four-chamber views) to demonstrate optimal transseptal positioning. These didactic lectures on transseptal puncture are then followed

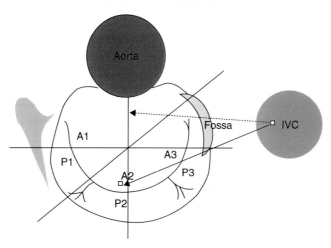

Figure 15.5 Anatomic map of the atrial septal structures relevant to the mitral valve is demonstrated. IVC = inferior vena cava; A1–3 = 1st through 3rd scallops of the anterior mitral valve leaflet; P1–3 = 1st through 3rd scallops of the posterior mitral valve leaflet; Fossa = fossa ovalis of the atrial septum; LAA = left atrial appendage. The dashed red line indicates the standard transseptal puncture direction, which gives an anterior transseptal course. The solid blue line indicates the transseptal puncture direction needed for the MitraClip® procedure, gaining perpendicularity over the line of coaptation of the mitral valve.

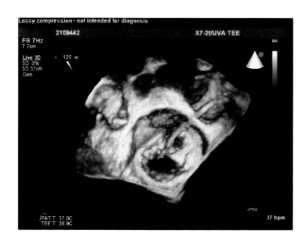

Figure 15.6 Three-dimensional transesophageal echocardiographic image of the mitral valve is shown. Note the anterior transseptal course of the MitraClip® delivery system which in this patient is perpendicular to the line of coaptation of the mitral valve.

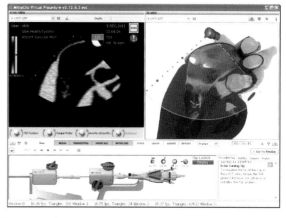

Figure 15.7 The computer simulation program used for MitraClip® training, MitraClip® Virtual Procedure, Abbott Vascular.

up by practice using computer simulation of the transseptal puncture guided by TEE (Fig. 15.7, MitraClip® Virtual Procedure simulator program, Abbott Vascular).

Guidance of the procedure is also done by TEE, and it is important for the trainees to understand 2D imaging prior to 3D imaging. Two-dimensional TEE imaging remains superior in its physical and temporal resolution. We use a case presentation format to illustrate the relevance of the four-chamber, intercommissural (or two-chamber), LVOT (or three-chamber), and transgastric views. We emphasize to the trainees the value of reconstructing the 2D images into 3D in their own heads as well as understanding the pathologic mechanism of the MR. We then repeat the case study but from using 3D TEE to understand its

value and optimal efficiency. These didactic lectures are followed up by hands-on practice with a physical simulator, the actual MitraClip® and MitraClip® delivery system working within a heart model. (Hands-on MitraClip® Simulator, Abbott Vascular; Fig. 15.8,) This physical simulator gives trainees a tactile familiarity with the MitraClip® delivery system and its mechanical controls. Trainees then practice steering and orienting the MitraClip® through the left atrium and relative to the line of coaptation of the mitral valve. The act of grasping the mitral valve leaflets with the MitraClip®, and salient echocardiographic points are discussed, followed by additional structured simulator training with both computer-based and physical models to reinforce the teaching points. This is then followed up by a

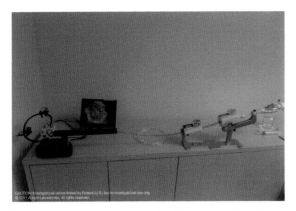

Figure 15.8 Physical simulator-used MitraClip® training, Abbott Vascular. Note three different microcameras simulating the three standard transesophageal echocardiographic (TEE) views used for the MitraClip® procedure, which can be then projected on the video monitor.

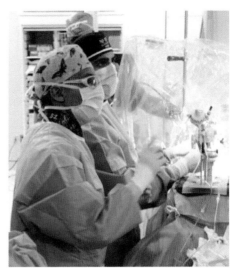

Figure 15.9 Image taken from a MitraClip® training course live case at the University of Virginia, in which both interventional cardiologist (foreground) and cardiac surgeon work collaboratively. Note that standing by the surgeon's left shoulder is the noninvasive imaging cardiologist.

didactic lecture on MitraClip® deployment, delivery system removal, and decision about a second clip.

We then discuss dealing with the complications that can be associated with the MitraClip® procedure, including those related to the transseptal puncture, left atrial injury, entanglement in mitral chords, partial clip detachment, and creation of mitral stenosis. In each of these cases, we demonstrate the recognition of the complication from the echocardiographic standpoint.

We round up the didactic lectures with discussions on postprocedure care, from a vascular access management, to medical therapy, and anesthetic recovery standpoints.

Of particular interest and value in training is live case observation and discussion. The MitraClip® procedure, with its measured pace and hemodynamic stability, particularly lends itself well to in-person teaching by both the noninvasive imager and operator involved in the case. This allows trainees to better understand the creation of the 3D TEE images by the imaging team, as well as the communication that occurs between imager and operator of the case. The live case teaching format also allows trainees to realize the flow of the procedure, with the operator being able to emphasize the points in the case that deserve focus and deliberation (i.e., transseptal puncture location, MitraClip® arm angulation, leaflet insertion assessment, etc.). The live case is also sandwiched by pre-procedure case review and post-procedure case debrief, emphasizing the team approach to the case (Fig. 15.9).

REFERENCES

1. Ailawadi G, Trento A, Mack M, et al. Initial north american experience of mitraclip® procedure performed by cardiac surgeons. Mitral Conclave 2011.
2. Lim S, Ailawadi G. Training cardiac surgeons to do percutaneous mitral valve repair. Transcatheter Ther 2011.
3. Holmes DR Jr, Mack MJ. Transcatheter valve therapy a professional society overview from the american college of cardiology foundation and the society of thoracic surgeons. J Am Coll Cardiol 2011; 58: 445–55.
4. Mack MJ, Holmes DR Jr. Rational dispersion for the introduction of transcatheter valve therapy. JAMA 2011; 306: 2149–50.
5. St Goar FG, Fann JI, Komtebedde J, et al. Endovascular edge-to-edge mitral valve repair: short-term results in a porcine model. Circulation 2003; 108: 1990–3.

Special techniques for functional mitral regurgitation
Olaf Franzen, Stephan von Bardeleben, and Susanna Price

Successful interventional treatment of functional mitral regurgitation (MR) requires a detailed understanding of the underlying pathomechanisms. This holds true for the interventionalist as well as for the echocardiographer. The basic pathomechanic concept postulates that regional or global remodeling of the left ventricle can lead to an outward displacement of one or both papillary muscles. As a consequence, the attached chordae tendineae tether the leaflets into the left ventricle ("apical displacement of the leaflets") (1). This mechanism, often in combination with annulus dilatation, reduces the area of coaptation between the leaflets and can finally lead to a loss of coaptation. However, this underlying basic concept can be much more complex in the individual patient. The extent and pattern of ventricular and annular dilatation, the shape and distribution of the papillary muscles and chordae tendineae, the shape and length of the leaflets and the presence and distribution of leaflet indentations as well as the actual closing force play a role in the development and degree of secondary mitral regurgitation (1). Some of these factors, as well as the MR itself, respond dynamically to exercise, filling volume, and pressure (2–4). The complete echocardiographic assessment of all individual factors and their interpretation is still an unsolved problem, especially when it comes to the subvalvular apparatus. Nevertheless, some helpful categorization has been suggested and can be identified by echocardiography (5). One of the most important concepts is the differentiation between more widely versus localized tethering of the leaflets. In this chapter these entities are referred as symmetric and asymmetric tethering. During the treatment of MR with the MitraClip® therapy, these principal pathoanatomic patterns as well as local anatomic variations can be addressed by special techniques.

SYMMETRIC AND ASYMMETRIC TETHERING

Symmetric Tethering

The displacement of the papillary muscles can cause symmetric tethering as for example in some cases, global dilatation of the left ventricle due to dilated cardiomyopathy. Apical infarction can cause symmetric or asymmetric tethering (6). Symmetric tethering can displace the complete line of coaptation rather symmetrically into the ventricle. In a normal heart, the anterolateral and posteromedial papillary muscles or groups of papillary muscles are situated more or less under the adjacent commissure. In severe dilatation of the left ventricle they may not only be displaced toward the apex but also be situated more eccentric (lateral or medial) in relation to the adjacent commissure (Fig. 16.1). Even severe left ventricular (LV)

dilatation not always induces relevant outward displacement of the papillary muscles (1). The extent and effect of the eccentric displacement may be dependent on the shape of the papillary muscles as well as on the extent and pattern of annulus dilatation. As a final consequence, the mobility of the anterior mitral leaflet (AML) and posterior mitral leaflet (PML) may be restricted, and the free margin of the posterior and anterior leaflet may be displaced apically (7). As the PML is rather short, the echocardiographic appearance of apical displacement might be a posteriorly retracted PML. In some patients with severe LV dilatation the P1 segment of the leaflets may be retracted laterally and the P3 segment medially. This lateral and medial retraction can lead to incomplete closing along the indentations on both sides of the P2 segment with two major jets originating from line of coaptation on the lateral and medial side of the P2. However, in most patients with symmetric tethering the major jet originates from the central part of the line of coaptation and may extend to the medial and lateral sides in various degrees.

Asymmetric Tethering

In a posterior myocardial infarction, only the posteromedial papillary muscle may be displaced apically (Fig. 16.2). As a result, leaflet tenting is asymmetric and affects predominantly the P3 and A3 segments and also the medial halves of the P2 and A2 segments (8). It is mentioned before this pattern may vary according to the position and shape of the papillary muscles and chordae tendineae (Fig. 16.3). In asymmetric papillary muscle displacement, MR typically originates from the line of coaptation adjacent to the medial part of the P2 segment and the central part of the line of coaptation. A regurgitant jet may also originate from the posteromedial commissure. As the medial posterior leaflet may also be displaced laterally, the margin of the indentation between the P3 and P2 segments may be pulled apart and a jet may originate from there.

Modest Tethering with Severe Annulus Dilatation

Left ventricular dilatation not always induces severe papillary muscle and apical leaflet displacement. The main "driving" mechanism of functional MR can also be annulus dilatation, which in extreme cases can even cause a gap between the leaflets (Fig. 16.4). The relative small distance from the line of coaptation to annular plane entails technical consideration described later in this chapter.

As the patterns of papillary muscle and chordae distribution cannot be sufficiently examined with echocardiography, the underlying pathoanatomy of functional MR must be inferred

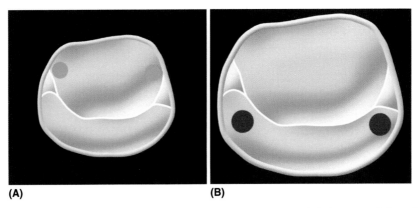

Figure 16.1 Normal position of the papillary muscles under the commissure (*Left*) and papillary muscle displacement, which may lead to symmetric apical displacement of the tips of the leaflets (*Right*).

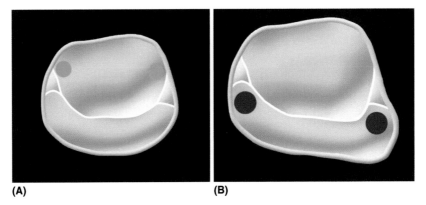

Figure 16.2 Normal position of the papillary muscles under the commissure (A) and displacement of posteromedial papillary muscle due to an aneurysm of the posterior wall. Additional eccentric annulus dilatation, the consequence may be asymmetric tethering predominantly in the medial parts of the mitral valve (B).

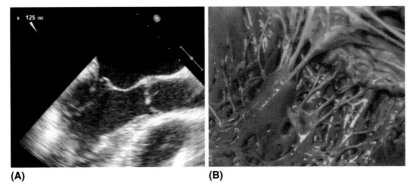

Figure 16.3 Patient with posterior wall aneurysm, transesophageal left ventricular outflow tract view (A) demonstrating severe apical displacement but almost no transapical displacement of the anterior mitral leaflet, possible explanation seen in the anatomic photograph (B) showing the posteromedial papillary muscle group with a long head (asterisk) free from the wall giving rise to chords of the anterior mitral leaflet and a posterior "muscle band" (arrows) closely attached to the posterior wall giving rise to the posterior leaflet.

from the position and mobility of the leaflets; the morphology, size and contractility of the left ventricle; the size of the mitral annulus; and the origin of MR. Optimally, the echocardiographic findings should fit in one of the three mentioned categories. The medical history (e.g., posterior infarction) of the patient should make the findings plausible. Although identification of the underlying mechanism is mandatory for optimizing the planning of the procedure, the principle of the MitraClip® procedure remains that the leaflets should coapt exactly at the origin of MR. Therefore, the anatomy of both leaflets at the origin of the MR, their spatial relation to each other, and the mitral annulus determine the technical and strategic considerations.

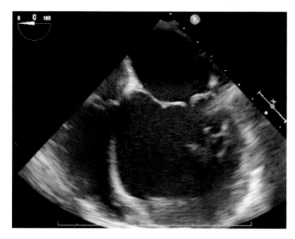

Figure 16.4 Transesophageal 4-chamber view, severe dilatation of the left ventricle in dilated cardiomyopathy in this case with moderate tethering on the strut chord of the anterior mitral leaflet but almost no tethering of the posterior mitral leaflet. Annulus dilatation entails a gap between the leaflets.

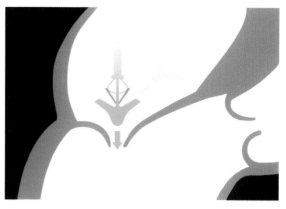

Figure 16.6 The green shaft orientation correctly bisects the angle between the leaflets while the red incorrect shaft orientation is too parallel to the AML.

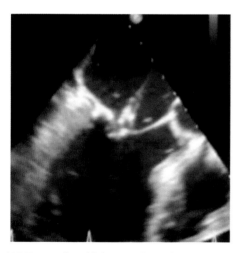

Figure 16.5 Transesophageal left ventricular outflow tract view with the shaft bisecting the angle anterior and posterior mitral leaflets.

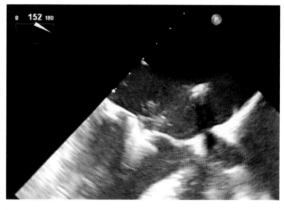

Figure 16.7 Transesophageal left ventricular outflow tract view, the incorrect shaft orientation is "favoring" the posterior mitral leaflet allowing the anterior mitral leaflet to slip off the clip arm.

GENERAL TECHNICAL CONSIDERATIONS
Optimal Angle Between the Leaflets and the Shaft of the MitraClip® System

In order not to favor one of the mitral leaflets, the shaft of the MitraClip® system should bisect the angle between PML and AML (Fig. 16.5). Even if the inter-atrial septum has been punctured in an optimal position, the shaft is often not optimally oriented toward the mitral valve. Typically, the shaft is more in parallel with the AML and more perpendicular to the PML (Fig. 16.6). Such orientation is not optimal for the subsequent grasping process. Upon retraction of the clip, the PML will be lifted up with the distal end of the posterior clip arm, precluding optimal leaflet insertion, while the tip of the anterior clip arm might not have close contact with the AML (Fig. 16.7). As a consequence, the AML tends to slip from the anterior clip arm. In most cases use of the plus (+) knob on the steerable

guide can optimize shaft orientation. This maneuver should only be performed when the clip is still in the left atrium and should be closely monitored with TEE. It must be mentioned that use of the plus (+) knob brings the clip closer to the mitral valve; therefore, it is preferable if the septal puncture site is not low. This is one of the reasons why many interventionalists try to avoid a puncture height of less than 4 cm.

Dynamic Adjustment of Anterior/Posterior Orientation During Clip Retraction

In principle, there are two strategies during the retraction of the clip toward the mitral leaflets. One strategy is, after optimal adjustment, to keep the anterior-posterior orientation fixed during retraction. If the given orientation is unfavorable, it can be adjusted and fixed again in order to try another grasp. The advantage of this technique is that the same

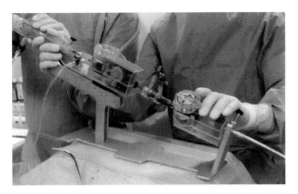

Figure 16.8 Primary operator retracts the handle and adjusts the anterior–posterior orientation while secondary operator controls the grippers and the actuator knob.

physician can retract the handle, drop the grippers, and close the clip arm positioner. The disadvantage is that in certain leaflet configurations it is almost impossible to have a correct grasp with both leaflets inserted well. The other strategy is to adjust the anterior-posterior orientation during the retraction of the clips toward the leaflets (Fig. 16.8). The grasping is facilitated especially in cases of adverse anatomy. In theory there might be a higher risk for the clip to get entangled in the chords. This risk may be amplified if the plus (+) knob has been used before because then the height difference by anterior-posterior movement is more pronounced. However, in experienced hands this technique is safe if used carefully; in some cases it might be the only chance to have a successful grasp in an unfavorable leaflet configuration, like, for instance, a posteriorly orientated PML or very long (>6 mm) coaptation length.

Loading the Leaflets onto the Clip Arms

In functional MR there is complete chordal support of the mitral leaflets. This makes it possible to carefully retract the clip toward the leaflets and load the leaflets onto the clip arms. Usually, this does not aggravate the MR. After the leaflets rest on the clip arms (Fig. 16.8), there is time to recheck the perpendicularity of the clip arms relative to the coaptation line and also to verify that the clip position is optimal in relation to the jet origin. When the optimal position and orientation of the clip has been verified, efforts should be taken to optimize the TEE images such that the dropping of the grippers and the closing of the clip can be fully visualized and stored in an echo-loop log. In case of later doubt about the leaflet insertion, rechecking this grasping process in the stored echo loop might be the most helpful way to verify optimal leaflet insertion.

Optimal Angle of the Clip Arms Before Dropping the Grippers

While the process of uploading the leaflets onto the clip arms can be performed with an inner angle between the clip arms of 140°, this might be not the optimal angle of the clip arms

before the grippers are dropped. If the gripper lever is lowered as far as possible and the grippers are completely dropped, the inner angle between the grippers is 60°. So the clip arms need to be closed each by another 40° before the leaflets start to get fixed between clip arms and grippers. The tips of the clip arms move during this closing process in the direction of the left atrium while the joint between the clip arms remains in the same position in the left ventricle. If the tips of the clip arms are already close to the annular plane before beginning the closing process, they might end in a supra-annular position. As a consequence, the uploaded leaflets might slip away from the shaft and less of the leaflets are inserted in the clip. In such a situation an advancement of the clip into the left ventricle can improve leaflet insertion. In leaflets with a short coaptation length this effect might be more pronounced. It can be advantageous to close the clip arms to an inner angle of 100° to 80° and then reassure in echocardiography that the tip of the leaflets still reach the shaft of the clip delivery system before the grippers are dropped and the clip is closed under TEE control. As mentioned before, the position of the tip of the posterior clip arm is also dependent on the angle between shaft and leaflets. Therefore, a retraction of the clip and an adjustment of the angle might be needed.

Short Coaptation Length and Gap Between the Leaflets

According to the valve suitability criteria from the EVEREST trials, the coaptation length of both leaflets should be at least 2 mm (9). With the first experience in Europe it became clear that also patients with less coaptation length could be treated successfully (10). Even patients with a systolic gap between the leaflets can be treated with good leaflet insertion if parts of the leaflets are still pointing toward the left ventricle ("virtual coaptation length"). In these cases it is very important to carefully optimize the angle between the shaft and leaflets as well as the clip angle before dropping the grippers. In the combination of a gap between the leaflets and almost no virtual coaptation length, the width of the gap determines if the valve is still suitable for MitraClip® therapy. In exceptional cases even a valve with a 10 mm central gap can be treated successfully. The first clip is placed not in the center of the gap but a little to the side of it, where the gap is smaller. It is retracted toward the leaflets with an inner angle between the clip arms of about 80–100°. The AML is uploaded completely; the posterior clip arm needs to be behind the PML. Then the clip is carefully retracted further and simultaneously steered posteriorly. This drags the AML in the direction of the posterior annulus and also brings more of the PML onto the posterior clip arm. As the distance between the leaflets is now also smaller in the center of the gap, a second clip can usually be placed successfully. Although this technique has been repeatedly used with success by the authors it is only recommended in exceptional cases because of a possibly unpredictable risk of tearing the AML. The long-term results of this technique and the impact of the increased anterior-posterior tension have not been elucidated yet.

Very Long Coaptation Length

In the majority of patients the coaptation length does not exceed 4–5 mm. However, in some patients echocardiography may measure coaptation lengths of more than 8 mm. A membrane between the paramedical chords might be the reason for such an echocardiographic appearance. Grasping the leaflets can be very difficult in these patients as the clip arms are only 8 mm long. If the clip is retracted with an inner angle of 120° toward the leaflets, the parts of the leaflets contributing to the coaptation length need to be furled in order to reach the body of the leaflets with the clip arms. Often in this situation at least one of the leaflets rolls in and finally slips off the opposing clip arm. In order to avoid this, the clip must be retracted with an inner angle of about 80°–100°. If the tips of the clip arms reach the bodies of the leaflets, the angle of the clip can again be opened further to allow more contact with the body of the leaflets. Typically in this situation with a lot of leaflet tissue furled, the leaflets tend to lift from the clip arm in systole before they are finally fixed between the grippers and the clip arms. Therefore in patients with sinus rhythm, administration of adenosine might facilitate the grasping process. The described maneuver applies force to the chords and leaflets during retraction; therefore, tearing of the leaflets or chordal rupture may occur in fragile leaflets.

Posteriorly Orientated Posterior Leaflet

In a posterior wall aneurysm the tip of the restricted posterior leaflet may extend during systole even more posterior than the annulus (Fig. 16.3A). Typically, this is accompanied by the echocardiographic appearance of an anterior extension of the posterior mitral annulus ("heart failure ridge"). The angle between AML and PML can be as small as approximately 90° at the point where the leaflets coapt. In this leaflet configuration, dynamic anterior-posterior adjustment during retraction of the clip can be very helpful. The posterior clip arm is retracted between PML and posterior wall. A relatively small inner angle (120–80°) between the clip arms might be needed to do so. If the posterior clip arm is between the posterior wall and the posterior leaflet, a careful anterior shift and opening of the clip arms might help also to upload the AML onto the anterior clip arm. This anterior shift should be performed very carefully as it lifts the PML away from the posterior wall and therefore applies tension to the chords that support the PML. When this maneuver has been performed successfully it is important to close the clip arms up to 80° and verify that both leaflets come into the V of the clip arms and touch the shaft of the clip. Only then should the grippers be dropped and the clip closed under careful echocardiographic control to ensure good leaflet insertion.

Short PML

Although in a prolapse the PML is often long, it is mostly rather short in functional MR. Since the length of the grippers is 5 mm, the posterior leaflet should have at least a length of 6 mm to guarantee stable position of the clip. In cases with such a short posterior leaflet, it can be helpful to upload the leaflets onto the clip arms and close the clip to 60°. Often it is necessary to slightly re-advance the clip into the left ventricle to avoid positioning the tip of the posterior clip arm higher than the posterior annulus. Finally, the tip of the posterior clip arm is steered very close under the posterior annulus by a posterior torque of the steerable guide before the grippers are dropped and the clip is closed. This maneuver secures maximal insertion of the posterior leaflet. In order to verify at least 5 mm of leaflet insertion, it can be helpful to measure the length of the posterior leaflet and compare it with the posterior leaflet left outside the clip after the clip is fully closed.

Jet from Indentations

Indentations can be mainly found in the PML between the scallops. Consequently, many patients will have two indentations in their PML. The length of the segments and therefore the position of the indentations can vary as can the depth of the indentation. In its maximum form of manifestation the indentation reaches up to the annulus. There may also be more than only two indentations and, depending on the position of the papillary muscles, the segments might have incomplete coaptation along the indentations. In such cases a jet can originate from an indentation, for example as in some forms of tethering caused by aneurysms of the posterior wall. (cf. asymmetric papillary muscle displacement above). If a significant part of the MR originates from the indentation, MitraClip® treatment may not be successful. The result can be difficult to predict. Therefore, such cases are often judged unsuitable for MitraClip®. It seems to be not reasonable to place a clip along the indentation as this might distort the valve with the consequence of even more severe MR. A clip between AML and PML first con the central part and, if needed, on the other side of the indentation might lift up both leaflets and bring the segments closer together, also along the indentation.

Jet from the Medial Commissure

In functional MR following a posterior myocardial infarction, the jet may originate from the medial commissure. A larger jet originating between the central segments of the mitral valve usually accompanies this finding. If the jet from the medial commissure is small, the risk–benefit ratio of treating it might be clearly on the side of risk. Only a significant jet from the medial commissure is worth treating. Three-dimensional echocardiography should be used to assess the perpendicular position of the clip at the line of coaptation close to the commissures. As it is not possible to use an LV outflow tract view for grasping atypical views demonstrating opposing AML and PML are needed.

Two Distant Jets on the Sides of the Central Posterior (P2) Segment

In severe symmetric tethering of the leaflets the "deepest" point of the closure line might be close to the insertion of the strut chords of the AML. Under general anesthesia the jet origin may be even restricted to these deepest points of the line of coaptation. However, if the patient's blood pressure is normal or high, this type of MR may appear as MR originating from all the length of the line of coaptation. It might be the best strategy to place a clip at each of these points, sometimes resulting in a triple orifice. The resulting opening area of the mitral valve is usually acceptable if the annulus is enlarged. In thickened leaflets or if the AML is very restricted it might occur that the leaflets between the clips do not separate in diastole. As a result, the remaining mitral valve opening area might be too small. In valves with many paramedical chords at the leaflet margin close to the strut chords, it may be difficult to successfully place the clip on the optimal location. The posterior clip arm might tend to be placed into a nearby indentation. This should be remembered, especially in cases where it seems to be impossible to grasp both leaflets at the same time. The structure of the chords can be more complex at the medial and lateral end of the P2 segment, which might carry a higher risk to get entangled in the mitral chords.

REFERENCES

1. Otsuji Y, Levine RA, Takeuchi M, Sakata R, Tei C. Mechanism of ischemic mitral regurgitation. J Cardiol 2008; 51: 145–56.
2. Magne J, Lancellotti P, Piérard LA. Exercise-induced changes in degenerative mitral regurgitation. J Am Coll Cardiol 2010; 56: 300–9.
3. Lancellotti P, Gérard PL, Piérard LA. Long-term outcome of patients with heart failure and dynamic functional mitral regurgitation. Eur Heart J 2005; 26: 1528–32.
4. Lapu-Bula R, Robert A, Van Craeynest D, et al. Contribution of exercise-induced mitral regurgitation to exercise stroke volume and exercise capacity in patients with left ventricular systolic dysfunction. Circulation 2002; 106: 1342–8.
5. Levine RA, Schwammenthal E. Ischemic mitral regurgitation on the threshold of a solution: from paradoxes to unifying concepts. Circulation 2005; 112: 745–58.
6. Yosefy C, Beeri R, Guerrero JL, et al. Mitral regurgitation after anteroapical myocardial infarction: new mechanistic insights. Circulation 2011; 123: 1529–36.
7. Godley RW, Wann LS, Rogers EW, Feigenbaum H, Weyman AE. Incomplete mitral leaflet closure in patients with papillary muscle dysfunction. Circulation 1981; 63: 565–71.
8. Watanabe N, Ogasawara Y, Yamaura Y, et al. Geometric differences of the mitral valve tenting between anterior and inferior myocardial infarction with significant ischemic mitral regurgitation: quantitation by novel software system with transthoracic real-time three-dimensional echocardiography. J Am Soc Echocardiogr 2006; 19: 71–5.
9. Feldman T, Wasserman HS, Herrmann HC, et al. Percutaneous mitral valve repair using the edge-to-edge technique: six-month results of the EVEREST phase I clinical trial. J Am Coll Cardiol 2005; 46: 2134–40.
10. Franzen O, Baldus S, Volker R, et al. Acute outcomes of mitraclip® therapy for mitral regurgitation in high-surgical-risk patients: emphasis on adverse valve morphology and severe left ventricular dysfunction. Eur Heart J 2010; 31: 1373–81.

17 The European experience since CE approval

Corrado Tamburino, Gian Paolo Ussia, and Valeria Cammalleri

Percutaneous repair of mitral regurgitation (MR) with the MitraClip® System (Abbott Vascular, Abbott Park, Illinois, USA) is a novel interventional technique developed as alternative to surgical approaches for the patients considered at high risk for conventional cardiac surgery. It is the most commonly used percutaneous procedure for MR therapy and currently the only transcatheter device which received the CE mark in Europe.

The first man in whom the MitraClip® procedure was performed was in 2003 and so far, more than 5000 procedures have been performed in selected centers in the United States (under the EVEREST trial) (1–3) and in Europe (under the ACCESS trial and commercial use). The sum of clinical data currently available for the MitraClip® System includes results derived from the EVEREST trials performed in North America and from the clinical studies following commercial approval in Europe (see Table 17.1).

Data from the real-life experience show that patients commonly treated in Europe present a higher surgical risk profile, more complex mitral valve anatomy and mainly functional MR, when compared with patients enrolled in the EVEREST trial.

The first published European experience with the MitraClip® System has been provided by Franzen et al.(4), showing that the percutaneous edge-to-edge procedure is feasible in patients at high surgical risk primarily determined by an adverse mitral valve morphology and/or severe left ventricular (LV) dysfunction. The study included 51 patients (mean age 73 ± 10 years, 67% men) with a mean logistic EuroSCORE of 28 ± 22 (range 2–86), STS-score of 15 ± 11 (range 1–43) and 47% with a logistic EuroSCORE <20, but with specific risk factors not included in the score system. Functional MR was presented in 69% of cases, while the remaining 31% suffered from organic MR. LV ejection fraction (EF) was 36 ± 17%. Thirty-five patients (69%), named EVEREST –, had LV characteristics and/or a mitral valve morphology that would have excluded them from enrolment in the EVEREST trials, whereas the others who could have been included in the EVERST Trial were defined as EVEREST +. Specific exclusion criteria present among the EVEREST – group were the following: LV end-systolic diameter >60 mm and an LV EF <20% in 34% and 29% of patients respectively, a mitral valve orifice area <4 cm² in 31%, a coaptation length <2 mm 34%, a flail width >15 mm in 11% of patients, and a flail gap >10 mm in one patient; 34% of patients had more than one and up to three of these features. A successful MitraClip® implantation was obtained in 49 patients (96%): 69% had a single clip, 29% received two clips, and one patient three clips. Mean device and fluoroscopy times were 105 ± 65 minutes and 44 ± 28 minutes, respectively. Procedure-related reduction in MR severity was one grade in 31%, two grades

47%, and three grades in 18% of patients. A clinical improvement at discharge was reported in 90% of patients: NYHA functional class ≥III in 98% before and 33% after the procedure (P < 0.0001). No procedure-related major adverse events and no in-hospital mortality were observed in this very high surgical risk cohort.

The preliminary Italian experience (5), including 31 patients [age 71 (IQR 62–79) years, 71% >65 years, male 81%] treated in Ferrarotto Hospital in Catania and San Raffaele Hospital in Milan, demonstrated satisfactory results in a high surgical risk population with congestive heart failure and depressed LV function. Patients were selected for the procedure if they met basic criteria for intervention from the European Society of Cardiology Task Force recommendation on the management of valvular heart disease. In addition to meeting guidelines criteria, patients were high-risk candidates for mitral valve surgery including cardiopulmonary bypass. High risk defined by a logistic EuroSCORE >20% and other external parameters, was established based on the consensus of the local heart team, including an independent cardiologist and a cardiac surgeon. Patient selection for the procedure was performed according to the EVEREST anatomical criteria. The primary acute safety endpoint was freedom from major adverse events at 30 days, defined as the composite of death, myocardial infarction, non-elective cardiac surgery for adverse events, renal failure, transfusion of >2 units of blood, ventilation for >48 hours, deep wound infection, septicemia, and new onset of atrial fibrillation. The primary efficacy endpoint was acute device success defined as clip implant with reduction of MR to ≤2+. Etiology of MR was functional in 58% of patients, whereas the remaining 42% had an organic degenerative disease. Logistic EuroSCORE and STS score were 14.3 ± 11.9 and 10.3 ± 8.8%, respectively; 45% of patients presented a history of coronary heart disease and 36% history of congestive heart failure. The MitraClip® procedure was successfully performed in all patients, with one clip implanted in 61% and two clips 39% of cases. Acute device success was observed in 96.8% of patients (95% CI 81.5–99.8). No procedural death was observed. At 30 days two patients experienced major adverse events (one death and one intra-procedural cardiac tamponade requiring surgical drainage and blood transfusion) resulting in a primary safety endpoint of 93.6% (95% CI 77.2–98.9). At 30 days, of the 28 patients with MR being 4+ before the procedure, 18 (58%) had MR graded as trivial to mild (0 to 1+), 9 (29%) had MR graded as mild to moderate (1 to 2+), and one patient had MR graded as moderate to severe (2 to 3+). All three patients with MR being 3+ before the procedure had an

MR graded as trivial to mild (0 to 1 +) at 30 days (Fig. 17.1). In addition, reduction in left ventricular diameters and annular septal-lateral dimension has been reported. These echocardiographic results were also accomplished by a significant clinical improvement at 30 days of follow-up. At baseline most of the patients (87%) were in New York Heart Association (NYHA) functional III/IV, whereas 13% were in I/II; at 30 days all patients (100%) were in NYHA class I/II.

A smaller series of nine high risk patients (78% male, age 75.9 ± 9.0 years) treated with the MitraClip® System for ≥3+ in Netherlands, was reported by Van den Branden et al. (6). The mean logistic EuroSCORE of the study population was 33.8 ± 9.0% and all patients had functional MR (56% ischemic and 44% non-ischemic) associated with a severe LV dysfunction. A significant impairment of the clinical status of these patients was reported: 89% were in NYHA functional class III and 11% in IV class. The clip was implanted successfully in all

nine patients. Partial clip detachment, diagnosed 24 hours post procedure, occurred in one patient, who underwent a successfully second clip placement five days later. One patient developed inguinal bleeding. Eight patients (89%) were discharged with a reduction in MR severity to ≤2 (p = 0.002); at 30 days 78% presented MR grade to ≤2 (p = 0.001). NYHA functional class improved from median 3 to 2 (p = 0.04) and the quality-of-life (QoL) index improved from 62.9 ± 16.3 to 49.9 ± 30.7 (p = 0.12).

Another similar experience, differing from the EVEREST trials in patient characteristics, was that published by Pleger et al. (7). This study included 33 patients, who underwent MitraClip® procedure in Germany, with an increased surgical mortality risk, as assessed by an STS score of 24 ± 4% and EuroSCORE of 41 ± 7%. At 30 days the MR grade significantly decreased from 2.9 ± 0.2 to 1.7 ± 0.7 (p <0.0001) and NYHA functional class improved from 3.38 ± 0.59 to 2.2 ± 0.4 (p < 0.001). Accordingly, the six-minute walk distance improved from 194 ± 44 to 300 ± 70 m (p < 0.01). No death occurred at 30 days. Two patients developed a left atrial thrombus, one patient required ventilation for >12 hours, and one patient experienced significant access site bleeding.

A retrospective European multicenter report of Franzen et al. (8) confirmed favorable outcomes in high-risk patients with end-stage heart failure and marked left ventricular dysfunction, treated with the MitraClip® System. This study included 50 heart failure patients (mean age 70 ± 11 years, 76% men) with an LV EF ≤25% and MR of at least grade 3+. All patients were on optimal medical and device treatment. Twenty-eight (56%) suffered from ischemic cardiomyopathy, whereas 22 (44%) had non-ischemic etiology. All patients had functional MR, were in NYHA functional class III (54%) or IV (46%), and the mean logistic EuroSCORE was 34 ± 12%. A total of 53 MitraClip® procedures were performed; one or more clips were implanted in 50 procedures (48 patients), for an

Table 17.1 Studies Evaluating the MitraClip® Device

Study	Population	N
EVEREST I (Feasibility)	Feasibility patients	55
EVEREST II (Pivotal)	Pre-randomized patients	60
EVEREST II (Pivotal)	Non-randomized patients (High Risk Study)	78
EVEREST II (Pivotal)	Randomized patients (2:1 Clip to Surgery)	279: 184 Clip, 95 Surgery
REALISM (Continued Access)	Non-randomized patients	675
ACCESS Europe	Non-randomized patients	681
Commercial use	Commercial patients	3546
Total		5279 + 95 surgery

Data complete to April 20, 2012.

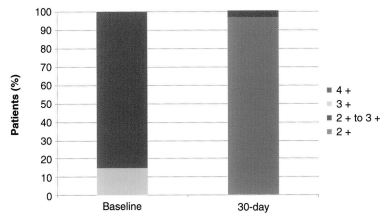

Figure 17.1 Baseline and 30-day mitral regurgitation. *Source*: From Ref. 5.

acute procedural success rate of 94%. Severity of MR was reduced in all successfully treated patients and 92% were discharged with MR ≤2+. Thirty-day mortality was 6%; cumulative survival at 6 months was 81.2%. At 6 months, 87% had MR ≤2+ and 72% of patients were in NYHA class I or II (Fig. 17.2). Moreover, improvement in measures of MR, left ventricular dimensions, six-minute walk distances, and NT-proBNP plasma levels has been reported. The authors proved that in this study population, survival was significantly impacted by NYHA functional class such that NYHA-III and NYHA-IV patients had 6-month survival estimates of 96 and 64%, respectively (8).

A recent Italian report by Ussia et al. (9) confirmed that the clinical and echocardiographic benefits obtained with MR reduction, following MitraClip® implantation, are accomplished by a significant QoL improvement, even if the reduction of MR is not complete at follow-up. The study population consisted in 39 consecutive patients (age 72 ± 11 years, male 82%), on optimal medical therapy at the time of the procedure, who received the SF-12v2 questionnaire before MitraClip® procedure and 6 months after the device implantation. The high risk of the cohort was demonstrated by a mean logistic EuroSCORE and an STS score of 20 ± 6% and 11 ± 5%, respectively; 82% of patients had >65 years; 69% referred a history of congestive heart failure and 15% of patients had a previous cardiac surgical intervention. Twenty-six patients (64%) presented with functional disease and 14 patients (36%) with organic degenerative MR. Acute procedural success was observed in all patients (100%) and there was no procedural mortality. Three patients experienced minor procedural complications, which were two inguinal hematomas and one lateral cervical hematoma caused during placement of the central venous catheter. A significant MR reduction was achieved immediately after the procedure and after 6 months: at follow-up 86% and 14% of patients had MR ≤1+ and MR 2+, respectively. Mean pre-procedural SF-12v2 scores showed a severe impairment of perceived QoL, both for physical and mental scores; after six months a striking improvement in physical (physical component summary; PCS 35.44 vs. 44.67, <0.0001) and mental (MCS 38.07 vs. 46.94, <0.0001) aspect of QoL was observed. In addition, physical and mental status improvement was higher in patients with functional MR (Fig. 17.3). NYHA functional class improved in all patients, from 2.9 ± 0.6 at baseline to 2.0 ± 0.7 (<0.0001) at discharge, and 1.5 ± 0.5 at 6 months (p = 0.001 when compared with discharge and <0.0001 when compared with baseline).

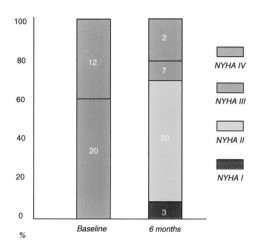

Figure 17.2 Distributions of New York Heart Association (NYHA) functional class at baseline and 6 months after MitraClip® implantation. *Source*: From Ref. 8.

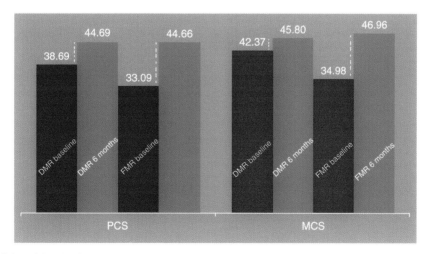

Figure 17.3 Results of physical (PCS) and mental (MCS) scores before and at 6 months in patients with degenerative (n = 15) and functional MR (n = 17). Physical and mental status upgrading was higher in patients with functional MR. *Abbreviations*: DMR, degenerative mitral regurgitation; FMR, functional mitral regurgitation. *Source*: From Ref. 9.

Recently, a prospective European multicenter study of the feasibility and safety of the MitraClip® procedure in nonresponders to cardiac resynchronization therapy (CRT) has been published, reporting improved functional class, increased LV EF, and reduced ventricular volumes in about 70% of the study patients (10). Fifty-one symptomatic CRT patients (nonresponders), consecutively treated with the MitraClip® device, were enrolled at seven European institutions. All patients were previously treated with CRT for at least six months and remained in NYHA functional class III or IV despite pharmacological optimization, with chronic functional MR ≥3+, due to LV dysfunction. An overall 30-day mortality of 4.2% was reported, whereas mortality during 14 months of follow-up was 19.9 per 100 person-years (95% CI: 10.3–38.3). Nonsurvivors had more compromised clinical baseline conditions, longer QRS duration, higher mean value of NT-proBNP, more dilated heart, more previous valvular surgery, and a much higher logistic EuroSCORE and STS score (10).

Since its introduction in Europe, patients treated with MitraClip® device have been enrolled in the ACCESS post-market registry, of which the preliminary results stated the high surgical risk of patients treated in Europe (11). The ACCESS patients (n = 257, age 73 ± 10 years, men 65%) had a logistic EuroSCORE of 20 ± 18%, low ejection fraction (LV EF <40% in 55%) and mostly had functional MR (78%, ischemic in 38%, and non-ischemic in 40%). Coronary artery disease was reported in 62%, previous cardiac surgery in 37% and moderate to severe renal failure in 43% of patients. The procedure was successful in 99%, with one clip implanted in 58%, two clips in 39% and three clips in 2% of cases. Thirty-day events reported were 2.7% death; 0.4% stroke; 0.4% myocardial infarction; 2.7% renal failure; 3.9% bleeding complications, and no pericardial tamponade. At 6 months 80% of patients had MR ≤2+ and 71% were in NYHA functional class I/II, compared with 16% of I/II class at baseline (p < 0.0001). Freedom from death resulted of 87.5%, whereas freedom from mitral valve surgery was 96% at 6 months. In addition, significantly improved QoL and six-minute walk test distance were observed (11).

Since the introduction of the MitraClip® a series of different case reports have been published, testing the use of the device in various situations. Ussia et al. assessed the feasibility of the percutaneous edge-to-edge procedure under deep conscious sedation using remifentanil hydrochloride (GlaxoSmithKline and Abbott as ULTIVA®) in a patient who had serious contraindications to general anesthesia (12). Three reports from different European institutions have been published about percutaneous double-valve interventions for aortic stenosis (AS) and MR, concluding that these procedures in the same patient are feasible options in selected cases (13–15). This dual approach may be safe and effective in patients with coexisting severe AS and MR at high risk for cardiac surgery; in addition, MitraClip® implantation can be used as a bailout therapy in case of new severe MR after aortic bioprosthesis deployment Fig. 17.4 (13). Franzen et al. used a percutaneous approach with MitraClip® system to treat successfully a tricuspid regurgitation

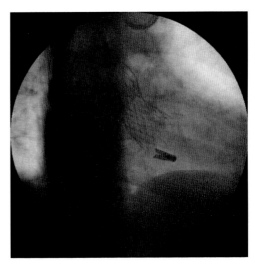

Figure 17.4 Fluoroscopy view showing the MitraClip® device and the CoreValve Revalving System (CRS; Medtronic Inc., Minneapolis, MN, USA).

in congenitally correct transposition of the great arteries (16). A German paper reported a case of a patient treated percutaneously with two MitraClip® devices and with left atrial appendage closure in the same procedure (17). Percutaneous mitral valve repair was also used as a bail-out strategy for patients with severe mitral regurgitation after cardiac surgery (18) and three female patients underwent previously coronary artery bypass grafting, tricuspid valve replacement, and aortic valve replacement combined with tricuspid valve repair at the University Heart Center, Hamburg. Postoperatively, severe functional MR impeded hemodynamic stabilization, therefore, to avoid early redo surgery associated with disproportional operative risk, an interventional approach with MitraClip® repair was chosen after interdisciplinary discussion (18).

An interesting study of Schillinger W et al. (19) investigated the impact of the learning curve on outcomes of 75 consecutive patients treated with MitraClip® System in three subsequent periods (25 patients each). Median total procedure time and device time decreased from 180 and 105 minutes in period 1–95 and 55 minutes in period 3 (P < 0.005 each). There was an excess of total safety events in period 1 (n = 16) that decreased in periods 2 and 3 (n = 6 and 3, P = 0.0003). Acute procedural success was 80% in periods 1 and 2, and 92% in period 3 (P = 0.46). At 6 months, improvement in durability and completeness of mitral valve repair was reported: 89.4% of patients in period 3 and 65.0% in period 1 had MR ≤2+ at 6 months (P = 0.03) (19).

The European data according to other smaller clinical experiences demonstrate that patients treated worldwide with the MitraClip® System have, in general, higher surgical risk profile than those enrolled in the EVEREST trials (Fig. 17.5). Although the EVEREST trials provide good results about the efficacy, safety and mid-term durability of the MitraClip® device (1–3), these data do not reflect the real characteristics of the patients treated

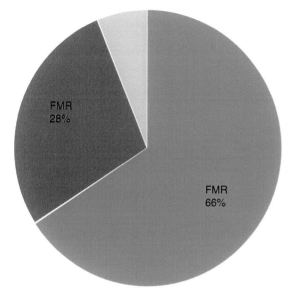

FMR
28%

FMR
66%

Figure 17.5 Commercial MitraClip® implant experience in Europe according to the etiology of mitral regurgitation. *Abbreviations:* DMR, degenerative mitral regurgitation; FMR, functional mitral regurgitation; M, mixed. Data as of October 10, 2011 by Abbott Vascular.

in the real life. In the randomized trial (3) the predominant valvulopathy treated was degenerative MR (73% both in device and in surgical group), in patients without contraindications for surgery, with a mean LV EF of 60 ± 10.1% and 60.6 ± 11% in device and in surgical group, respectively. The trial data are also in contrast with the real clinical practice which includes a larger range of complex anatomical conditions, ample proportion of subjects with functional MR, with left ventricle dysfunction and heart failure, who represent a more challenging subset of patients in whom surgical results are less satisfactory.

REFERENCES

1. Feldman T, Wasserman HS, Herrmann HC, et al. Percutaneous mitral valve repair using the edge-to-edge technique: six month results of the EVEREST phase I clinical trial. J Am Coll Cardiol 2005; 46: 2134–40.
2. Feldman T, Kar S, Rinaldi M, et al. Percutaneous mitral repair with the mitraclip® system: safety and midterm durability in the initial EVEREST endovascular valve edge-to-edge repair study cohort. J Am Coll Cardiol 2009; 54: 686–94.
3. Feldman T, Foster E, Glower DG, et al. Percutaneous repair or surgery for mitral regurgitation. N Engl J Med 2011; 364: 1395–406.
4. Franzen O, Baldus S, Rudolph V, et al. Acute outcomes of mitraclip® therapy for mitral regurgitation in high-surgical-risk patients: emphasis on adverse valve morphology and severe left ventricular dysfunction. Eur Heart J 2010; 31: 1373–81.
5. Tamburino C, Ussia GP, Maisano F, et al. Percutaneous mitral valve repair with the mitraclip® system: acute results from a real world setting. Eur Heart J 2010; 31: 1382–9.
6. Van den Branden BJ, Post MC, Swaans MJ, et al. Percutaneous mitral valve repair using the edge-to-edge technique in a high-risk population. Neth Heart J 2010; 18: 437–43.
7. Pleger ST, Mereles D, Schulz-Schönhagen M, et al. Acute safety and 30-day outcome after percutaneous edge-to-edge repair of mitral regurgitation in very high-risk patients. Am J Cardiol 2011; 108: 1478–82.
8. Franzen O, van der Heyden J, Baldus S, et al. Mitraclip® therapy in patients with end-stage systolic heart failure. Eur J Heart Fail 2011; 13: 569–76.
9. Ussia GP, Cammalleri V, Sarkar K, et al. Quality of life following percutaneous mitral valve repair with the mitraclip® system. Int J Cardiol 2012; 155: 194–200.
10. Auricchio A, Schillinger W, Meyer S, et al. Correction of mitral regurgitation in nonresponders to cardiac resynchronization therapy by MitraClip® improves symptoms and promotes reverse remodeling. J Am Coll Cardiol 2011; 58: 2183–9.
11. Maisano F, Franzen O, Baldus S, et al. MitraClip® therapy demonstrates favourable mid-term outcomes in ACCESS-EUROPE heart failure patients with left ventricular ejection fraction. Preliminary report from the 6-month ACCESS-EU analysis cohort. EuroIntervention 2011; 7(Suppl M).
12. Ussia GP, Barbanti M, Tamburino C. Feasibility of percutaneous transcatheter mitral valve repair with the MitraClip® system using conscious sedation. Catheter Cardiovasc Interv 2010; 75: 1137–40.
13. Barbanti M, Ussia GP, Tamburino C. Percutaneous treatment of aortic stenosis and mitral regurgitation in the same patient: first human cases description. Catheter Cardiovasc Interv 2011; 78: 650–5.
14. Ong SH, Beucher H, Mueller R, et al. Percutaneous double-valve interventions for aortic stenosis and pure mitral regurgitation. Am J Cardiol 2011; 108: 893–5.
15. Chan PH, Alegria-Barrero E, Patterson T, et al. Successful dual-valve transcatheter therapy for severe aortic stenosis and mitral regurgitation. Int J Cardiol 2012; 157: e35–7.
16. Franzen O, von Samson P, Dodge-Khatami A, et al. Percutaneous edge-to-edge repair of tricuspid regurgitation in congenitally corrected transposition of the great arteries. Congenit Heart Dis 2011; 6: 57–9.
17. Füller M. Cardiology news: percutaneous mitral valve repair and interventional left atrial appendage closure. MMW Fortschr Med 2011; 153: 33–5.
18. Franzen O, Seiffert M, Baldus S, et al. Percutaneous mitral valve repair as a bail-out strategy for patients with severe mitral regurgitation after cardiac surgery. J Thorac Cardiovasc Surg 2011; 142: 227–30.
19. Schillinger W, Athanasiou T, Weicken N, et al. Impact of the learning curve on outcomes after percutaneous mitral valve repair with mitraclip® and lessons learned after the first 75 consecutive patients. Eur J Heart Fail 2011; 13: 1331–9.

18   An interventionalist's approach to the practical use of TEE guidance
Howard C. Herrmann

MitraClip® repair of mitral regurgitation (MR) is an investigational therapy that has promise, particularly in high-risk patients (1,2). It is a unique procedure in that much of the technique involves echocardiographic guidance and assessment of the mitral valve, requiring collaboration in the cardiac catheterization laboratory between an imaging expert and the interventionalist. The need for echocardiography speaks as much for the attributes of non-invasive imaging as it does for the limitations of fluoroscopy which cannot identify soft tissue landmarks or structures. Fluoroscopy is also incapable of monitoring catheter contact with cardiac structures, of monitoring device position relative to soft tissue structures (such as the mitral valve), and cannot instantaneously assess blood flow to monitor efficacy and complications. Although echocardiography also has limitations, namely the need for multiple views, dedicated operators, and anesthesia, it has become indispensable for this procedure.

Other chapters in this book describe the echocardiographic approach and views for all of the aspects of MitraClip® edge-to-edge repair. In this chapter, the goal is to more clearly describe the imaging approach from the point of view of an interventionalist and the early lessons learned at our institution which helped facilitate this unique collaboration. In the earliest procedures utilizing this novel technology, it was not clear which modality would be best. We, and others, initially tried transthoracic (TTE), transesophageal (TEE), and intracardiac (ICE) echocardiography. We quickly discovered that more was not always better and that the use of multiple imaging modalities added to procedure time without improving the results. We ultimately learned to rely on a small number of standard TEE imaging planes.

LESSONS LEARNED FROM EARLY EXPERIENCE
The goal of adjunctive imaging is to improve procedural safety and efficacy. The use of echocardiography adds time to the procedure and as stated above required us to streamline multiple modalities to TEE alone and minimize the number of standard imaging planes (3). Similarly, it is important to minimize adjunctive procedures, such as diagnostic angiography and baseline echocardiographic assessments. Probably, the single most important lesson from the earliest procedures was the evolution of communication between the interventionalist and the echocardiographer. We quickly discovered that echocardiographers think from inside the esophagus, whereas catheterizers think from outside of the patient. This can lead to miscommunication in terms of left-right, anterior-posterior, superior-inferior orientation if it is not clear whether an operator is describing a direction relative to

the valve, the patient, or the screen. The entire team must speak the same language and utilize a common, standardized, anatomically based vocabulary. In this regard, it can be helpful to utilize imaging aids (diagrams, printed images from the specific patient) that are appropriately labeled and taped below the monitor bank for easy reference. It is also absolutely essential that the echocardiographic images are visible in front of the catheterizer, either on the monitor bank or with a separate slave monitor. It is impossible for the catheterizer to manipulate the clip delivery system (CDS) while looking over his or her shoulder at the echo machine.

Further measures to reduce procedure time include a pre-procedure strategy conference or review. This allows the interventionalist and echocardiographer to discuss the operative plan, including which view(s) will be helpful during the procedure, where the ideal placement should be for the first clip (e.g., lateral or medial portion of P2-A2), and agreement on the plan for procedure conduct. In addition to the team speaking the same language, it is also important for only one person (usually the interventionalist) to direct the procedure by asking for the needed view and not be responding to whatever the echocardiographer shows or decides to look at. The potential for the interventionalist to be provided with information overload (X-plane, multiple omniplane views, proximal isovelocity surface area, and pressure half-time measurements) at times that he or she is concentrating on steering the clip in a single view has to be avoided through good communication and direction. Thus, the interventionalist needs to understand the views and information available, and may need additional TEE training if it was not available during cardiac fellowship (3,4). Even then, additional training for the interventional physician specific to the MitraClip® procedure is useful.

The benefits of all of the tips described above are evident in our single-center learning experience for device time (Fig. 18.1). Most procedures now can be performed with an average device time of 90–120 minutes. A similar learning curve has been demonstrated in multiple centers, facilitated by using an echocardiographic script (Table 18.1) (3).

TRANSSEPTAL GUIDANCE
The indications for transseptal catheterization have expanded in recent years. Initially, it was utilized for the diagnosis of mitral gradients when the capillary wedge pressure was unreliable or in the presence of a mechanical aortic prosthesis and for aortic gradients when the valve could not be crossed or for intraventricular gradient measurement. More recently, the explosion in structural heart interventions and electrophysiology procedures has created new indications for transseptal left heart access (5).

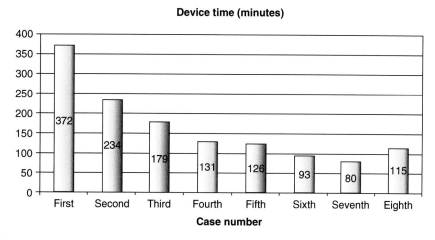

Figure 18.1 Hospital of the University of Pennsylvania single-center learning experience.

Table 18.1 Multicenter Learning Experience (from Ref. (3)) Device Time for Successful (30 Days) MitraClip® Procedures

Initial Procedure	Device Time (min)[a], Median	Device Time (min), Range
5 initial sites, first round (n = 6)	198	92–372
5 initial sites, second round (n = 6)	145	123–320
5 new sites (n = 5)	132	75–174

[a]Device time refers to the time from steerable guide catheter insertion to removal of clip delivery system (first or second in a procedure with 2 deployed MitraClips®).

Along with this increasing use of an old procedure has come a realization that not all transseptals are created equal. There are different transseptal puncture locations that facilitate the various purposes of left atrial access.

Many experienced interventionalists rely on fluoroscopic landmarks (with or without dye injections) and hemodynamic measurements to facilitate the transseptal puncture. However, there are a number of reasons to recommend echocardiographic guidance. First among these is the safety provided by confirmation of the needle location prior to puncture. In addition, the use of echocardiographic guidance allows the early identification of complications. Finally, the preciseness of puncture location has become essential for many procedures, including PFO closure, LAA occlusion, and MitraClip® insertion. Although TTE, ICE, and TEE can all be used to facilitate transseptal puncture, the excellent visualization and preciseness in multiple planes provided by TEE makes this modality the ideal one for MitraClip® insertion (3–5).

The ideal location for the transseptal puncture for MitraClip® edge-to-edge repair is posterior on the fossa ovalis as the mitral valve's line of leaflet coaptation is posterior to the fossa. This allows for the CDS to be inserted coaxial to the valve and avoids the "S" turn from anterior to posterior prior to turning down onto the valve from above. In addition, the puncture location must be sufficiently superior to allow for the caudal turn on to the valve as well as provide sufficient height above the grasp point to allow the upward tension on the clip that lets the leaflets fall into it.

The plane of the atrial septum runs from 1 o'clock to 7 o'clock (as viewed from the feet with the patient lying supine). The fossa ovalis is posterior and caudal to the aortic root and anterior to the free wall of the right atrium. The fossa ovalis is approximately 2 cm in diameter and is bounded superiorly by a ridge (the limbus). This anatomy can be distorted by left atrial enlargement in which the septum becomes flatter and more horizontal and the fossa ovalis itself tends to lie more inferior/caudal. Similarly, severe tricuspid regurgitation due to pulmonary hypertension will change the distance from the needle and sheath's entry into the right atrium from the inferior vena cava and thereby the distance and curve to the septum (5). It is important to understand the fossa anatomy when trying to enter the left atrium in a specific location. For example, if one turns the transseptal needle clockwise in order to puncture more posteriorly, the needle will move inferiorly as well (see next paragraph). Understanding these trade-offs for an exact puncture location is key for successful MitraClip® procedures.

We have developed a diagrammatic aid that describes the anatomy from the "catheterizer's view" to be helpful in thinking through the ideal transseptal puncture location (Fig. 18.2). This diagram illustrates the location of the mitral valve, transseptal needle, and septum superimposed on the TEE and valve nomenclature. The basic echo views utilized during the transseptal puncture (shown as red lines on Fig. 18.2) are shown in Figure 18.3. The important trade-offs between superior and posterior locations described above are further illustrated in Figure 18.4. As one turns the needle posteriorly to better align

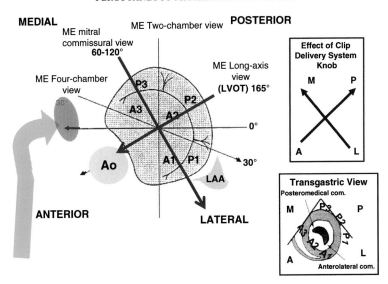

Figure 18.2 Echocardiographic aid for catheterizer, the catheterizer's view (shown from below, patient's right side). *Notes:* Green arrow represents the path of transseptal sheath and needle. Blue box is the fossa ovalis. Red lines correspond to basic TEE views shown in Figure 18.3. *Abbreviations:* Ao, aorta; LAA, left atrial appendage; LVOT, left ventricular outflow tract; ME, mid-esophageal.

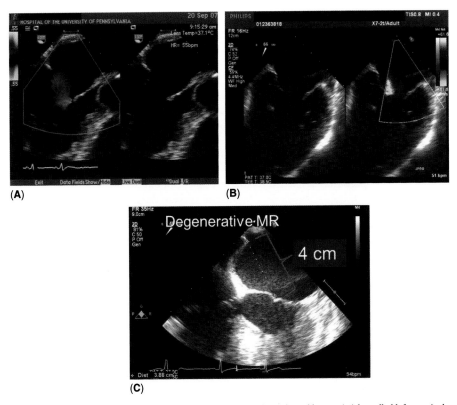

Figure 18.3 Basic TEE views used during transseptal puncture and guidance. (A) Mid-esophageal long-axis (also called left ventricular outflow tract) view (150–180). (B) Mid-esophageal mitral commissural (also called intercommissural) view (60–120). (C) Four-chamber view (0).

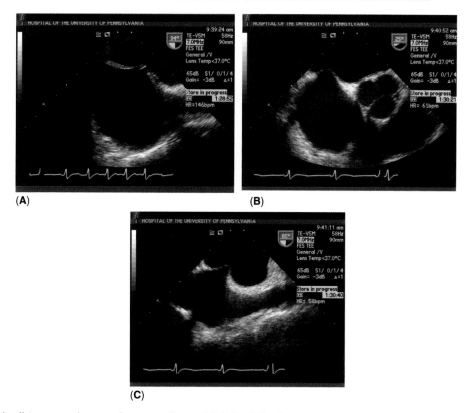

Figure 18.4 Trade-offs in transseptal puncture location are illustrated. (A) Bicaval view demonstrating superior needle tenting. (B) Anterior-posterior view demonstrating somewhat posterior (distance from the aortic valve) tenting. (C) Loss of superior position with an attempt to move the needle more posterior.

with the mitral valve's line of leaflet coaptation, there is an obligate movement further inferiorly along the rim of the fossa ovalis. These trade-offs need to be considered in compromising on the final puncture location. Finally, the four-chamber view must be used to confirm adequate height above the intended grasp point of the leaflets to allow for clip excursion during the device pull-back from below the leaflets to the grasping point (Fig. 18.3C). In this regard, the ideal height is approximately 4 to 5 cm above the leaflets (3). However, the height may need to be less in ischemic disease where the leaflets are pulled or tented lower into the ventricular chamber or higher in bileaflet prolapse cases where the line of coaptation may be above the plane of the mitral annulus.

Subsequent to the initial MitraClip® procedures performed in 2005, three-dimensional (3D) TEE was introduced into routine clinical use. This has allowed for on-line acquisition of a 3D dataset without the need for ECG or respiratory gating utilizing a phased array transducer with 512 elements. Options for imaging include parallel imaging of two planes ("X-plane"), live 3D volume, and color full-volume acquisitions. This modality has added important features to MitraClip® procedures, particularly during clip guidance (described in the next section). However, it also allows for better understanding of

the transseptal puncture location. In this regard, it is useful to consider the "surgeon's view" of the mitral valve in which one imagines standing in the left atrium near the head of the patient and looking down on the mitral valve (Fig. 18.5). In this construct, it is easier to understand the anterior-posterior trade-off for the transseptal puncture (Fig. 18.6).

GUIDANCE OF THE CLIP DELIVERY SYSTEM

Once a successful and localized transseptal puncture has been performed, the CDS is introduced through the transseptal sheath and steered with echocardiographic guidance toward the middle scallops of the mitral valve. As emphasized above, this requires perfect communication between the echocardiographer and interventionalist using a minimum of simplified views with iteration between the views (4). The conduct of the procedure should be dictated by the interventionalist who will be making knob adjustments on the CDS and will want to see the effect of each adjustment in multiple views. Although some operators utilize the X-plane view to see the effect of clip movement simultaneously in two views, others prefer to iterate between the views, and yet others will use real-time 3D imaging for the initial maneuvering. I personally, prefer 3D imaging for the gross adjustments to get close

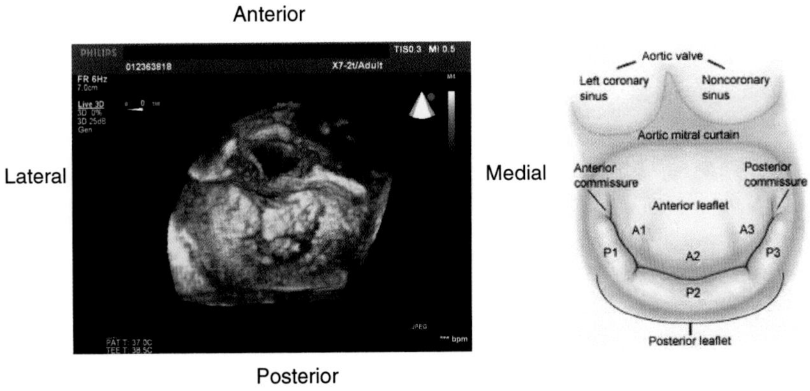

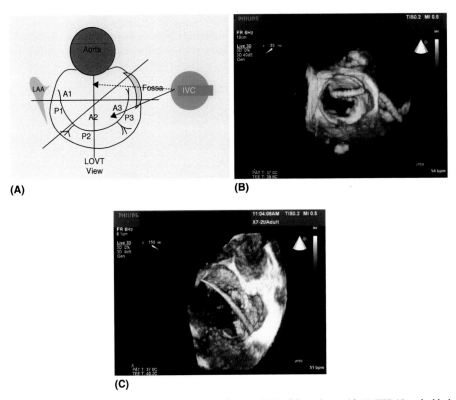

Figure 18.5 The "Surgeon's View" provided by 3D real-time TEE imaging.

Figure 18.6 The directionality of the transseptal puncture illustrated in the "Surgeon's View" from above with 3D TEE. Note the black arrow (**A**) that will position the clip delivery system (CDS) anterior to the valve necessitating an "S" turn back and down to the leaflets (**B**). A more posterior puncture location (dotted arrow in **A**) better aligns the CDS with the valve's line of leaflet coaptation (**C**).

to the valve and then frequently switch to 2D with its superior resolution for more fine adjustment when I am getting close to the proper position (video 18.1). Similarly, I tend to use 3D to see gross clip alignment after opening the clip and 2D iterations for fine tuning and cross checking. The key views for these maneuvers have already been discussed and are illustrated in Figures 18.2, 18.3A, and 18.3B. The importance of having ease of visualization of the echocardiographic images for the interventionalist and the evolution over time is illustrated in Figure 18.7.

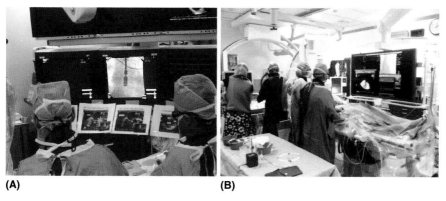

Figure 18.7 Catheterization laboratory setup for MitraClip® procedure. In our earliest procedures (*above*), the fluoroscopic image was in the front and center with echocardiographic views taped to the monitor and a slave echo monitor off to the side (not seen in this picture). In our newest lab (*below*), the echo images become fully integrated into a digital high-definition monitor bank with the echo image larger and more central than the fluoroscopic image confirming the important role of imaging in this procedure.

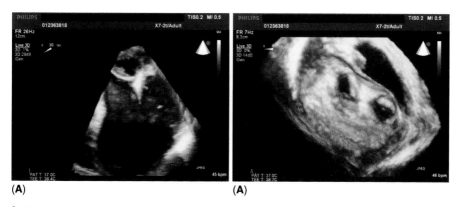

Figure 18.8 (A) Leaflet insertion assessed with a 3D TEE. (B) Confirmation of creation of a double orifice with transgastric TEE.

During the course of the procedure, we will utilize different echocardiographic views (3,4). Clip guidance toward the valve is frequently done initially in a 3D surgeon's view followed by fine tuning in the 2 key 2D TEE views (left ventricular outflow tract; LVOT and intercommissural). The clip is opened in the left atrium and aligned perpendicular to the leaflets first in 3D and then confirmed in the 2D LVOT view as well as in the transgastric view. Once the clip is inserted into the left ventricle, the 2D LVOT and transgastric views again are utilized to confirm the perpendicularity and lack of rotation during advancement. The grasp is routinely performed in the LVOT view. Final assessment of leaflet insertion is facilitated by 3D interrogation (Fig. 18.8A) and confirmation of location and creation of a double orifice in transgastric short axis with 2D or 3D imaging (Fig. 18.8B).

Finally, hemodynamic and Doppler gradients are evaluated to ensure the absence of mitral stenosis, particularly if a second clip insertion is contemplated (6).

CONCLUSIONS

In summary, echocardiography is the dominant imaging modality required for successful MitraClip® procedures. It is necessary for the echocardiography and interventionalist to develop a good working relationship, combined understanding of the procedure, common working vocabulary, and plan for the procedure. The typical steps and preferred views are described in Table 18.2. A successful procedure requires a unique collaboration to develop new tools for the "imaging catheterizer" and appreciation of the technical aspects of the procedure by the "interventional echocardiographer."

Table 18.2 Typical Steps and Views in MitraClip® Repair

Procedure Step	Transsesophageal Echocardiographic View(s)
1. Transseptal puncture	Basal short axis with bicaval and anterior-posterior imaging 4-chamber for height assessment Optional: confirmation in 3D
2. Clip manipulation	LVOT and intercommissural views (X-plane option) Real-time 3D
3. Clip orientation	3D surgeon's view Confirm in LVOT view (both in LA and LV) and with transgastric view
4. Grasp	LVOT view
5. Assessment of leaflet insertion and dual orifice	Multiple views (LVOT, transgastric, 3D)

Abbreviations: LA, left atrium; LV, left ventricle; LVOT, left ventricular outflow tract.

REFERENCES

1. Feldman T, Wasserman H, Herrmann HC, et al. Percutaneous mitral valve repair using the edge-to-edge technique: 6 month results of the EVEREST phase I clinical trial. J Am Coll Cardiol 2005; 46: 2134.
2. Feldman T, Foster E, Glower D, et al. For the EVEREST II investigators. percutaneous repair or surgery for mitral regurgitation. New Engl J Med 2011; 364: 1395–406.
3. Silvestry FE, Rodriguez L, Herrmann HC, et al. Echocardiographic guidance and assessment of percutaneous repair for mitral regurgitation with the evalve mitraclip®: lessons learned from EVEREST 1. J Am Soc Echocardiogr 2007; 20: 1131–40.
4. Silvestry FE, Kerber RE, Brook MM, et al. Echocardiography-guided interventions (ASE recommendations for clinical practice). J Am Soc Echo 2009; 23: 213–31.
5. Bannan A, Herrmann HC. Transseptal catheterization in the adult. In: Hijazi Z, Feldman T, Cheatham JP, Sievert H, eds. Complications During Percutaneous Interventions for Structural and Valvular Heart Disease. London: Informa, 2009: 304–310.
6. Herrmann HC, Kar S, Siegel R, et al. Effect of percutaneous mitral repair with the mitraclip® device on mitral valve area and gradient. EuroIntervention 2008; 4: 437–42.

19 Echocardiographic guidance of MitraClip® mitral valve repair
Frank E. Silvestry

INTRODUCTION

Edge-to-edge mitral valve repair aims to improve mitral leaflet coaptation and to reduce or eliminate significant mitral regurgitation (MR) by approximating the middle scallops of the mitral valve, thus creating a double orifice for diastolic inflow (1–6). The surgical edge-to-edge repair technique is approximated by the percutaneous transcatheter MitraClip® system, in which a clip is placed on the mitral valve via a steerable transseptal system (7–11). The MitraClip® is a polyester fabric-covered cobalt–chromium implantable clip with two arms which can be opened and closed with a steerable-guiding mechanism. A larger steerable guide catheter with a steerable clip delivery catheter is used, allowing for precise placement of the clip in the desired location on the mitral valve. The device has been shown to be effective in selected patients with either degenerative (both prolapsed leaflets and flail leaflets) or functional MR due to ischemic or dilated cardiomyopathy (9,12–14). The MitraClip® has been used most extensively to successfully treat mitral regurgitation arising from the central aspect of the mitral valve, at the A2 and P2 scallops. Alternative uses, such as commissural clip placement, have been reported as well, but the greatest experience is with the creation of a double-orifice mitral valve with approximation of A2-P2.

Each part of the MitraClip® system is comprehensively imaged with transesophageal echocardiography (TEE), and this procedure relies upon TEE for step-by-step real-time procedural guidance as detailed below (15–17). The procedure is performed under general anesthesia and typical procedure times are approximately two hours. An antegrade transseptal approach is used with the device first axially aligned and positioned at the central (A2-P2 segments) portion of the mitral valve, then the clip arms are aligned perpendicular to the line of coaptation using a sophisticated guiding and positioning system, and a combination of echocardiographic and to a much lesser degree fluoroscopic guidance. Echocardiography, and specifically TEE, is the primary imaging modality used at all stages of the percutaneous mitral clip procedure, with minimal use of fluoroscopy. When a second clip is placed to create a wider edge-to-edge repair, fluoroscopy may play a greater role in procedure guidance. Virtually, every step of the MitraClip® procedure is guided by TEE in real time (Tables 19.1 and 19.2). Patient selection for MitraClip® mitral repair and MR severity assessment by transthoracic echocardiography and TEE is covered previously (see previous sections covering these topics).

This TEE-guided procedure requires a close and intense collaboration between echocardiographer and interventionalist, and is unlike any other interventional echo procedure. Dedicated echocardiography personnel are required to guide this procedure. A number of lessons were learned early in the collective collaborative experience of performing this procedure at multiple centers (16). Table 19.1 lists the standard views used and general imaging recommendations. For example, a standardized vocabulary based on internal mitral valve anatomic landmarks is used to facilitate clear communication during the procedure. Images from the TEE are displayed on the main screens of the room display along with hemodynamic data and fluoroscopy (Fig. 19.1 A and 19.1 B). A pre-procedure strategy meeting is conducted to plan the procedure and standardized imaging views are used. A highly realistic training simulator ("MitraClip® Virtual Procedure simulator") has been developed to simulate all of the required imaging steps and goals, as well as iterative manipulation of the system (Fig. 19.2). During the live case, the practice is to allow the interventionalist to "drive" the procedure and ask for a change in the image only when they are ready for a different view. Most centers typically rely on real-time three dimensional transesophageal ultrasound systems for the rapid and effective placement of the clip, although the vast majority of the imaging used during the case uses the biplane or X-plane image display of two different simultaneous images, and not rendered 3D volumes per se. Rendered real-time 3D imaging has allowed for improvement in several of the steps of the procedure as well as rapid detection of complications (15,18–20).

KEY ALIGNMENT AND POSITIONING OBJECTIVES

Positioning of the MitraClip® relative to the mitral orifice and leaflets is achieved with iterative adjustments of the guide catheter and clip delivery system using torque, translation, and adjustments of the systems steering knobs. During the procedure, the three primary positioning objectives (Table 19.3) may be recalled using the acronym "HAP" which stands for Height above the mitral valve, Axial alignment, and Perpendicular clip arm positioning. Further detail of each of these objectives is listed in each of the sections that follow below.

TRANSSEPTAL CATHETERIZATION

During the transseptal puncture, TEE is essential in establishing the ideal site of puncture. Precise positioning of the transseptal catheter is essential to successful positioning of the MitraClip® guide and delivery catheter. The primary views used for this step are the mid-esophageal short-axis view (30–60° multiplane angle) and bicaval (90–120° multiplane angle) view at the level of the aortic valve (Fig. 19.3 A and 19.3 B). These can be simultaneously displayed with biplane or X-plane imaging using a 3D ultrasound system. Rendered 3D images of the fossa are typically not used for this step. The transseptal puncture should

Table 19.1 Echocardiography for MitraClip® Procedure

Reliance on standard views for each procedural step
    Bicaval view
    Short axis at base
    Intercommissural: 2 chamber
    4 Chamber
    5 Chamber
    Left ventricular outflow track (LVOT)
    Transgastric short axis
Use each echo view efficiently
    Eliminate unnecessary device maneuvers
    Eliminate unnecessary TEE probe maneuvers
    Do not rely on 3D imaging if no incremental information obtained
Interventional operator asks for views
    Drives the procedure based on specific imaging needs

Table 19.2 MitraClip® Procedure Steps Guided by Echocardiography (TEE)

1. Patient selection
2. Assessment of pre procedural MR severity
3. Transseptal catheterization (height, posterior location)
4. Entry of guide and clip delivery system into LA: avoidance of contact with left atrial structures
5. Axial alignment of clip delivery system over mitral valve (anterior-posterior, medial-lateral, clip trajectory is parallel to mitral inflow)
6. Alignment of clip arms perpendicular to line of coaptation
7. Advance into LV prior to grasping
8. Grasping of leaflets
9. Assessment of leaflet insertion into clip after it is closed
10. Assessment of residual MR and measurement of gradients PRIOR to release of clip
11. Clip release from delivery system
12. Steering of clip delivery system out of LA: avoidance of contact with atrial structures
13. Placement of second clip if needed
14. Assessment of transseptal shunt after removal of guide
15. Monitor for complications

be performed through the posterior aspect of the fossa with the system directed toward the mitral line of coaptation, to facilitate ideal positioning of the clip delivery system. During transseptal puncture, TEE identifies the position of the needle tip by detecting tenting created on the septum. Tenting implies the site of needle entry and its trajectory, and only occasionally is direct imaging of the needle tip used. The transseptal puncture site should be approximately 3.5–4.0 cm above the mitral valve coaptation plane, and this distance is often referred to as "height," and represents the H in the HAP key positioning acronym. It is important to place the distal tip of the clip more than 1.0 cm above the leaflets to facilitate adequate clearance for grasping, and the site of transseptal entry directly determines this distance. Height, therefore, refers to the distance between transseptal entry and mitral coaptation point. This is best demonstrated by the mid esophageal four-chamber view (Fig. 19.4). A greater distance (3.5–4.0 cm) above the leaflets is desirable when treating degenerative MR where the leaflets prolapse or flail backward into the atrium. A smaller distance (i.e., 3.5 cm) is used when treating functional MR where the leaflets are tethered and pulled into the left ventricle (LV) by the ventricular remodeling. If the position of the transseptal catheterization is suboptimal, the transseptal sheath and needle may be repositioned prior to puncturing the septum. Ideal transseptal location is critical to the success of the procedure.

ENTRY OF THE GUIDE CATHETER INTO THE LEFT ATRIUM, ADVANCING THE CLIP DELIVERY SYSTEM TOWARD THE MITRAL VALVE, AND AXIAL ALIGNMENT OF THE SYSTEM

Once the correct transseptal puncture has been made and the septum has been dilated, the 24-F guide catheter is inserted. The guide should sit at least 0.5–1.0 cm in the left atrium (LA) across the atrial septum, and the hyper echoic tip is clearly visible on 2D and 3D TEE imaging (Fig. 19.5 A and 19.5 B). Once the guide is in the LA, the mitral clip delivery system is introduced and steered down toward the mitral

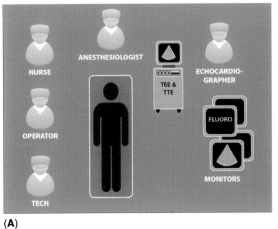

(A)

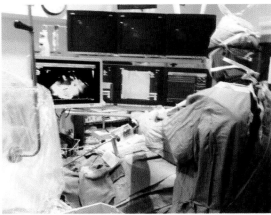

(B)

Figure 19.1 (A and B) Lab setup diagram and photograph of procedure with attention to echo images on the monitor.

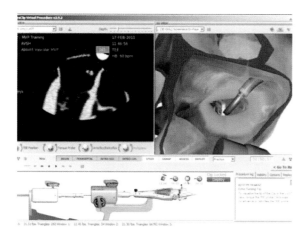

Figure 19.2 Screen shot from MitraClip® virtual procedure software simulator. *Source*: Courtesy of Abbott.

Table 19.3 Key Positioning Objectives for the MitraClip® Procedure (The "HAP" Rules)

Height above valve
   Tension on chordae needed
      Distal tip of Clip ≥1.0 cm above leaflet
Axial alignment
   Both medial-lateral and anterior-posterior planes
   Clip trajectory is axial
   Clip positioned at the origin of the MR jet
Perpendicular arms
   Perpendicular to line of coaptation

valve plane (Fig. 19.6 A–D). Care must be taken to avoid contact with the lateral and superior aspects of the LA, and the tip of the clip is "followed" as it is introduced into the LA. The clip is angled down toward the mitral leaflets, aiming for the central portion of the valve. The tip of the clip introduced into the LA must be visualized at all times to avoid contact with atrial structures. In particular, the system may naturally be directed toward or into the left pulmonary veins and carefully steered to avoid contact with the LA prominence and appendage.

Once oriented toward the valve, axial alignment can be performed using the intercommissural (50–70° multiplane angle) views demonstrating medial—lateral alignment and the LV outflow tract (LVOT; 120–160° multiplane angle) view demonstrating posterior–anterior alignment (Fig. 19.7). Axial alignment ensures that the shaft of the delivery system is parallel to the direction of mitral inflow, and most importantly that the trajectory of the clip as it is advanced is parallel to the direction of mitral inflow. Real-time three-dimensional TEE (3D zoom with a large field of view) covering the entire mitral valve and septum quickly facilitates the gross orientation of the clip as it provides an en face view of the mitral leaflets and approaching clip (Fig. 19.8 A and 19.8 B), but biplane imaging with the intercommissural view and LVOT view as described above is essential to confirming ideal axial alignment prior to proceeding to opening the clip.

POSITIONING THE CLIP ABOVE THE REGURGITANT ORIFICE AND ORIENTATION OF THE CLIP ARMS

The optimal position of the clip delivery system is immediately above the regurgitant orifice, which serves as a "target" of the clip. Color Doppler flow mapping with "color compare" side by side imaging allows placement of the clip above the origin of MR while visualizing the clip in 2D (Fig. 19.9). The target orifice is chosen using the maximal phase-invariant signature

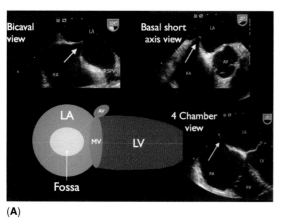

(A)

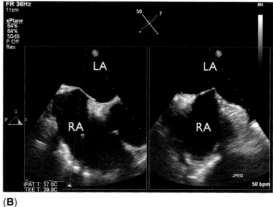

(B)

Figure 19.3 (A) Transseptal catheterization views used; (B) tenting demonstrated by X-plane in short axis and bicaval views.

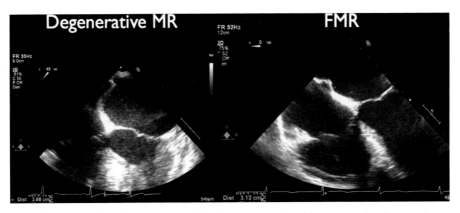

Figure 19.4 Mid-esophageal 4-chamber view demonstrating "height" differences for DMR and FMR.

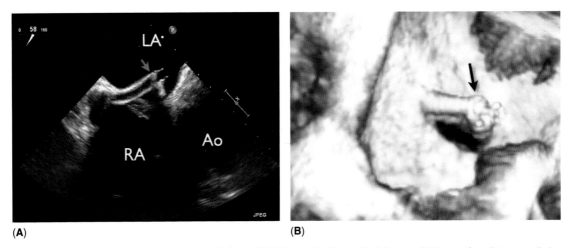

(A)   **(B)**

Figure 19.5 (A) A 2D image of guide catheter with hyper echoic tip; (B) 3D image of guide entering left atrium (LA) across fossa (LA perspective).

algorithm (PISA) effect and widest vena contracta. Once axially alignment confirmed, and positioning over the maximal MR jet origin is visualized, the clip is then fully opened in the LA (180°). The arms of the clip should then be aligned perpendicular to the line of coaptation (Fig. 19.10A-C). This is typically performed first in the LVOT view. In this view, the clip arms open to 180° should appear to be of equal length (Fig. 19.10A). If clip arms are not of equal length, then the clip is turned until both arms appear equal. Perpendicular alignment is also assessed with real-time 3D zoom imaging, creating an en face view of the mitral valve and open clip. If 3D is not available, the transgastric short-axis view may be used for this purpose as well (Fig. 19.10 B and 19.10 C). Perpendicular alignment of the clip arms is crucial to maximizing leaflet insertion into the clip and preventing the unlikely possibility of partial leaflet detachment.

GRASPING OF THE MITRAL LEAFLETS AND ASSESSMENT OF LEAFLET INSERTION

As viewed from the LVOT view (120–160° multiplane angle), the clip arms are then partially closed to approximately 120° prior to crossing the mitral leaflets and entering the LV (Fig. 19.11A). Here, 3D zoom imaging (or alternatively the transgastric short-axis view) permits a rapid confirmation that the arms of the mitral clip device remain perpendicular to the line of coaptation as the delivery system may rotate due to stored torque as it is advanced into the ventricle. Once the delivery system is in the LV, with the clip arms are opened to approximately 120°, the system is pulled back toward the LA, simultaneously grasping the mitral leaflets with the clip (Fig. 19.11B). After grasping, the device grippers which hold the leaflets in place while the clip is being closed are lowered toward the valve. The LVOT view is typically used for leaflet grasping,

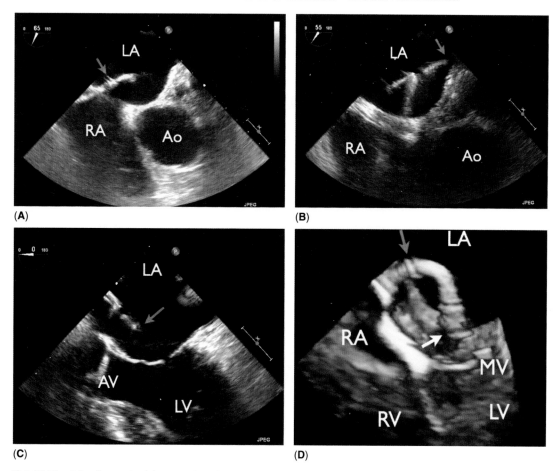

Figure 19.6 (A) Tip of the clip entering left atrium through guided echocardiography. (B) Tip of the clip well visualized in superior left atrium (LA). (C) Tip of the clip oriented toward mitral valve in 5-chamber view. (D) Live 3D view of open clip as well as tip of guide in LA in 4-chamber view.

or biplane imaging with both the LVOT view and intercommissural view. Capture of both leaflets must be verified while the clip is being closed. If either leaflet is inadequately captured, the clip is reopened and re-advanced into the LV and the process is repeated. A careful assessment of leaflet insertion is performed to ensure that each leaflet is adequately captured in the clip (Table 19.4). This requires careful 2D multiplane assessment focusing on one leaflet at a time with the clip closed to approximately 60°.

ASSESSMENT OF MITRAL VALVE FUNCTION AFTER GRASPING
Once both leaflets are satisfactorily grasped and leaflet insertion is deemed ideal, an assessment of residual MR with color Doppler mapping is performed (Fig. 19.11 C and 19.11 D). Machine settings including Color Doppler gain and Nyquist limit should be identical to those used for the pre-procedure assessment. Attention to the patient's volume status and blood pressure is important, and approximation of pre-procedure loading conditions is performed if these parameters have changed. It is important to carefully screen for an eccentric

regurgitant jet as MR can be redirected significantly after clip placement.

Quantitation of any residual MR may be more complicated with the creation of two orifices and the mitral inflow volume required for volumetric (quantitative) Doppler MR estimation cannot be obtained due to the creation of a double diastolic orifice. In the absence of significant aortic regurgitation, LV forward flow can be calculated as flow through the outflow tract using the continuity equation, and LV stroke volume calculated from 3D derived estimates of end-diastolic and end-systolic volumes. The difference between the two (stroke volume − forward flow) represents the regurgitant volume, although this method is time consuming and may be best suited to long-term follow up. During the procedure in the catheterization lab, color Doppler echocardiography using semi-quantitative techniques based on regurgitant jet dimensions may be best suited for real-time intraprocedural assessment.

Similarly, the PISA approach for calculating the effective regurgitant orifice area (EROA) has not been validated for

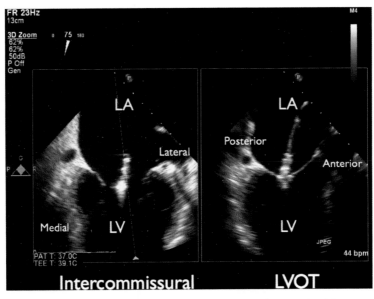

Figure 19.7 Biplane imaging for axial alignment (intercommissural and left ventricular outflow tract views) demonstrating trajectory of system.

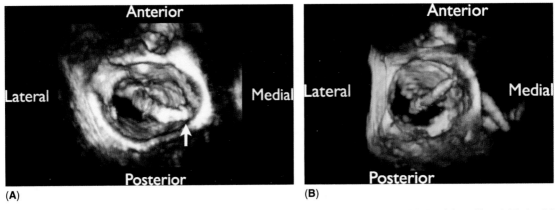

Figure 19.8 3D Zoom view of system in left atrium (LA) with en face view of mitral valve demonstrating (A) tip of the guide and (B) tip of the clip oriented to A2-P2.

multiple regurgitant jets that may exist post MitraClip® with the double-orifice geometry created with this device. Accurate assessment of the EROA by PISA may not be possible due to clip shadowing artifact as well.

If two jets are present, important to realize that Color Doppler jet area mapping may overestimate the corresponding regurgitant volume (21). If color Doppler jet mapping is felt to be acceptable with regard to MR reduction or elimination, a careful hemodynamic assessment is then performed including pulse wave Doppler interrogation of all pulmonary veins. As with native valve regurgitation, an integrated approach is essential.

Once MR assessment is complete, it is important to measure transvalvular gradients and estimate the mitral valve area to

exclude mitral stenosis, and especially when two clips have been deployed. This is accomplished by measuring the transvalvular gradient with continuous wave Doppler (Fig. 19.12) and planimetering the two orifices using en face 3D or transgastric short-axis views. Three-dimensional assisted planimetry may be performed using Q lab software included on the 3D ultrasound machine. Clinically significant mitral stenosis has not been seen with the MitraClip® procedure as a result of careful pre-procedure screening of patients (pre-procedure mitral valve area by planimetry >4.0 cm) and with careful Doppler and planimetered double-orifice MVA assessment during the procedure *prior* to clip release, especially when two clips are used (22,23). If MR reduction is satisfactory and the transmitral gradients are acceptable (mean gradient ≤4 to 5 mmHg),

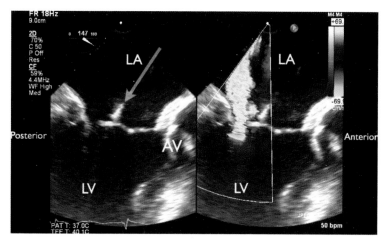

Figure 19.9 Clip over color Doppler jet (color comparison of identical view).

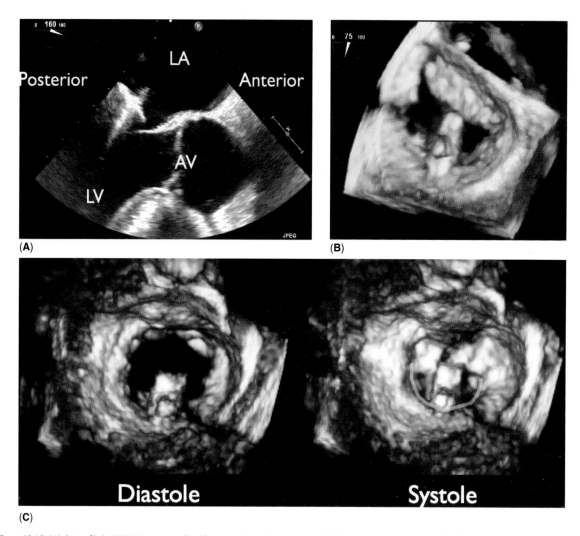

Figure 19.10 (A) Open clip in LVOT view. Arms should appear of equal length in the LVOT view when clip open to 180°. (B) 3D en face views demonstrating open clip aligned perpendicular to line of coaptation, and (C) same view in diastole and systole.

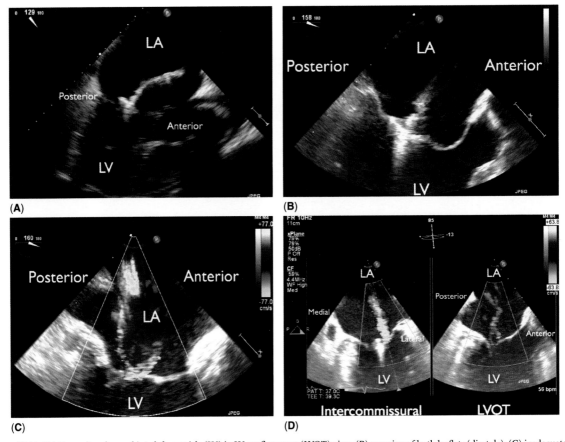

Figure 19.11 (**A**) Open clip advanced into left ventricle (LV) in LV outflow tract (LVOT) view; (**B**) grasping of both leaflets (diastole); (**C**) inadequate MR reduction mandated repositioning of clip; and (**D**) moderate residual MR lateral to the first clip; decision made to place the second clip.

Table 19.4 Leaflet Insertion Guide

Use systematic assessment of leaflet insertion with Clip closed to
  approximately 60°
Use imaging to verify satisfactory grasp of the leaflets observing the
  following:
  Leaflet immobilization and a double-orifice valve
  Limited leaflet mobility relative to the tips of both clip arms
  Decrease in MR
  An improper grasp will allow one or both leaflets to move freely
  Closing and deploying the Clip in this situation may result in loss
  of leaflet capture and insertion (partial clip detachment)
If clip is not in the proper position, release the leaflets and reposition the
  Clip for grasping

the clip is fully deployed by detaching it from the delivery system. At this point, a final TEE assessment of MR is performed by color Doppler jet mapping, measurement of vena contracta width, PISA EROA determination (if possible), and pulmonary vein flow assessment. Final gradients are recorded using continuous wave Doppler as well.

PLACEMENT OF A SECOND CLIP

If there is significant residual regurgitation and the source of the residual regurgitation is felt to be amenable to correction with the placement of a second clip, a second clip may be deployed using a similar overall approach but using the first clip as a reference point. A second clip creates a wider edge-to-edge repair and may address MR that is medial or lateral to the first clip placement site (Fig. 19.13). When placing a second clip, fluoroscopy may take a greater guidance role in the procedure, where the first clip serves as a fluoroscopic landmark for initial positioning. Axial alignment, clip arm orientation, and grasping are still completely guided by TEE in an identical fashion as the first clip. In assessing the degree of residual MR, it is again important that the volume status and systolic blood pressure approximate normal values for the patient. This is particularly important in patients with functional MR, which is afterload dependent.

Using 3D echocardiography, it is possible to observe the mitral valve en face from both atrial (Fig. 19.14 C and 19.14 D) and ventricular perspectives, documenting the dual orifices created by the clip(s). Three-dimensional full volume with

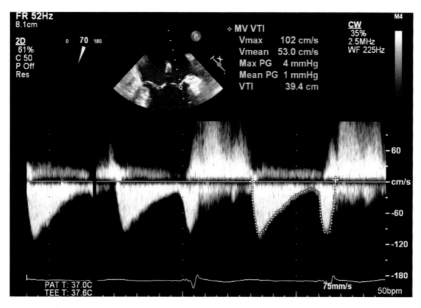

Figure 19.12 Measurement of transmitral gradients with continuous wave Doppler prior to deciding to release and/or place the second clip.

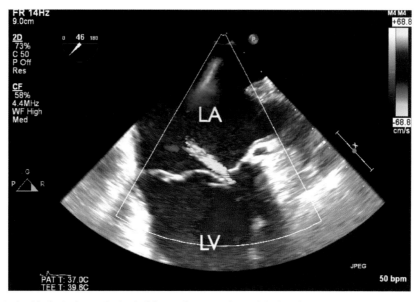

Figure 19.13 Final residual mitral regurgitation (mild) post placement of second clip lateral to original clip (compare with Fig. 19.11 D).

color mapping also provides delineation of the site(s) of any residual regurgitation, along with standard biplane imaging.

DETECTION OF COMPLICATIONS AND ASSESSMENT OF RESIDUAL ATRIAL SHUNT

Real-time TEE also provides a method for early detection of the potential complications of clip placement including the thrombus formation on the system, the unlikely occurrence of a perforation of the atrial wall when introducing the clip into the LA, resulting in pericardial effusion, partial detachment of the clip after initial seating and leaflet or chordal tears caused by repeated attempts to grasp the leaflets. The assessment of residual atrial septal shunting post transseptal catheterization is also performed (Fig. 19.15).

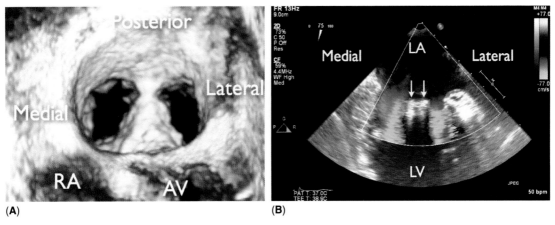

(A)   **(B)**

Figure 19.14 (**A**) 3D zoom double-orifice mitral valve post clip placement and (**B**) intercommissural view demonstrating double orifice and two clips (arrows).

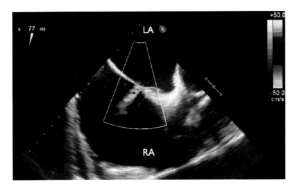

Figure 19.15 Residual atrial septal defect due to transseptal puncture.

CONCLUSION

Mitral valve repair with the MitraClip® system is a safe and effective real-time TEE-guided procedure that requires close collaboration between interventionalist and echocardiographer for its success. Reliance upon standardized imaging views and vocabulary, and a streamlined goal-oriented imaging protocol facilitate rapid and efficient placement of the clip on the mitral valve, creating a percutaneous edge-to-edge mitral repair in patients with functional and degenerative mitral regurgitation.

REFERENCES

1. Maisano F, Redaelli A, Pennati G, et al. The hemodynamic effects of double-orifice valve repair for mitral regurgitation: a 3D computational model. Eur J Cardiothorac Surg 1999; 15: 419–25.
2. Alfieri O, Maisano F, De Bonis M, et al. The double-orifice technique in mitral valve repair: a simple solution for complex problems. J Thorac Cardiovasc Surg 2001; 122: 674–81.
3. Block PC. Percutaneous mitral valve repair for mitral regurgitation. J Interv Cardiol 2003; 16: 93–6.
4. Maisano F, Caldarola A, Blasio A, et al. Midterm results of edge-to-edge mitral valve repair without annuloplasty. J Thorac Cardiovasc Surg 2003; 126: 1987–97.
5. Alfieri O, Maisano F, Colombo A. Percutaneous mitral valve repair procedures. Eur J Cardiothorac Surg 2004; 26(Suppl 1): S36–7; discussion S7-8.
6. Maisano F, Vigano G, Blasio A, et al. Surgical isolated edge-to-edge mitral valve repair without annuloplasty: clinical proof of the principle for an endovascular approach. EuroIntervention 2006; 2: 181–6.
7. St Goar FG, Fann JI, Komtebedde J, et al. Endovascular edge-to-edge mitral valve repair: short-term results in a porcine model. Circulation 2003; 108: 1990–3.
8. Fann JI, St Goar FG. Percutaneous aortic valve replacement and mitral valve repair. Future Cardiol 2005; 1: 393–403.
9. Feldman T, Wasserman HS, Herrmann HC, et al. Percutaneous mitral valve repair using the edge-to-edge technique: six-month results of the EVEREST Phase I clinical trial. J Am Coll Cardiol 2005; 46: 2134–40.
10. Condado JA, Acquatella H, Rodriguez L, et al. Percutaneous edge-to-edge mitral valve repair: 2-year follow-up in the first human case. Catheter Cardiovasc Interv 2006; 67: 323–5.
11. Feldman T, Herrmann HC, St Goar F. Percutaneous treatment of valvular heart disease: catheter-based aortic valve replacement and mitral valve repair therapies. Am J Geriatr Cardiol 2006; 15: 291–301.
12. Feldman T, Foster E, Glower DD, et al. Percutaneous repair or surgery for mitral regurgitation. N Engl J Med 2011; 364: 1395–406.
13. Feldman T, Glower D. Patient selection for percutaneous mitral valve repair: insight from early clinical trial applications. Natl Clin Pract Cardiovasc Med 2008; 5: 84–90.
14. Feldman T, Kar S, Rinaldi M, et al. Percutaneous mitral repair with the mitraclip® system: safety and midterm durability in the initial EVEREST (endovascular valve edge-to-edge repair study) cohort. J Am Coll Cardiol 2009; 54: 686–94.
15. Silvestry FE, Kerber RE, Brook MM, et al. Echocardiography-guided interventions. J Am Soc Echocardiogr 2009; 22: 213–31; quiz 316-7.
16. Silvestry FE, Rodriguez LL, Herrmann HC, et al. Echocardiographic guidance and assessment of percutaneous repair for mitral

regurgitation with the evalve mitraclip®: lessons learned from EVEREST I. J Am Soc Echocardiogr 2007; 20: 1131–40.

17. Zamorano JL, Badano LP, Bruce C, et al. EAE/ASE recommendations for the use of echocardiography in new transcatheter interventions for valvular heart disease. Eur J Echocardiogr 2011; 12: 557–84.

18. Altiok E, Becker M, Hamada S, et al. Real-time 3D TEE allows optimized guidance of percutaneous edge-to-edge repair of the mitral valve. JACC Cardiovasc Imaging 2010; 3: 1196–8.

19. Daimon M, Shiota T, Gillinov AM, et al. Percutaneous mitral valve repair for chronic ischemic mitral regurgitation: a real-time three-dimensional echocardiographic study in an ovine model. Circulation 2005; 111: 2183–9.

20. Swaans MJ, Van den Branden BJ, Van der Heyden JA, et al. Three-dimensional transoesophageal echocardiography in a patient undergoing percutaneous mitral valve repair using the edge-to-edge clip technique. Eur J Echocardiogr 2009; 10: 982–3.

21. Lin BA, Forouhar AS, Pahlevan NM, et al. Color doppler jet area overestimates regurgitant volume when multiple jets are present. J Am Soc Echocardiogr 2010; 23: 993–1000.

22. Herrmann HC, Rohatgi S, Wasserman HS, et al. Mitral valve hemodynamic effects of percutaneous edge-to-edge repair with the mitraclip® device for mitral regurgitation. Catheter Cardiovasc Interv 2006; 68: 821–8.

23. Herrmann HC, Kar S, Siegel R, et al. Effect of percutaneous mitral repair with the mitraclip® device on mitral valve area and gradient. EuroInterv 2009; 4: 437–42.

20　A critical appraisal of edge-to-edge repair with the MitraClip®
Peter C. Block

Multiple publications in the surgical literature have described the open surgical double-orifice technique, described originally by Otto Alfieri, and its place in the surgical armamentarium for repair of mitral regurgitation (MR). The technique has appeal since it can decrease cardiopulmonary bypass time, but its surgical application has been limited. Among surgeons there is debate as to its usefulness as a stand-alone operation because most surgeons using the technique combine it with a surgical mitral annuloplasty in hopes of achieving a better, longer-lasting reduction in MR. Thus no large registries of patients undergoing stand-alone double-orifice technique surgery have been published and no randomized trials in the surgical literature have compared the technique with other forms of surgical MR repair. One must conclude from the surgical literature that there is efficacy of the double-orifice technique in selected patients (1) but widespread adoption of the technique even with associated annuloplasty has not occurred. Instead a variety of repair techniques, especially for degenerative (prolapse) valve disease have proliferated and evolved. Successful, long-term outcomes for treatment of degenerative MR with multiple repair techniques now dominate the surgical literature.

Against this background, the transcatheter, percutaneously placed MitraClip® device was developed to mimic the double-orifice technique. Its development was based on the hope that a transcatheter edge-to-edge repair technique could treat MR without need for surgery, replace surgical intervention in selected patients with degenerative or functional MR, reduce MR adequately to relieve the symptomatic and congestive effects of MR, and would have good long-term outcomes making it suitable even for younger patients. The EVEREST trials, which comprised a Phase I registry, a single arm High-Risk trial, and a randomized (against surgery) EVEREST II trial were an unprecedented study of a new, essentially untested, technology (the MitraClip®) versus a well-established surgical approach with known mid- and long-term follow up results. Uniquely, both surgical and MitraClip® outcomes were evaluated by a central echocardiographic Core Laboratory, which allowed an independent evaluation of both outcomes. The analyses revealed information not previously reported either in the cardiology or cardiac surgical literature. A short summary of the outcome is that initial safety results in the Phase I EVEREST I trial were reflected in safety outcomes in the randomized EVEREST II trial. Safety outcomes in the MitraClip® group were superior to surgery. However, efficacy of the MitraClip®, though statistically non-inferior, has left clinicians with a mixed report (Table 20.1). Thus, any critical appraisal of transcatheter mitral repair using the MitraClip®,

and what its use is (or will be) in patient care, must answer the following questions.

1. Is treatment with the MitraClip® truly safe and efficacious?
2. How much can the MitraClip® reduce MR; is the reduction enough to improve symptoms and reduce ventricular dysfunction; and how does this compare with surgical repair?
3. Does the MitraClip® have adequate enough outcomes to make it suitable for younger patients with degenerative MR?
4. Given the data available from the literature, which patients are best treated with the MitraClip® at present, and will patient selection broaden in the future?

IS TREATMENT WITH THE MITRACLIP® SAFE AND EFFICACIOUS?

The EVEREST II trial was a prospective randomized (2:1) study that compared percutaneous mitral valve repair using the MitraClip® system with surgical therapy (either surgical mitral valve repair or mitral valve replacement). Patients were included who had 3+ or 4+ MR and who were also candidates for surgical repair/replacement. The primary efficacy and safety endpoints were central to the outcome of the trial. Efficacy was judged by freedom from death, mitral valve surgery (or re-operation), or residual 3 or 4+ MR at 12 months. The primary safety endpoint was defined as a composite of major adverse events at 30 days. The prespecified major adverse event list was populated by commonly accepted adverse events: death, major stroke, re-operation, urgent/emergent cardiac surgery, myocardial infarction, renal failure, deep wound infection, need for mechanical ventilation for more than 48 hours, new onset of permanent atrial fibrillation, sepsis, gastrointestinal complication requiring surgery, and need for any transfusion of more than 2 units.

The 2:1 randomization scheme between MitraClip® therapy and mitral surgery (repair or replacement) was straightforward. The follow-up mandated echocardiographic Core lab and clinical follow-up at baseline, 30 days, 6, 12, 18 months and yearly through 5 years. This made EVEREST II unique in that all outcomes were evaluated by an impartial Core laboratory (2).

The results of the Phase I EVEREST I trial (a registry) foreshadowed the fact that the safety endpoint of the randomized EVEREST II trial would be met. In the first EVEREST I publication reporting 27 patients there were no procedural complications and only four 30-day major adverse events: clip detachment

Table 20.1 EVEREST II Subgroup Analyses

Subgroup	Surgery Better	Crosses Line of Unity
All patients	•	
Sex		
Male	•	
Female		•
Age		
>70 yrs		•
<70 yrs	•	
MR Category		
Functional		•
Degenerative	•	
Left Ventricular		
Function		
<60%		•
>60%	•	

Source: Data from Ref. (5).

from one leaflet in three patients who underwent elective valve surgery and one patient who had a post-procedural stoke that resolved (3). In an ensuing report of 107 patients, 9% had a major adverse event, which included one non-procedural death and 10 patients with clip detachment from one leaflet, but no clip embolization. Sixty-six percent of patients successfully treated were free from death, mitral valve surgery, or MR >2 at 12 months (4).

Thus the randomized EVEREST II trial supported the early safety signals. In the "intention-to-treat" analysis 15% of the MitraClip® group had major adverse events at 30 days compared to 48% of the surgical cohort. Adverse events were driven in both groups by transfusion, but transfusion need was more than 4 times more common in the surgical group (44.7% vs. 13.3%). Death (2.1%), re-operation (1.1%), stroke (2.1%), and urgent/emergent surgery (5%) occurred in the surgical group and most events occurred in the surgery post-clip group. Thus the safety superiority endpoint of MitraClip® therapy was easily met. A modified analysis substituting "major bleeding requiring transfusion >2 units" for "all transfusions >2 units" produced quite similar results. If the need for transfusion was excluded, the rates of major adverse events at 30 days was still lower in the MitraClip® group than in the surgical cohort though the p value was not significant at 0.23 (5).

The efficacy analysis of the MitraClip® in EVEREST II is more complex. In an "intention-to-treat" analysis rates of residual MR (of grade 3 or greater) and death were similar in the Mitra-Clip® and surgical group. However, surgery for residual MR was more common in the MitraClip® group than in the surgical cohort (20.4% vs. 2.2%). The primary efficacy endpoint was predefined as a combination of freedom from death, freedom from surgery for mitral valve dysfunction, and freedom from MR grade 3+ or 4+ at 12 months. Only 55% of the MitraClip® patients achieved this result compared with 73% in the surgical cohort (5). Thus the expectation that surgical treatment would

be more effective, but that the use of the MitraClip® would be safer, was borne out.

HOW MUCH CAN THE MITRACLIP® REDUCE MR; IS THE REDUCTION ENOUGH TO IMPROVE SYMPTOMS AND REDUCE VENTRICULAR DYSFUNCTION; AND HOW DOES THIS COMPARE TO SURGICAL REPAIR?

In the EVEREST II trial, survival with reduction in MR to less than 2+ at one year occurred in 55% of patients treated with the MitraClip® in the "intention-to-treat" analysis (in which any mitral valve surgery following the clip procedure is counted as a failure). Note that surgical MR repair (or replacement) in this analysis resulted in 73% of patients achieving that goal. If 2+ or less MR is chosen as an endpoint, MitraClip® repair results in an additional 27% of patients for a total of 82%. However, surgical therapy clearly produces a better reduction in the amount of MR with 96% of patients having 2+ or less MR after repair/replacement (5).

Arguably a reduction to MR of 2+ or less is not adequate to improve symptoms and ventricular dysfunction, but the EVEREST results indicate otherwise—at least in the short term. In EVEREST II, quality-of-life scores in patients with reduction of MR to 2+ or less slightly favored MitraClip® therapy over surgery. Changes from baseline were significantly improved in both the physical and mental component summary in both groups at 1 year but in the surgical group (perhaps not surprisingly) patients did not have improvement in the physical component summary at 30 days but did at a later follow-up.

Reduction in MR to 2+ or less in the MitraClip® group produced significant changes from baseline in left ventricular volume measurements. Left ventricular ejection fraction changed –3% in the MitraClip® group and –7% after surgical therapy—both statistically significant from baseline and also between groups (5). Nevertheless, the question that must be raised is whether a reduction of MR to 2+ or less in a patient with 3 to 4+ MR enough to improve ventricular performance; especially, if that can be achieved by nonsurgical, percutaneous transcatheter therapy. In short the answer to that question is "yes." Ventricular function in both the MitraClip® group and the surgery cohort improved. However, whether the difference in improvement in the amount of MR between the two therapies makes a clinical difference in mortality outcomes, for example, is unknown. To design a trial to answer that question would be impractical if "hard" outcomes are chosen as endpoints due to the low rate of events that would surely occur in the first years of such a trial. Choosing "softer" endpoints such as quality-of-life measurements, NYHA class improvement, six-minute walk testing, and so on makes much more sense, but it seems likely that subtle differences in MR grade (between 1+ and 2+ for example) would result in minor differences in these endpoints. The number of patients needed to evaluate the differences would be large, making such a trial unlikely to be conducted.

Nevertheless, the data from EVEREST II showing improvement in left ventricular dimensions after MitraClip® placement support an interesting potential clinical strategy. If a patient with severe MR is severely limited by heart failure symptoms and wishes a better quality-of-life with no regard for long-term outcomes (associated end-stage renal failure, neoplasm in partial remission, etc.), MitraClip® placement and reduction in MR to less than 2+ would achieve that result without surgery. For an individual patient that makes sense. The intriguing issue is whether the reductions in hospitalizations observed in the single arm High-Risk trial could be proven in a randomized trial. That would make MitraClip® therapy a good public health strategy for such patients.

DOES THE MITRACLIP® HAVE ADEQUATE OUTCOMES TO MAKE IT SUITABLE FOR YOUNGER PATIENTS WITH DEGENERATIVE MR?

Surgical repair of degenerative MR has gained widespread acceptance as data have accumulated that medical therapy, possibly even for moderate MR, is less effective. Reports from the Mitral Regurgitation International Database, a registry created for multicenter study of MR with echocardiographically diagnosed flail leaflet as a model of pure, organic MR showed clear benefit of surgery over medical management (6). Patients were relatively young (age 64 ± 11 years), ejection fraction was maintained, and more than half were in NYHA functional class I or II. During a median follow-up of nearly 4 years, linearized event rates/year for medical management were 5.4% for atrial fibrillation, 8.0% for heart failure, and 2.6% for death. Mitral valve surgery had a perioperative mortality of <1% and during follow-up was independently associated with reduced risk of death (adjusted hazard ratio 0.42). Such studies and others support early surgical consideration in patients with MR due to flail leaflets for whom surgical repair is feasible (7).

In the face of good surgical outcomes, treatment with the MitraClip® in young patients with degenerative MR faces several hurdles. The two most important are presence of residual MR, and the lack of even mid-or long-term follow-up of patients treated with the MitraClip®. Surgical reports of long-term outcomes up to 10 years after repair of degenerative MR show freedom from recurrent moderate or severe MR at 10 years can be 80% ± 5%. The presence of recurrent MR seems associated with a higher mortality and a re-repair for degenerative disease is warranted (8). The same holds for patients with functional MR in which survival by Kaplan–Meier analysis was 76.4% at three years and 65.1% at five years with 0 to 2+ MR postoperatively versus 61.3% and 35.8% with 3+ to 4+ MR (9). To further complicate this issue most surgical reports of follow-up after mitral valve repair split the amount of recurrent or residual MR into 2+ or less versus >2+. The majority of patients treated successfully with the MitraClip® have 2+ or less MR. An understanding of what 2+ or less residual MR has on long-term follow-up is impossible to impute from these data (notwithstanding the different populations of patients in the surgical and MitraClip® literature). Until the results of EVEREST II are followed for at

least 5 years, it seems premature to consider that younger patients who likely will have excellent surgical outcomes for degenerative MR repair should be better treated with the MitraClip®. To suggest treatment with the MitraClip® would presume that a percutaneous, transcatheter edge-to-edge repair (if successful) can produce a good outcome without later deterioration in MR status. The surgical consensus is that an edge-to-edge repair should be done with an annuloplasty in all instances to ensure a good long-term result and that a surgical edge-to-edge repair alone will fail (10). Nevertheless there are other tantalizing data emerging from the 2-year follow-up of the EVEREST II trial. In comparing patients in need of an operation (or re-operation) among those receiving the MitraClip® versus surgically treated patients there is a clear difference in "freedom from surgery" within the first six months, since patients with a failed MitraClip® procedure underwent MR surgery. However, after 6 months the percentage of patients free from surgery in both groups remains nearly constant—indicating that at least up to two years the edge-to-edge MitraClip® repair is not failing. Why this should be so is intriguing. One explanation is that the follow-up of MitraClip® patients is simply too short, and that an operation for recurrent MR may be necessary for most of them in the future. Another is that the MitraClip® is not identical with a suture-based operative edge-to-edge repair and such comparison is meaningless. The MitraClip® may produce a more robust edge-to-edge bridge that is less likely to fail and the fibrous ingrowth stimulated by the MitraClip® may additionally serve to stabilize the posterior annulus, keeping it from dilating. These two factors might produce a better long-term reduction in MR than a suture-based surgical edge-to-edge repair. However, these are speculative thoughts and the results from ongoing long-term follow-up of EVEREST II are needed.

One might also consider that an attempt at MitraClip® therapy is justified to avoid a thoracotomy, and accepting more residual MR as a consequence. If residual MR is 2+ or more or if there is clip detachment from one leaflet, surgery could be performed later. Preserving conventional surgical options in this scenario would be critical. Reports (11,12) describe surgical treatment at varying intervals up to 5 years after the MitraClip® procedure. The indications for mitral valve surgery after treatment with the MitraClip® included clip detachment from one leaflet, residual or recurrent MR >2+, atrial septal defect, device malfunction during implantation in one patient, and incorrectly diagnosed mitral stenosis in one patient. The EVEREST investigators reported that 87% of the operated patients underwent the same surgical procedure planned before surgery, but about one-sixth of patients with planned repair underwent mitral valve replacement as late as five years after clip implantation. Although successful repair was performed in the majority of patients after the MitraClip® procedure, not all had a repair as planned. While considering younger patients for MitraClip® therapy, one must accept that MR will likely not be reduced as completely as at surgery. In case of MitraClip® failure, mitral repair may, in a minority of cases, not be possible.

GIVEN THE DATA AVAILABLE FROM THE LITERATURE, WHICH PATIENTS ARE BEST TREATED WITH THE MITRACLIP® AT PRESENT, AND WILL PATIENT SELECTION BROADEN IN THE FUTURE?

The landmark EVEREST II trial was the first and (so far) only randomized trial of a percutaneous, transcatheter therapy for treatment of MR versus surgical therapy. In summary, EVEREST II showed the following:

1. MR was more effectively reduced by surgery at hospital discharge, and at 1- and 2-year follow-up (though in comparing the two therapies rather than pre-post MR in each group, the reductions were similar).
2. Clinical improvement with the MitraClip® was significant and sustained over 2 years.
3. As a result of greater MR reduction with surgery, reduction in left ventricular end-diastolic volumes was greater in the surgical group than in the MitraClip® group (though patients who underwent MitraClip® therapy also had significantly reduced left ventricular dimensions compared with baseline).
4. MitraClip® therapy was associated with more frequent additional procedures for treatment of MR.
5. Even if "transfusion need" is excluded from the analysis, surgery for MR is associated with more adverse events and thus is not as safe.

Thus, the results of EVEREST II and the fact that long-term outcomes of MitraClip® therapy (even if successful) are not yet available; both present the clinician caring for patients with MR a mixed portfolio of outcomes (Table 20.2). The bottom line question that must be applied to patients being considered for MitraClip® therapy is whether a therapy which is less effective, but safer is acceptable. In a report from the Cleveland Clinic surgical repair of degenerative (prolapse) MR provides an operative risk of <0.1% and 15-year survival of 76%, superior to the age- and sex-matched U.S. population (13). At 10 years, freedom from mitral reoperation was 97%, and 77% had no or 1+ MR. Given such excellent results of surgical repair of degenerative (prolapsed) MR, it is difficult to support the use of the MitraClip® in younger patients in whom long-term outcomes

are a major part of a therapeutic decision. Surely there are exceptions: patients with comorbid conditions that make surgery a higher risk; those who refuse surgery or transfusions; previous thoracotomy and so on. But on balance, it seems prudent, with the data now available, to consider surgery a better option for many patients who are good operative candidates with degenerative MR.

The EVEREST II trial was designed to compare the results of treatment of degenerative and functional MR. However, the majority of patients randomized had degenerative MR. A lot more information have emerged from sub-group analyses within EVEREST II itself and also from the accompanying single-arm High-Risk trial. In exploratory hypothesis generating subgroup analyses, for patients with age >70 years, functional MR, and left ventricular systolic dysfunction surgery was not superior to MitraClip® therapy. Such patients are likely better served by MitraClip® therapy. Remember that patients enrolled in EVEREST I and EVEREST II had to be surgical candidates. But associated with these trials was a High-Risk trial in which the MitraClip® was placed in patients with an STS Score or an estimated operative mortality rate of >12% (14). The 30-day mortality rate in these patients was significantly less than the anticipated surgical mortality rate, and one-year mortality rate was better than that of a matched group of medically treated patients. Of note is that beneficial results occurred in both patients with degenerative and functional MR. The data from the High-Risk trial are perhaps the most important as they will help us in understanding how MitraClip® therapy will be used in the future. Patient selection for MitraClip® therapy in Europe (the device was commercialized there in 2008) has concentrated on patients with high surgical risk and patients with functional MR—both groups which have limited surgical options and which were not studied in the EVEREST II randomized trial. Despite the rapid growth of the MitraClip® experience in Europe, European outcomes data have been reported only from a limited number of registry reports (15–18). Most patients selected for MitraClip® therapy in those reports were at high surgical risk, with congestive heart failure and depressed left ventricular function. These reports showed favorable outcomes. Adverse events were uncommon and the degree of MR was improved in most patients. Left ventricular dimensions, 6-minute walk distances, and plasma BNP levels have all been shown to improve (17). Reports from Europe indicate a success rate of >90% with use of more than one clip in one-third of patients or more. Thirty-day mortality was <5% in patients with surgical EuroScores of 29–44% (15,16). In the United States, the REALISM continued access registry has followed completion of enrollment in the U.S. pivotal trial, and has enrolled additional high surgical risk patients. The REALISM registry collects data from U.S. centers with continued access to the MitraClip® therapy. It is a continuation of the EVEREST II trial but patients, instead of being randomized to MitraClip® versus surgery, are screened for enrollment to either a high-risk or non–high risk arm. Follow-up is for five years. Contributors to the high-risk arm of REALISM have

Table 20.2 Factors Favoring Surgery or MitraClip® Therapy

Favoring surgical repair	Favoring MitraClip®
MR more effectively reduced	Clinical improvement better at 30 days
Left ventricular volumes less	Safer (fewer adverse events, less transfusion)
Fewer repeat procedures	Non-operative candidates
Good long-term outcome	Better for high-risk surgical patients
Best for degenerative MR	Better for functional MR
	Better for patients with low LVEF

enrolled elderly high-risk patients, mostly with functional MR, who have anatomical criteria suited for the MitraClip®. The results of REALISM, longer-term outcomes from clinical use in Europe, and longer-term outcomes from the EVEREST High-Risk trial will then allow greater insight into the usefulness of MitraClip® therapy in patients who arguably are, and will be, the most in need for this transcatheter technology.

REFERENCES

1. Maisano F, Vigano G, Blasio A, et al. Surgical isolated edge-to-edge mitral valve repair without annuloplasty: clinical proof of the principle for an endovascular approach. EuroIntervention 2006; 2: 181–6.

2. Foster E, Wasserman HS, Gray W, et al. Quantitative assessment of severity of mitral regurgitation by serial echocardiography in a multicenter clinical trial of percutaneous mitral valve repair. AJC 2007; 100: 1577–83.

3. Feldman T, Wasserman HS, Herrmann HC, et al. Percutaneous mitral valve repair using the edge-to-edge technique: six-month results of the everest phase I clinical trial. JACC 2005; 46: 2134–44.

4. Feldman T, Kar S, Rinaldi M. Percutaneous mitral repair with the MitraClip® system: safety and midterm durability in the initial everest (endovascular valve edge-to-edge repair study) cohort. JACC 2009; 54: 686–94.

5. Feldman T, Foster E, Glower DD, et al. For the EVEREST II investigators. percutaneous repair or surgery for mitral regurgitation. NEJM 2011; 364: 1395–406.

6. Grigioni F, Tribouilloy C, Avierinos JF, MIDA Investigators. Outcomes in mitral regurgitation due to flail leaflets a multicenter European study. JACC Cardiovasc Imaging 2008; 1133–41.

7. Johnston DR, Gillinov AM, Blackstone EH, et al. Surgical repair of posterior mitral valve prolapse: implications for guidelines and percutaneous repair. Ann Thorac Surg 2010; 89: 1385–94.

8. Suri RM, Schaff HV, Dearani JA, et al. Recurrent mitral regurgitation after repair: should the mitral valve be re-repaired? J Thorac Cardiovasc Surg 2006; 132: 1390–7.

9. Crabtree TD, Bailey MS, Moon MR, et al. Recurrent mitral regurgitation and risk factors for early and late mortality after mitral valve repair for functional ischemic mitral regurgitation. Ann Thorac Surg 2008; 85: 1537–42.

10. Cohn LH. Percutaneous mitral valve repair with the edge-to-edge technique: a surgeon's perspective. JACC 2005; 46: 2141–2.

11. Argenziano M, Skipper E, Heimansohn D, et al. EVEREST investigators. surgical revision after percutaneous mitral repair with the MitraClip® device. Ann Thorac Surg 2010; 89: 72–80.

12. Rogers JH, Yeo KK, Carroll JD, et al. Late surgical mitral valve repair after percutaneous repair with the MitraClip® system. J Card Surg 2009; 24: 677–81.

13. Johnston DR, Gillinov AM, Blackstone EH, et al. Surgical repair of posterior mitral valve prolapse: implications for guidelines and percutaneous repair. Ann Thorac Surg 2010; 89: 1385–94.

14. Perlowski A, Feldman TE. The EVEREST pecutaneous mitral leaflet repair trials. Cardiac Interv Toady 2011.

15. Treede H, Schirmer J, Rudolph V, et al. A heart team's perspective on interventional mitral valve repair: percutaneous clip implantation as an important adjunct to a surgical mitral valve program for treatment of high-risk patients. J Thorac Cardiovasc Surg 2012; 143: 78–84.

16. Franzen O, Baldus S, Rudolph V, et al. Acute outcomes of MitraClip® therapy for mitral regurgitation in high-surgical-risk patients: emphasis on adverse valve morphology and severe left ventricular dysfunction. Eur Heart J 2010; 31: 1373–81.

17. Franzen O, van der Heyden J, Baldus S. MitraClip® therapy in patients with end-stage systolic heart failure. Eur J Heart Failure 2011; 13: 569–76.

18. Tamburino C, Ussia GP, Maisano F. Percutaneous mitral valve repair with the MitraClip® system: acute results from a real world setting. Eur Heart J 2010; 31: 1382–9.

21 Technique for surgical removal of the MitraClip®
Lori Soni and Michael Argenziano

INTRODUCTION

After the promising results of the MitraClip® in the Endovascular Valve Edge-to-Edge Repair STudy (EVEREST) (1) phase I safety and feasibility trial in 2005, the phase II trial, EVEREST II, evaluated the performance of endovascular mitral repair with the MitraClip® in comparison to conventional mitral surgery (2). In Europe, the MitraClip® has been commercially available since 2008, and ACCESS-Europe is an ongoing observational study of these patients. As of 2011, more than 3,200 MitraClips® have been implanted in Europe and the United States (3).

As the clinical use of the MitraClip® increases in Europe, and as additional clinical experience is gained in the United States through continued access and compassionate use protocols, questions remain about the role of this technology in patients who are also candidates for surgical repair. Given the proven efficacy, safety, and durability of current surgical mitral repair techniques, the introduction of a newer, percutaneous approach raises questions. In order for percutaneous techniques to become a reasonable alternative, they must have a risk–benefit profile that matches the safety and efficacy of currently available surgical approaches. This is especially true for young, healthy patients, in whom the risks of surgery are minimal and the importance of repair success and durability is paramount.

With regard to the question of safety, the EVEREST trials have shown low procedural morbidity. The efficacy of the procedure (percentage of patients treated definitively by the Mitra-Clip® device), although lower than that observed with standard surgical approaches, is reasonable in the early experience with this first-in-class device, and is improving with increased operator experience, technologic refinements, and maturation of patient selection criteria.

One argument advanced by proponents of the MitraClip® system is that the procedure is successful in a significant proportion of patients and should be offered as a first-line treatment, with surgical treatment reserved for percutaneous treatment failures. The strength of this argument, of course, depends on whether a failed percutaneous procedure somehow "burns bridges," increasing the risk or decreasing the success rate of subsequent mitral repair surgery.

SURGERY AFTER MITRACLIP®: INDICATIONS AND RESULTS

Delivered through a percutaneous femoral venous transseptal approach, the MitraClip® can be used to grasp the leaflets and evaluate MR reduction by transesophageal echocardiography prior to clip deployment. If mitral regurgitation (MR) is not sufficiently, the clip can be repositioned prior to deployment or withdrawn. There are four indications for surgical intervention after the clip procedure: (i) failure to deploy the MitraClip®, (ii) clip deployment with acute procedural failure, (iii) clip deployment with delayed procedural failure, and (iv) procedure-related complications requiring surgery.

The first indication, failure to deploy the clip, may be due to several reasons including procedure failure (defined as greater than 2+ MR after clip deployment) or inability to grasp the leaflets at the desired location with the clip. The second indication, clip deployment with acute procedural failure, may be due to procedure failure, partial clip detachment, or iatrogenic injury to the valve. The third indication, clip deployment with delayed procedural failure, is due to failure noted after patient discharge, with recurrence of MR or partial clip detachment. The fourth indication, procedure-related complications, has included surgical intervention due to persistent atrial septal defect from transseptal puncture (4,5) or cardiac tamponade due to iatrogenic transmural aortic puncture (4).

We and others have reported experience with surgical repair after failed MitraClip® procedures (5–8). To date, most of the published series have focused on surgical intervention after clip failure in the short term, and only one addresses surgical results after late failure. The feasibility and success of secondary surgical mitral valve repair after percutaneous intervention are described in few case series with small numbers of patients (4–8).

Although few initial reports from the EVEREST I and II trial cohorts suggested preservation of surgical repair options (4,7) in patients with failed clip procedures, more recent reports have identified cases in which repair options were compromised (5,6). Several authors have noted leaflet injury upon clip explant (4,6). Although in most cases these leaflet disruptions have been minor and have been repaired with simple or running sutures, in other cases clip injury to the valve leaflets or chordal entrapment has led to a more complex repair or even valve replacement (5,6). When longer periods have elapsed from clip implant to explant, a fibrous bridge encasement has been noted to form over the clip (4,8). This tissue bridge has been removed with sharp dissection, but there have been reports of leaflet injury or the need for chordal transsection in order to remove the encasing tissue.

Although leaflet or chordal damage induced by the clip has prevented valve repair in some cases, in most patients failed MitraClip® deployment has not materially changed the eventual operation performed. The results of the EVEREST II trial demonstrated a 22% crossover from MitraClip® to surgery at two years (3). Thus, with increasing adoption of MitraClip® therapy in patients similar to those in EVEREST II, that is, younger patients with structural valve disease, it might be expected that there continue to be patients with previous MitraClips® who require surgical intervention. However, as experience improves, anatomic predictors of success are refined, and the MitraClip® is increasingly used in elderly, high surgical risk patients, the negative impact of failed MitraClip® therapy on valve surgery outcome will likely decrease. The predominant use of the MitraClip® in the elderly and high-risk patient cohorts in Europe, where the device is commercially available, supports this prediction.

ANATOMY AND PATHOLOGY OF CLIP ADHERENCE AND REMOVAL

The extent to which the clip may be encased in tissue will depend on the degree of healing commensurate with clip duration. A closer look at the histologic evaluation of the explanted MitraClip® has demonstrated several stages of the healing response (9). In the acute interval at <30 days, there is a thin layer of fibrin and platelets covering the device surface. After seven days, acute inflammatory cells are replaced by a mixture of chronic inflammatory cell infiltrate including macrophages, lymphocytes, plasma cells, and occasional giant cells. In the subacute interval from 31 to 90 days, granulation tissue covers the device with fibrin in various stages of organization. In the subacute phase, there is early collagen deposition, and some of the explanted devices are noted to have tissue bridge formation between the two arms. In the chronic interval form 91 to 300 days, the device is encapsulated with type III and type I collagen. Acute inflammatory cells are no longer observed. In the long-term interval from 301 to 1878 days, the fibrous capsule covering the device is composed of predominantly type I collagen.

The mitral valve is composed of two leaflets, anterior and posterior, that are scalloped in appearance. The scallops demarcate the three segments, denoted as A1 and A2; A3 and P1; P2 and P3. The most lateral scallop near the anterolateral commissure is A1 and P1 while A3 and P3 are situated near the posteromedial commissure and A2 and P2 constitute the middle scallop. The anterior leaflet constitutes one-third and the posterior leaflet constitutes two-thirds of the valve circumference (10).

The leaflets are connected by chordae tendineae, fibrous strings of connective tissue, to the anterior and posterior papillary muscles. The anterior papillary muscle is supplied by blood flow from the left anterior descending and the circumflex artery and is less prone to infarction as compared with the posterior papillary muscle which is supplied by the right coronary or a dominant circumflex artery (11). Primary chordae tendineae attach directly to the leaflet free edges while secondary and tertiary chordae tendineae connect to the ventricular surface of the leaflet closer to the annulus (12). The anterior mitral valve annulus is composed mostly of collagen while the posterior annulus is more muscular in composition. The annulus may have a cord or a sheet-like appearance.

Several important structures lie in close proximity to the mitral valve and may be injured during mitral valve surgery. The aortic annulus lies anterior to the mitral valve runs parallel to the anterior annulus of the mitral valve. The right and left fibrous trigones lie on both edges of the anterior mitral

annulus. To be more specific, the right fibrous trigone lies at the intersection of the membranous septum and the annulus of the mitral, tricuspid and aortic valves (11). The left trigone lies between the left coronary cusp of the aortic valve and the anterior mitral valve annulus. Both the AV node and the bundle of His lie in the vicinity of the right trigone. The left circumflex artery lies adjacent to the posterior mitral valve annulus, and the extent of this relationship depends on the dominance of the vessel.

MITRACLIP® REMOVAL

The operative approach depends on the patient's body habitus and previous surgical history. The options include median sternotomy with bicaval and aortic cannulation, ministernotomy or minithoracortomy with peripheral venous cannulation, and central or peripheral arterial cannulation. Antegrade cardioplegia is administered with or without retrograde. After institution of cardiopulmonary bypass, the aorta is cross-clamped. Most surgeons open the left atrium just anterior to the right pulmonary veins.

Depending on the duration since clip placement, a tissue bridge of varying thickness may cover the clip. The tissue bridge may be removed with sharp dissection so that the clip is clearly visualized. The clip is structured such that the native leaflets are sandwiched between two parts, the arm and the gripper. The arm abuts the ventricular surface of the leaflet while the gripper abuts the atrial surface of the leaflet. The lock is located in the center on the atrial side of the clip (Figs. 21.1, 21.2). By stabilizing one end of the clip with forceps and placing forward pressure on the lock, the mechanism is released resulting in the separation of the arm and the gripper thus freeing the leaflet. The forward pressure may be applied using a forceps or the tip of a Frazier suction catheter (7). An alternative technique includes placing a suture through the loops of the lock harness (7). The suture is then snared. Upward tension can be applied on the suture while a forward motion is applied by advancing the snare toward the lock (Fig. 21.3).

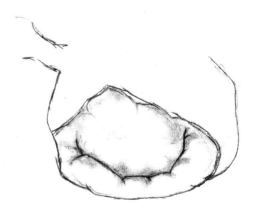

Figure 21.1 Mitral valve. Source: Courtesy of Jeffrey Jiang.

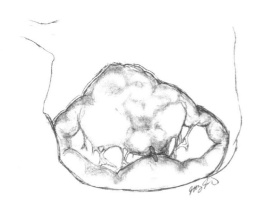

Figure 21.2 MitraClip® in situ. Source: Courtesy of Jeffrey Jiang.

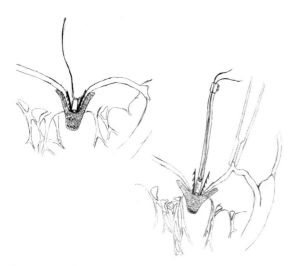

Figure 21.3 Technique for MitraClip® removal with a suture placed through the locking mechanism, snared, and then the tourniquet is advanced with a forward motion while counter-traction is maintained with the suture. *Source:* Courtesy of Jeffrey Jiang.

Small defects will often be noted in the leaflet at the location of clip explant. There have been reports of the creation of more significant clefts or tears in the leaflet at clip explant (5,6). These are more important when they involve the anterior mitral leaflet because, unlike the posterior leaflet the anterior leaflet is not usually resected in structural leaflet repairs. Anterior leaflet injuries can be usually be repaired with simple sutures, (4) although we have repaired small leaflet defects with patches of autologous pericardium. After the clip is explanted and any damaged leaflets resected or repaired, the valve may usually be repaired or replaced as clinically indicated.

CONCLUSIONS

Surgical intervention in patients with previous MitraClip® deployment or attempted deployment presents a novel challenge for cardiac surgeons. Because the real and perceived risks of MitraClip® treatment are different from surgical approaches, the timing of intervention, extent and nature of mitral valve pathology, and patient comorbidities may be different from those usually encountered by surgeons. On the one hand, the low morbidity of the percutaneous approach may prompt earlier intervention in patients who are unwilling to consider surgical treatment. Conversely, the percutaneous procedure may be applied to very high-risk patients who might not otherwise be deemed as appropriate surgical candidates. In the first circumstance, the surgeon operating on a failed MitraClip® may be faced with a more complex repair than usual, in a patient for whom avoidance of prosthetic valve replacement is of great importance. In the second situation, although the importance of repair is much diminished, the surgeon is often challenged by comorbidities that often preclude surgery as an option. In other words, a failed MitraClip® as an indication for surgery can present a surgeon with one of two unwelcome options: a young patient with complex mitral anatomy who desires repair, and an elderly, sick patient who may be too ill to get through open heart surgery.

Despite these considerations, the fact is that the patients who we believe to be the best candidates for MitraClip® therapy—the elderly, those with high or prohibitive risk for surgery, and those with mitral pathologies with imperfect surgical remedies (such as functional MR)—do benefit from avoiding surgery, and will not likely pursue surgical options even in the face of MitraClip® failure. Of all the surgical procedures performed for failed clips, truly emergent indications for surgery have been rare. Instead, most patients with failed clips in the trials have been left clinically where there were before clip deployment. Thus, for patients who are not good surgical candidates, either because of their risk or of their valve pathology, a failed clip will not lead to surgery in most cases. In the cases that go to the operating theater, the increasing worldwide experience suggests that in the vast majority of patients, the MitraClip(s)® can be removed without disrupting the remainder of the surgical procedure.

REFERENCES

1. Feldman T, Wasserman H, Herrmann H, et al. Percutaneous mitral valve repair using the edge-to-edge technique: six-month results of the EVEREST phase I clinical trial. J Am Coll Cardiol 2005; 46: 2134–40.
2. Feldman T, Foster E, Glower D, et al. Percutaneous repair or surgery for mitral regurgitation. N Engl J Med 2011; 364: 1395–406.
3. Feldman T. Percutaneous repair for MR: follow up and longer term outcomes. Transcatheter Cardiovascular Therapeutics (TCT) Angioplasty Summit. Korea: Seoul, 2011: 27–29.
4. Argenziano M, Skipper E, Heimansohn D, et al. Surgical revision after percutaneous mitral repair with MitraClip® device. Ann Thorac Surg 2010; 89: 72–80.

5. Geidel S, Ostermeyer J, Lass M, Schmoeckel M. Complex surgical valve repair after failed percuteaneous mitral intervention using the MitraClip® device. Ann Thorac Surg 2010; 90: 277–9.

6. Conradi L, Treede H, Franzen O, et al. Impact of MitraClip® therapy on secondary mitral valve surgery in patients at high surgical risk. Eur J Cardiothorac Surg 2011.

7. Dang N, Aboodi M, Sakauchi T, et al. Surgical revision after percutaneous mitral valve repair with a clip: initial multi-center experience. Ann Thor Surg 2005; 6: 2338–42.

8. Rogers J, Yeo K, Carroll J, et al. Late surgical mitral valve repair after percutaneous repair with the MitraClip® system. J Card Surg 2009; 24: 677–81.

9. Ladich E, Michaels M, Jones R, et al. Pathological healing response of explanted MitraClip® devices. Circulation 2011; 123: 1418–27.

10. Akhter S. The heart and pericardium. Thorac Surg Clin 2011; 21: 205–17.

11. Cohn LH, LH E. Cardiac Surgery in the Adult, 3rd edn. New York: McGraw-Hill, 2011.

12. Sellke FW, Ruel M. Atlas of Cardiac Surgical Techniques. Philadelphia: Saunders Elsevier, 2010.

22   Special considerations for mitral valve repair after clip therapy
Subhasis Chatterjee, David A. Heimansohn, and John C. Alexander

BACKGROUND

Mitral valve (MV) repair is accepted worldwide as the treatment of choice for mitral regurgitation (MR) (1). Repair is preferred to replacement because of improved long-term survival as seen in propensity-matched groups (2). In an analysis of almost 60,000 patients from the Adult Cardiac Database of Society of Thoracic Surgeon, operated during 2000–2007 undergoing isolated MV surgery, MV repair for MR was accomplished in 69% of patients with an elective operative mortality of 1.2% (3). Surgical results for degenerative MV disease (4) are generally thought to be more durable than results for functional MR (5). Recurrent MR after MV repair surgery can still be treated by re-repair of the MV approximately half the time in surgical series (6). Repair has demonstrated survival benefits with improved ejection fraction and more favorable left ventricular (LV) remodeling (7). Despite the well-established role of surgery in MR, there is a significant unmet clinical need due to a sizable number of patients not referred for surgery mainly because of perceived operative risk (8). In octogenarians the 90-day mortality results approach 19% for MV repair and 32% for MV replacement even in published series from experienced centers (9).

The MitraClip® (Abbott Vascular, Menlo Park, California, USA) device is a viable option for selected high risk patients with MR. Unfortunately, there will still be patients who will need MV surgery after an unsuccessful MitraClip® procedure. In this chapter we will attempt to understand the types of MV injury that may occur after a MitraClip® procedure and describe its safe removal to preserve repair options. We will also analyze the most recent Endovascular Valve Edge-to-Edge REpair STudy (EVEREST) II randomized trial experience and previous surgical reports on mitral repair following MitraClip® procedure.

EVEREST II TRIAL EXPERIENCE

The EVEREST II trial has been reviewed extensively in other chapters (10). The trial dataset included a prospectively defined group of trial patients that received high-quality core lab echocardiography follow-up. This has been one of the criticisms of long-term surgical mitral repair trials with inconsistent and heterogeneous echocardiography follow-up and a focus on defining success as "Freedom from Reoperation" as opposed to "Freedom from Recurrent 3 to 4+ MR", or better yet, the EVEREST composite of one year freedom from the combined incidence of death, reoperation, or recurrent severe MR. In EVEREST II, enrolled patients were eligible for MV repair or replacement with either degenerative MR (anterior, posterior, and bileaflet disease), or functional MR. Patients

with active endocarditis, rheumatic valve disease, and mitral stenosis were specifically excluded. In the trial, surgeons were required to predict the likelihood of MV repair or replacement before randomization with the actual decision to repair or replace made at the time of surgery. Both the device (89%) and surgical control (86%) arms of the trial had a high overall repair rate. In the device group (n = 178), a total of 158 patients received a MV repair (138 by MitraClip® and 20 had surgical MV repair post device) while 17 received a mitral valve replacement (MVR) post device placement. In the surgical control group (n = 80), 69 patients received a MV repair and 11 a MVR. It did not appear that the surgeon's previous experience with surgical MV repair influenced the type of surgery in the EVEREST II surgical control group. The MV repair rates for the EVEREST II surgeons who had performed more than 25 MV repairs in the prior year (89% repair rate) were not statistically different from those who had less than 25 MV repairs performed the prior year (83% repair rate).

In analyzing EVEREST II, 37 out of the 158 patients or 23.4% crossed over from device to surgery. Of specific concern was the possibility that either valve injury or difficulty in device removal would compromise the ability to perform MV repair and result in MV replacement. In other words, does a MitraClip® procedure "burn a bridge" with regard to a future MV repair if needed? Would there be a significant number of patients eligible for MV repair surgery that would end up with an MVR after a failed MitraClip® procedure? This may not be a major consideration in a high-risk 80-year-old patient; however, it would be a major concern for a healthy 60-year-old patient who might consider MitraClip® instead of conventional mitral repair surgery. Patient and physician acceptance of less invasive coronary stenting over coronary bypass surgery for certain patients, for example, has been enhanced by reassurance that initial stenting does not compromise subsequent coronary surgery if necessary.

Table 22.1 lists the indications for surgery in EVEREST II. Valve injury by the device or difficulty in removing the device was noted in 11 of the 37 surgery post MitraClip® (SPMC) patients. However, the repair rate in the 11 patients where there was a report of valve injury or difficulty removing the device (45%) did not statistically differ from the repair rate in the 26 patients without mention of valve injury or difficult removal (58%, p = 0.72). Thus, the overall repair rate in both groups was lower than the 92% expected repair rate. Valve injury or difficulty removing the device did not have a significant influence on the repair rate. Finally, the surgeon has to be highly motivated and experienced to attempt MV repair after clip placement, especially when the clip has been in place for more than a month. It is analogous to re-repair situations when the anatomy is not completely revealed until surgery.

An additional concern was whether the duration of the implant influenced the ability to perform surgical MV repair. It was noted that the repair rate was 52% (14 of 27) when surgery was performed within 90 days of the MitraClip® procedure and 60% (6 of 10) when performed after 90 days of the procedure. Based on this small sample, it did not appear that the duration of the implant influenced the ability to still repair the mitral valve. There are reports of successful MV repair out to five years after the MitraClip® implant (11). When compared to primary surgery, SPMC was not associated with a higher modified major adverse event (major bleeding defined as >2 unit blood transfusion or surgical intervention) rate (37.8% in the n = 37 SPMC group and 50% in the n = 80 surgical control group, p = 0.2382, 95% CI 8.9–33.2). Finally, clinical success

(defined as freedom from death, reoperations, and MR >2 +) at 1 year was similar (SPMC = 86.2%, n = 29; control = 87.8%, n = 80) to the surgical control group.

Glower presented a detailed analysis of EVEREST II at the American Association of Thoracic Surgery in 2011 on the predictors of MV repair or replacement (12). It appeared that MVR rather than repair was strongly associated with anterior/bileaflet flail and prolapse. MV repair (MitraClip® or surgical, n = 225) when compared with MV replacement (post MitraClip® or de novo surgery, n = 30), anterior leaflet involvement was found to be higher (47%) in the replacement group compared with the repair group (28%, p = 0.037). It did not appear that age, prior cardiac surgery, functional MR, or surgical experience influenced the repair/replacement rate.

Freedom from subsequent MV replacement at one year was similar for both the groups. A hundred and fifty eight of the 178 (89%) MitraClip® patients and 67 of the 80 (84%) de novo surgery patients did not need MV replacement. However, it does appear that there is a trade-off. When comparing surgery post MitraClip® with de novo surgery, it was found that 8 out of 80 (10%) of de novo surgery patient underwent MVR when surgical MV repair was the planned preprocedure. In the SPMC group, 15/37 (41%, p < 0.001) underwent MVR when mitral repair was the planned preprocedure. Of this group, 5/37 (14%) were directly related to MV injury or the inability to successfully explant the device, and the remaining 10 had more complex valve pathology that was felt to be less amenable to a successful repair. Thus, in the 37 MitraClip® patients who underwent surgery, there was a 92% predicted repair rate and a 54% actual repair rate. In the 80 de novo surgery patients, there was also a 92% predicted repair rate and an 84% (p < 0.001 compared with 54% SPMC repair rate) actual repair rate. Figure 22.1 demonstrates that if we would estimate in a group of 100 mitral repair candidates with an expected 90% repair rate who all proceeded to MitraClip®, 20 patients would need SPMC. Of that group, 40% or 8 would end up with an MV replacement. If, on the other hand, they had all proceeded

Table 22.1 EVEREST I and II Indications for Surgery Post MitraClip® Within 12 Months

Indication	EVEREST I & EVEREST II Roll In % (n)	EVEREST II % (n)
No MitraClip® device implanted	28 (9)	46 (17)
Single leaflet insertion	31 (10)	24 (9)
Residual MR	6 (2)	14 (5)
Recurrent MR	22 (7)	8 (3)
Clinical symptoms despite MR reduction		8 (3)
Other (ASD, device malfunction, suspected MS)	13 (4)	
Total	100 (32)	100 (37)

Abbreviations: ASD, atrial septal defect; MR, mitral regurgitation; MS, mitral stenosis.

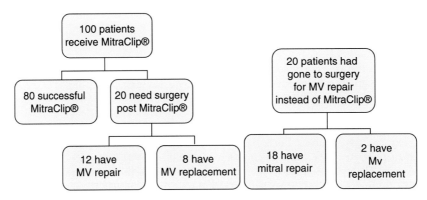

Figure 22.1 Calculations based on EVEREST II data of excess mitral valve replacement from MitraClip® placement.

to surgery, then of those 20 patients, only 2 would end up with a replacement. Thus, for every 100 patients receiving a Mitra-Clip® there would be an extra six MVRs than if they had all gone directly to surgery. There would, however, be one more death due to surgery. Practically speaking, for every 16 patients going for MitraClip® placement there would be one patient who received a MVR who would have received a surgical MV repair if that patient had gone directly to surgery. It is important to note that this calculation is based on one-year EVEREST II data. It will be more interesting to note the five year data to see the mid-term rate of SPMC over a larger time period to see how these calculations change.

The surgical literature supports a number of predictors of MV replacement or failure of MV repair including advanced patient age, gender, comorbidities, surgeon experience, endocarditis, specific anatomical features such as presence of anterior/bileaflet involvement, greater number of scallops involved, extensive mitral annular/leaflet calcification, and functional MR (13,14). Anterior leaflet prolapse is recognized as the major factor for recurrent MR and subsequent reoperation for recurrent MR (15). Thus, the same risk factor that makes surgical MV repair less durable appears to be the same risk factor that makes long-term success with percutaneous MV repair less likely.

ADDITIONAL SPMC SERIES
The first clinical report on SPMC comes from Dang (16) who reported on six patients with SPMC. Five patients underwent successful repair with leaflet resection, reconstruction, and ring annuloplasty and one required replacement. The mean time from clip placement to surgery was 55.5 days ± 55 days. Four patients had clip malposition and two had insufficient MR reduction. Each clip was able to be removed without difficulty. As this series reported an earlier phase of the EVEREST I trial, the learning curve may explain the higher frequency of clip malposition as a cause of SPMC compared with more recent reports. Geidel (17) demonstrated a complex valve repair after failed MitraClip® utilizing Gore-Tex neochords (Ethicon, Somerville, NJ) and ring annuloplasty 32 days after clip deployment. Minimally invasive MV repair through a right thoracotomy has also been successfully reported after MitraClip® placement with clip removal and MV repair (11).

The largest published series comes from the phase I EVEREST I Feasibility trial and the EVEREST II roll-in phase reported by Argenziano (18). Of the 107 trial patients, 32 (30%) required surgical intervention at a median follow-up of 386 days performed by 24 different surgeons at 19 institutions. The indications for surgery are listed in Table 22.1 . Of those who had surgery 88% had preoperative degenerative MR. Of the 32 patients who underwent surgery, 21 (64%) had MV repair and 11 (34%) had MV replacement. Importantly, after deciding on the planned surgical procedure (repair or replacement), 87% (27/31, unknown in one case) successfully underwent the planned procedure. Sixteen percent (4/27) underwent MV replacement when a repair was planned. The conclusion of this report was that 84% of patients who underwent SPMC with a planned MV repair were

able to have MV repair. This provided some level of reassurance for MitraClip® since about five out of six patients who were expected to have a MV repair were still able to receive that repair despite a failed MitraClip® placement. Why the exceptional initial results (84%) in the non-randomized EVEREST I group were much higher than the randomized EVEREST II repair rate (54%) despite the same group of surgeons is unclear based on the small sample size. The indications for SPMC in the two trials are similar and do not yield an obvious explanation for the difference. There may have been subtle differences such as the type of valves being clipped, the number of clips, or length of time to surgical intervention all of which could have influenced the prospects for repair.

Bleiziffer (19) and colleagues do sound a note of caution in a paper presented at the 2011 AATS. They report on six patients after MitraClip® (6.7%, six of 90) who presented with severe symptomatic MR and atrial septal defect (ASD) with surgical indication after a median of 24 days. All patients were treated with replacement with four demonstrating iatrogenic injuries to the MV prohibiting repair. The authors make the point that repair may not always be possible and in this series it was 0%. This may have been due to the higher risk of these patients compared with the EVEREST trials. It is unknown what proportion of the cases were planned as MV repairs and were converted to MV replacement or whether all of them were planned only for MV replacement due to clinical circumstances. It is interesting to note that all of the six patients had off-label indications for MitraClip® use.

TECHNICAL CONSIDERATIONS
Based on the patient, the TEE and the surgeon's experience, a decision to repair the MV after MitraClip® placement should be made. The timing of surgery after MitraClip® should be made based on the patient's clinical condition. The approaches and techniques to MV repair are well described and are a routine aspect of surgical practice. If there was no attempt at Mitra-Clip® deployment then the operation proceeds in a standard fashion. There are advantages to performing the primary implant in a hybrid operating room in such a situation or if there is acute hemodynamic deterioration during MitraClip® placement. If MitraClip® deployment has occurred the first surgical task is removal of the clip while preserving as much of the MV leaflets and subvalvular apparatus as possible. The technique for clip removal is described in Figure 22.2. Removal is technically challenging in the presence of significant scarring and requires diligence.

Patients who have had a previous sternotomy (21% of the entire EVEREST II cohort) may be preferentially approached from a less invasive right thoracotomy by surgeons comfortable with this approach. This approach can avoid sternal adhesions or functioning bypass grafts, which increase the operative risk of reoperative MV surgery. One of the authors (DAH) has performed eight SPMC procedures through this approach with six MV repairs. A minimally invasive, right small thoracotomy

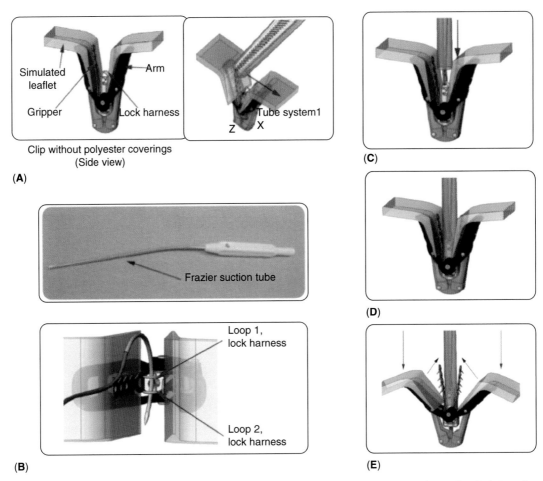

Figure 22.2 (**A**) Gripper lift technique. Pick up the tip of the gripper and raise it toward the center of the clip (red arrow direction). Once the gripper is raised, to the leaflet can be separated from the clip. (**B**) Clip unlock technique. Straighten the Frazier suction tube after the stylet has been removed. Use the needle end to pass the 2–0 suture (at least 30 cm long) through both loops of the lock harness. Remove the needle from the suture. (**C**) Use suction to assist advancing the 2–0 suture through the suction tube. Hold both ends of the suture, then advance the suction tube toward the clip. (**D**) Fully advance the suction tube into the clip while placing tension on sutures. The suture tension should unlock the clip. Clamp suture to maintain tension. (**E**) Using a blunt instrument, apply pressure (in the direction of red arrows) on atrial surface to open clip arms to approximately 90°. If the clip is difficult to open, squeeze the tips of arms together while maintaining suture tension and reapply pressure on atrial surface to open the clip arms to 90°. After opening the clip, lift the grippers (direction of blue arrows), extract the leaflet, and remove the clip. *Source:* Diagram courtesy of Abbott Vascular.

approach is a good option for those patients in need of a post clip MVP, and should be considered if the minimally invasive program is established and used for routine mitral repairs at the specific institution. As for reoperation, no data exist proving that it is a lower risk approach, but in the author's experience it can reduce the risk of injury to structures that would be at risk when approached through a prior sternotomy.

The benefit of the mini thoracotomy approach is best demonstrated by a clinical situation. An attempt to place the clip in a hybrid operating room was unsuccessful in an elderly male with functional MR. The clip procedure took five hours due to difficulty with deployment and release of the device. The patient had a heparin allergy and previous sternotomy for coronary bypass surgery. He was converted to emergent surgery

using a right mini-thoracotomy approach in the hybrid operating room. He had minimal pleural adhesions and required minimal pericardial dissection. An MV annuloplasty was performed using cardiopulmonary bypass and fibrillatory arrest. Although he did have a coagulopathy after bypass (INR = 13) and required transfusions for anticoagulation reversal, he did not suffer postoperative hemodynamic instability or any transfusion sequelae, for example acute respiratory distress syndrome or renal insufficiency. Had he had a redo sternotomy with major dissection of cardiac structures, bleeding after separation from bypass would likely have been more substantial and potentially fatal. Thus a mini-thoracotomy approach reduces tissue dissection, risk to previous grafts, and potentially avoids cross-clamping when a fibrillatory arrest approach is used which can be especially beneficial in patients with lower EF (20). The main contraindication to this approach would be aortic valve insufficiency greater than a mild degree.

An important technical point during surgery after SPMC is to look for ASD. The occurrence of an ASD post transseptal puncture is more likely as the entry site approaches the thinner tissue of the fossa ovalis and center of the atrial septum. If the puncture is near the lateral atrial wall, it is more likely to heal in the interim. The mini thoracotomy approach if preferred does allow a complete view of the atrial septum to identify and repair a residual ASD.

Technical factors that affect repair include the amount of involvement of scarring of the clip to the subvalvular apparatus. If many chords are scarred to the clip base, it is difficult, if not impossible, to repair, in our experience. Repair may also be more likely in cases of degenerative valve pathology, as frequently the leaflet tissue is excessive, and allows for resections and adjustments that cannot be safely performed in patients with functional valves that frequently have very thin small leaflets.

It is important to balance the risk of surgery with the actual benefit to the patient. While a MitraClip® procedure only addresses the MR, when traditional MV surgery is contemplated then concomitant coronary artery disease, aortic and tricuspid valve disease, and atrial fibrillation are also under consideration for correction. Indeed, 60% of all MV operations in the United States include either concomitant coronary artery bypass grafting (CABG) and/or aortic valve replacement (AVR) surgery (3). Thus, it is important to remember that the excellent results of the EVEREST II surgical arm (2% mortality) would not likely be duplicated if SPMC also included a high percentage of concomitant CABG and AVRs. Thus, it is critical to balance a surgical strategy of treating everything as opposed to treating the MR alone.

During planned concomitant AVR/MV repair, there are different surgical approaches depending on the situation. When we think there is a high likelihood of MV repair and there is no more than 1+ aortic insufficiency (AI), we perform the MV repair first and utilize a flexible annuloplasty band. This allows us to perform saline testing on the integrity of the MV repair. If there is more than 2+ AI, we may perform the AVR first and then proceed to the mitral repair which will allow saline testing now that the AI is fixed. Finally, if we believe that MV replacement is likely, we will remove the native aortic valve, then do the MV replacement, and then finish with the AVR. Concomitant CABG can be performed if indicated. Similar to others, we take an aggressive approach at the time of MV surgery toward concomitant tricuspid regurgitation, (21) atrial fibrillation, (22) and in patients without previous cardiac surgery, left atrial appendage removal (23). Active discussion between the surgeon and cardiologist(s) should guide the timing of surgery and the appropriate concomitant procedures at the time of SPMC. In general, if a MitraClip® outcome has not been successful, consideration should be given to early SPMC.

Consideration for MV replacement may be given based upon the preoperative TEE, anticipated complexity of MV repair, and

surgical experience; the clinical condition including age and comorbidities of the patient. If MV repair is not feasible in this higher risk group of patients then propensity-matched studies demonstrate that replacement has similar long-term survival to repair for degenerative MR (24). Chordal preserving bioprosthetic MVR is a reasonable choice for most patients who may have had a MitraClip® placement. Mechanical MVR may be a consideration in some patients depending on patient preference of whether a previous mechanical prosthesis is already in place. In our experience, in patients who have extensive leaflet destruction or when there was a significant degree of annular calcification present that we were less confident of the success of repair, we have not hesitated to proceed with replacement.

After removal of the clip, an accurate systematic assessment of the remainder of the valve leaflets is performed. There may be a small amount of leaflet tissue removed during the clip removal process in the region of the A2-P2 segment since the pathology is most commonly confined to this area in the patients enrolled with degenerative MR. These areas can be incorporated into standard quadrangular or triangular resection techniques of the anterior and/or posterior leaflets. The procedure would then be completed with a ring or band annuloplasty for which there are numerous choices according to surgical preference.

In cases of functional MR, it is generally the case that after successful clip removal, ring annuloplasty is sufficient. The surgeon would proceed with a standard functional mitral regurgitation (FMR) annuloplasty ring in their practice with consideration for rigid complete downsizing. It is interesting that in the U.S. component of the EVEREST trials there was a much higher enrollment of degenerative MR patients enrolled (73% in EVEREST II; 79% in EVEREST I and the roll-in EVEREST II registry). On the other hand, in the published European series, there is a much higher proportion of FMR patients as seen, for example, in an Italian series (25) (58%) from two leading centers and a single-institution German series (26) (69%). Indeed, almost 70% of the patients in the latter series would have been excluded from the EVEREST trials mainly due to LV dysfunction or severe abnormalities of the MV apparatus. The same group reported a 2.8% (six cases out of 215 patients implanted with MitraClip®) incidence of SPMC suggesting that with increasing implant experience the incidence of SPMC is reduced. MV repair was successful in four out of six patients with one death (27). There is a current National Institute of Health–sponsored clinical trial (clinical trials. gov identifier NCT00807040) that would be the first randomized trial in ischemic MR to determine optimal treatment: MV repair or replacement. This may help guide decision-making in the future for ischemic FMR patients and in SPMC for FMR.

Figure 22.3 illustrates an 82-year-old lady NYHA IV with severe FMR who had two clips placed. She had a one grade improvement in MR which disappeared within three months and she came to surgery in severe congestive heart failure despite maximal medical management. On intraoperative assessment, the clip had torn the anterior leaflet and surgical MVR with tricuspid valve repair, Maze procedure, and left atrial appendage amputation was performed. Similarly, in another 80-year-old with EF being 20% on inotropic support, it was felt that MVR was the more expeditious and safer procedure (Fig. 22.4). Finally, in one situation the clip had scarred into the chordae and papillary muscle that could not be safely removed without sacrificing the subvalvular apparatus and so MVR was performed. Each of these three patients tolerated the procedure without major complications.

Figure 22.5A demonstrates a case with two MitraClips® in place with persistent 3 to 4+ MR. During SPMC a posterior leaflet resection was performed (Fig 22.5B) with an annuloplasty band with excellent results.

CONCLUSION

The MitraClip® device is available in Europe after receiving CE Mark approval in 2008 and is under FDA consideration in the United States. As this device becomes more widespread in its use, surgeons will likely confront patients who need subsequent MV surgery after MitraClip® placement. It is important for surgeons, encountering patients with a MitraClip® who present for operation, to understand the technique for removing a MitraClip®. There are some suggestions that off-label use of the MitraClip® in Europe may make subsequent repair more difficult. Moreover, if the clinical application extends into younger or lower risk patients then the long-term impact of residual 2+ MR (27% in the EVEREST II MitraClip® group) may result in later MV surgery in a not insignificant number of patients. As a result, practical surgical strategies for dealing with this subset of patients will continue to evolve. It is likely

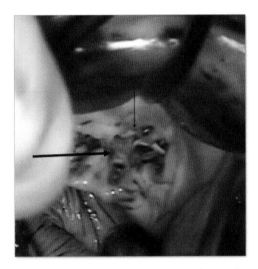

Figure 22.3 The operative view of MitraClip® attached to P2 of posterior leaflet that has torn off the anterior leaflet. Patient was treated with mitral valve replacement. Thick arrow = MitraClip® in place. Thin arrow = anterior leaflet tear.

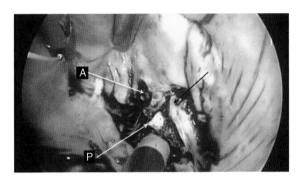

Figure 22.4 First clip demonstrates perforation of the anterior leaflet (A) and clip detached from the posterior leaflet (P). Arrows indicate the second clip attached to both leaflets.

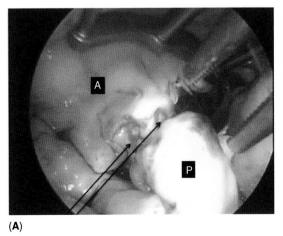

(A)

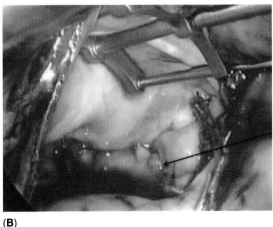

(B)

Figure 22.5 (A) Two MitraClips® (arrows) with attachment to anterior (A) and posterior (P) leaflets. (B) Posterior leaflet resection (arrow) and annuloplasty band repair after clip removal.

that these patients will benefit from being treated by experienced mitral repair surgeons to maximize their chance for a successful repair.

REFERENCES

1. Adams DH, Rosenhek R, Falk V. Degenerative mitral valve regurgitation: best practice revolution. Eur Heart J 2010; 31: 1958–67.
2. Moss RR, Humphries KH, Gao M, et al. Outcome of mitral valve repair or replacement: a comparison by propensity score analysis. Circulation 2003; 108: II–90.
3. Gammie JS, Sheng S, Griffith BP, et al. trends in mitral valve surgery in the United States: results from the society of thoracic surgeons adult cardiac database. Ann Thor Surg 2009; 87: 1431–9.
4. Gillinov AM, Cosgrove DM, Blackstone EH, et al. Durability of mitral valve repair for degenerative disease. J Thorac Cardiovasc Surg 1998; 116: 734–43.
5. Wu AH, Aaronson KD, Bolling SF, et al. Impact of mitral valve annuloplasty on mortality risk in patients with mitral regurgitation and left ventricular systolic dysfunction. J Am Coll Cardiol 2005; 45: 381–7.
6. Zegdi R, Sleilaty G, Latremouille C, et al. Reoperation for failure of mitral valve repair in degenerative disease: a single center experience. Ann Thorac Surg 2008; 86: 1480–4.
7. Suri RM, Schaff HV, Dearani JA, et al. Recurrent mitral regurgitation after repair: should the mitral valve be re-repaired? J Thorac Cardiovasc Surg 2006; 132: 1390–7.
8. Bach DS, Awais M, Gurm HS, Kohnstamm S. Failure of guideline adherence for intervention in patients with severe mitral regurgitation. J Am Coll Cardiol 2009; 54: 860–5.
9. Chikwe J, Goldstone AB, Passage J, et al. A propensity score-adjusted retrospective comparison of early and mid-term results of mitral valve repair versus replacement in octogenarians. Eur Heart J 2011; 32: 618–26.
10. Feldman T, Foster E, Glower DG, et al. Percutaneous repair or surgery for mitral regurgitation. New Engl J Med 2011; 364: 1395–406.
11. Rogers JH, Yeo KK, Carroll JD, et al. Late surgical mitral valve repair after percutaneous repair with the MitraClip® system. J Card Surg 2009; 24: 677–81.
12. Glower D, Ailawadi G, Argenziano M, et al. EVEREST II randomized clinical trial: predictors of mitral valve replacement in de novo surgery or after the MitraClip® procedure. J Thorac Cardiovasc Surg. 2012; 143(4 Suppl): S60–3.
13. Bolling SF, Li S, O'Brien SM, et al. Predictors of mitral valve repair: clinical and surgeon factors. Ann Thorac Surg 2010; 90: 1904–12.
14. Gillinov AM, Blackstone EH, Nowicki ER, et al. Valve repair versus valve replacement for degenerative mitral valve disease. J Thorac Cardiovasc Surg 2008; 135: 885–93.
15. David TE, Ivanov J, Armstrong S, Christie D, Rakowski H. A comparison of outcomes of mitral valve repair for degenerative disease with posterior, anterior, and bileaflet prolapse. J Thorac Cardiovasc Surgery 2005; 130: 1242–9.
16. Dang NC, Aboodi MS, Sakaguchi T, et al. Surgical revision after percutaneous mitral valve repair with a clip: initial multicenter experience. Ann Thorac Surg 2005; 80: 2338–42.
17. Geidel S, Ostermeyer J, Lass M, Schmoekel M. Complex surgical valve repair after failed percutaneous mitral intervention using the MitraClip® device. Ann Thorac Surg 2010; 90: 277–9.
18. Argenziano M, Skipper E, Heimansohn D, et al. Surgical revision after percutaneous mitral repair with the MitraClip® device. Ann Thorac Surg 2010; 89: 72–80.
19. Bleiziffer S, Stroh K, Gunther T, Voss B, Lange R. Does mitral valve clipping affect the opportunity for a subsequent valve repair. Presented at the American Association for Thoracic Surgery Meeting. 2011.
20. Umakanthan R, Leacche M, Petracek MR, et al. Safety of minimally invasive mitral valve surgery without aortic cross-clamp. Ann Thorac Surg 2008; 85: 1544–50.
21. Calafiore AM, Gallina S, Iaco AL, et al. Mitral Valve Surgery for Functional Mitral Regurgitation: Should Moderate-or-More Tricuspid Regurgitation Be Treated? A Propensity Score Analysis. Ann Thorac Surg 2009; 87: 698–703.
22. Melo J, Santaigo T, Aguiar C, et al. Surgery for atrial fibrillation in patient with mitral valve disease: results at five years from the international registry of atrial fibrillation surgery. J Thorac Cardiovasc Surg 2008; 135: 863–9.
23. Chatterjee S, Alexander JC, Pearson PJ, Feldman T. Left atrial appendage occlusion: lessons learned from surgical and transcatheter experiences. Ann Thorac Surg 2011; 92: 2283–92.
24. Gillinov AM, Blackstone EH, Nowicki ER, et al. Valve repair versus valve replacement for degenerative mitral valve disease. J Thorac Cardiovasc Surg 2008; 135: 885–93.
25. Tamburino C, Ussia GP, Maisano F, et al. Percutaneous mitral valve repair with the MitraClip® system: acute results from real world setting. Eur Heart J 2010; 31: 1382–9.
26. Franzen O, Baldus S, Rudolph V, et al. Acute outcomes of MitraClip® therapy for mitral regurgitation in high-surgical risk patients: Emphasis on adverse valve morphology and severe left ventricular dysfunction. Eur Heart J 2010; 31: 1373–81.
27. Conradi L, Treede H, Franzen O, et al. Impact of MitraClip® therapy on secondary mitral valve surgery in patients at high surgical risk. Eur J Cardiothorac Surg 2011; 40: 1521–8.

23 Gross and histologic findings after MitraClip® placement
Elena Ladich, Masataka Nakano, and Renu Virmani

INTRODUCTION

Mitral regurgitation (MR) affects 2–2.5 million people in the United States and is expected to rise to 4.8 million by 2030 because of population aging and growth (1). The most common causes of surgical MR in western countries are degenerative (DMR) including primary myxomatous disease, primary flail leaflets, and mitral annular calcification (60–70% of cases) followed by ischemic/functional MR (FMR) accounting for 20%. Other causes, including rheumatic disease, endocarditis, and collagen vascular diseases comprise the remainder (2).

In 1972, Perloff and Roberts proposed the concept of the mitral valvular complex emphasizing the integrated relationships between the mitral leaflets, chordae, annulus, and subvalvular apparatus including papillary muscles and left ventricle (3). Derangements in one or more of the components of the mitral valve complex may lead to MR. However, the primary disease mechanisms and cardiac pathology underpinning DMR and FMR are fundamentally different.

In DMR, the disease results from myxomatous changes in the mitral leaflets. A spectrum of pathologic changes has been observed in myxomatous degeneration of the mitral valve. In mild cases, the posterior mitral leaflet (usually the middle scallop) demonstrates myxoid thickening, increased length, and mild prolapse. In the more severe form, all scallops of the posterior mitral leaflet (PML) are involved with or without involvement of the anterior mitral leaflet (AML). Myxoid degeneration, valve thickening, and elongation are substantially more pronounced in severe cases (4). Histologically, there is expansion of the leaflet spongiosa layer by proteoglycans often with disruption of the collagenous fibrosa and ventricularis layers. Further, the normal pattern of chordal insertion is often effaced; chordae insert chaotically, producing poor leaflet support.

In contrast, chronic ischemic MR results from coronary artery disease with scarring of the left ventricle with resultant papillary muscle displacement and mitral annular dilatation. Papillary muscle displacement exerts traction on non-extensible chordae resulting in tethering and apically displaced leaflets (tenting), which leads to loss of coaptation and functional MR. Mitral leaflet morphology, however, is normal.

TREATMENT

Mitral valve repair is the procedure of choice for patients with MR because of the low perioperative mortality, improved survival, better preservation of postoperative left ventricular function, and lower long-term morbidity compared with valve replacement (5).

Mitral valve repair techniques include segmental valve resection, often accompanied by an annuloplasty ring, artificial chordae, and Alfieri edge-to-edge repair.

Percutaneous mitral valve repair techniques are attractive because they offer less invasive alternatives to surgery for the treatment of MR. Currently, a number of percutaneous therapies specifically developed for the mitral valves are in early stages of clinical practice or in clinical trials (6). The majority of these are modifications of surgical techniques already in use. The MitraClip® is a percutaneous approach that mimics the surgical repair technique of Alfieri for the treatment of functional and degenerative MR (7). The device is placed on the central portion of the anterior and posterior leaflets providing leaflet coaptation resulting in a double orifice. Over a period, the MitraClip® creates a fibrous tissue bridge between the two leaflets, potentially increasing the durability of the repair.

Although mitral valve repair techniques have advantages over surgical replacement, it may be reasonably anticipated that repaired mitral valves, whether employing percutaneous or surgical techniques, may require reoperation. Up to 10% of patients who undergo mitral valve repair will require late reoperation for recurrent mitral valve dysfunction (8). In a recent pathology study by our laboratory analyzing explanted Mitra-Clips®, 50 out of 337 patients were explanted and converted to surgery over a five-year period (9). In fact, the MitraClip® was designed to allow for device explant and conversion to surgical mitral valve repair or replacement if required.

Pathologic analysis of explanted devices removed at reoperation or autopsy provides an important opportunity to study the tissue reactions between the host and implanted device. This chapter provides an overview of gross and histologic findings observed in implanted MitraClip® devices and briefly summarizes relevant pathologic observations described for other types of implanted valvular devices.

DEVICE DESCRIPTION

The MitraClip® device (Fig. 23.1A) is a 4 mm-wide polyester covered "V" shaped cobalt–chromium device with two arms that open and close. The device arms can coapt up to 8 mm of each mitral leaflet—anterior and posterior—securing the leaflet tissue between an arm and a gripper. After a grasp, confirming good leaflet insertion and a functioning double orifice valve, the device is fully closed, locked, and detached from the MitraClip® delivery system. As a function of device positioning, the device is exposed to both the atrial and ventricular blood flow (Figs. 23.1B and 23.1C). To promote leaflet to leaflet healing and long-term tissue ingrowth the device is covered with a polyester fabric.

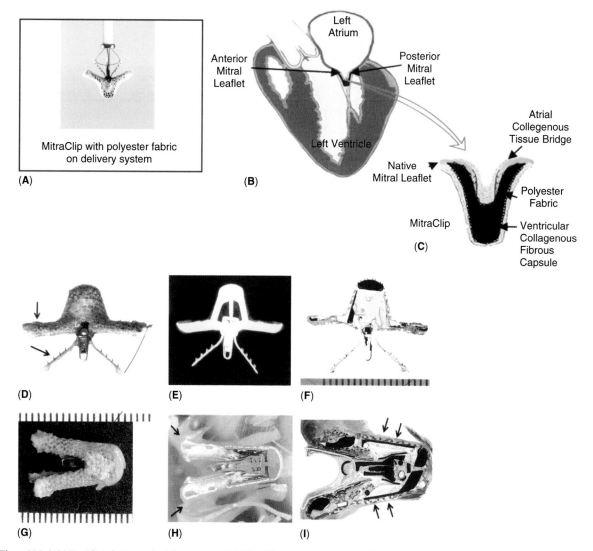

Figure 23.1 (**A**) MitraClip® device on the delivery system. (**B**) MitraClip® device placement within the mitral valve structure in the left ventricle. (**C**) Illustration of the tissue healing response around the device explant. (**D–I**) MitraClip® device in the open position with the arms (red arrow) retracted away from the leaflet grippers (black arrow) (**D**). Radiographic image (**E**) and photomicrographs of the histologic section (**F**). MitraClip® device in the closed position (**G**). Methacrylate-embedded device bisected in the sagittal plane with secured native leaflet tissue on either side (arrows) (**H**) and photomicrograph of the histologic section (**I**). Arrows indicate areas of fibrous capsule thickness measurements. Outlined yellow area between arms indicates tissue bridge area measurement. *Source:* From Ref. 9.

PRECLINICAL STUDIES

The MitraClip® was first tested in the porcine model prior to use in humans (10). The morphologic findings of excised Mitra-Clips® in pigs were studied at time intervals ranging from 4 to 52 weeks and largely predicted the histopathologic response later reported in human cases. As early as 4 weeks post implantation there was neointimal tissue growth on both surfaces of the device, confirmed by scanning electron microscopy. By 24 weeks, tissue formation was further developed with a tissue bridge connecting the two arms of the device (Fig. 23.2).

Interestingly, 71% of the pigs showed incorporation of adjacent chordae tendineae by tissue growth, similar to contact of chordae following prosthetic mitral valve replacement.

GROSS AND HISTOLOGIC ANALYSIS OF RETRIEVED HUMAN IMPLANTS AT SURGERY

Over a five-year period, 67 devices from 50 patients were explanted and submitted for histologic evaluation to our laboratory. Descriptive analysis as well as semiquantitative scoring of the cellular response were performed and reported

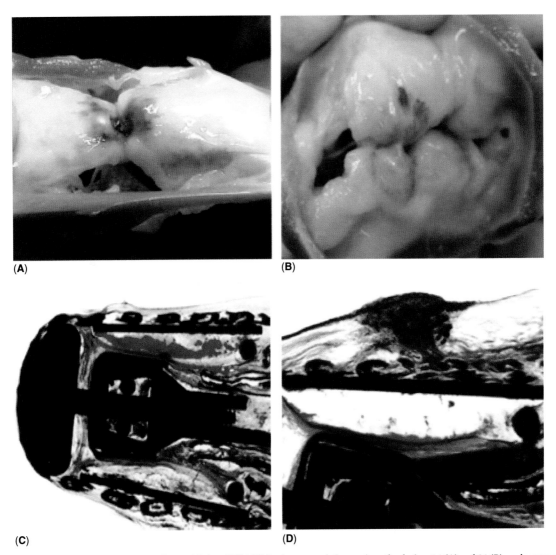

(A)

(B)

(C)

(D)

Figure 23.2 Gross and histologic images, porcine model. A and B highlight tissue growth (pannus) on the device at 4 (A) and 24 (B) weeks respectively. B shows nicely a tissue bridge formed between the two leaflets and the arms of the clip. Histological appearance of tissue growth in clip excised at 4 (C) and 24 weeks (D). At 4 weeks there is a thin layer of new fibrous tissue growth onto the fabric and device. (Stain H&E 2.5x) The tissue is thicker at 24 weeks and is composed of mature collagenous tissue (H&E 5x). *Source*: Reproduced with permission from Ref. 10.

as 0 = absent, 1 = mild, 2 = moderate, and 3 = severe. Collagen deposition was scored as 0 = absent, 1 = predominantly early collagen (type III), 2 = moderate maturity (type III to type I), and 3 = predominantly type 1. In cases where native valve tissue was present, leaflet tissue was also submitted for analysis. The number and reasons for device explantation are delineated by time frame in Table 23.1. As expected, the healing response varies based on implant duration and between individuals. A summary of the semiquantitative analysis of the cellular response is provided in Table 23.2.

Analysis of Surgically Explanted MitraClips®

The devices were analyzed in four time intervals (<30 days, 31–90 days, 91–300 days, and >301 days). By 30 days, the majority of devices showed some degree of pannus formation around the polyester cover. Initially, a thin layer of fibrin and platelets was present around the polyester fabric followed by the development of loosely organized connective tissue (Fig. 23.3). Neutrophils predominated in the first few days with a mixed chronic inflammatory cell infiltrate and scattered multinucleated giant cells around polyester cloth

Table 23.1 Patient Demographics of the MitraClip® Device Histologic Explant Cohort

	0–30 Days N = 7	31–90 Days N = 15[a]	91–300 Days N = 12[a]	>300 Days N = 16
Age in yrs (mean)	61.57 ± 13.8	61.67 ± 13.3	69.18 ± 14.1	61.94 ± 13.0
Percent male	57%	33%	36%	44%
>65 yrs	57%	52%	77%	56%
NYHA class III or IV	45%	33%	46%	37%
Etiology: DMR	86%	73%	92%	81%
Etiology: FMR	14%	27%	8%	19%
Reason for explant	7 residual MRs	7 Residual MRs 6 recurrent MRs 2 clinical symptoms	3 Residual MRs 5 recurrent MRs 4 clinical symptoms	3 Residual MRs 8 recurrent MRs 4 clinical symptoms 1 other surgery
Surgical outcome repair/replace	3/3[b]	8/7	7/5	10/6

[a]Patients with 2 devices implanted at 2 distinct time points were assigned to the longer implant duration interval. [b]One patient died during surgery.
Abbreviations: DMR, degenerative mitral regurgitation; FMR, functional mitral regurgitation; NYHA, New York Heart Association.*Source*: From Ref. 9.

Table 23.2 Assessment of the Cellular Response to the MitraClip® Device over the Four Explant Time Periods

Implant Duration (Days)	Devices Analyzed	Inflammatory Response Score		Fibrin Deposition Score	Granulation Tissue Score	Collagen Deposition Scorea	Ca++ Score	Fibrous Capsule Thickness (mm) 38 Devices	Tissue Bridge (mm2) 25 Devices
		Acute	Chronic						
0–30	n = 7	0.9 ± 1.1	1.0 ± 0.8	1.0 ± 0.6	0	0	0	0	0
31–90	n = 23	0.2 ± 0.7	1.7 ± 0.8	2.1 ± 1.0	1.6 ± 0.9	1.0 ± 0.6	0	0.25 ± 0.3	4.93 ± 2.7
91–300	n = 18	0	1.9 ± 0.9	0.9 ± 1.0	2.2 ± 1.0	2.5 ± 0.7	0	0.26 ± 0.2	5.83 ± 4.0
>300	n = 19	0	2.3 ± 0.6	0.6 ± 0.6	1.7 ± 0.8	2.6 ± 0.7	0	0.40 ± 0.3	7.39 ± 4.3

[a]Assessed by H&E staining and confirmed with Sirius Red in 3 samples.*Source*: From Ref. 9.

bundles present at later time-points. By 90 days, there was generally greater tissue coverage around the polyester cover and several devices demonstrated tissue bridges; in two patients a measurable tissue bridge was already present by days 41 and 54, respectively. Histologically, early collagen formation was seen focally covering the fabric intermingled with granulation tissue (Fig. 23.4). Between 91 and 300 days, fibrous encapsulation was more developed with complete fibrous encapsulation of several devices and tissue bridges observed in nearly half of the devices (Fig. 23.5). Several long-term explants (301–1878 days) demonstrated extensive tissue bridges completely incorporating the atrial surfaces of the anterior and posterior leaflets (Fig. 23.6). Histologically, fibrous tissue was composed predominantly of mature type I collagen, demonstrating maturation of collagen types over time. There was focal residual granulation tissue predominantly around the inner mechanical components but less than that observed at earlier time-points.

Differential rates of healing were noted histologically between the ventricular and atrial aspects of the device. As early as 30 days, loosely organized connective tissue was observed on the atrial aspect between the gripper arms. Overall the ventricular aspect demonstrated much less collagen deposition as observed at 31–90 days. This delay likely results from a greater turbulent flow in the left ventricle producing higher shear forces on the ventricular aspect of the device.

Analysis of Long-Term Autopsy Case (356 Days)

Grossly, the specimen consisted of an excised mitral valve with intact leaflets and surrounding atrioventricular myocardium. The anterior and posterior leaflets were connected with a single MitraClip® incorporated with smooth fibrous tissue growth resulting in an orifice on each side of the clip (Fig. 23.7). Histologically, there was complete incorporation of the polyester fabric by collagen-rich tissue growth that was continuous with the native leaflet surfaces as well as coverage around the insertion site of adjacent chordae tendineae, findings similar to those previously reported in the porcine model (Fig. 23.8). Areas around the internal components were filled with granulation tissue and chronic inflammatory cells with multinucleated giant cells within the polyester fabric bundles, an expected response to a foreign material (Fig. 23.9). Overall, the fibrous encapsulation of the device was consistent with the duration of implantation and similar to pathologic findings observed in the surgically explanted long-term MitraClip® explants.

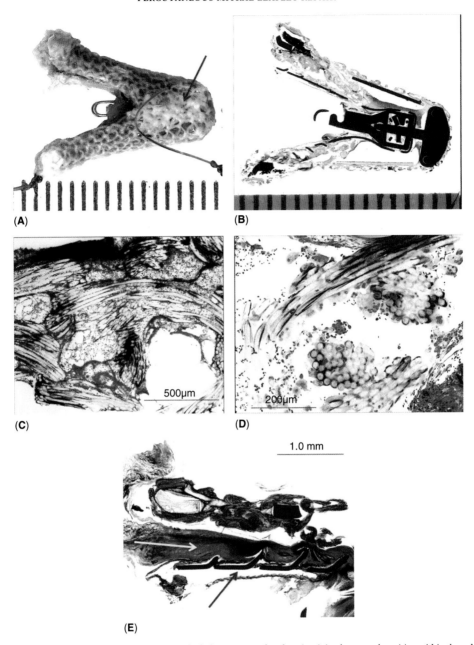

Figure 23.3 Acute explant group (<30 days): (A) Gross image, which demonstrates that there is minimal pannus deposition within the polyester fabric (red arrow) and (B) photomicrograph of the histologic section of a MitraClip® device explanted after 16 days. High magnification of the histologic section reveals unorganized fibrin deposition around the polyester bundles (C), and chronic macrophage and giant cell infiltration surrounding the polyester bundles (D). (E) Photomicrograph of the histologic section of native mitral valve leaflet inserted between the arm and gripper elements of the device (yellow arrow); the leaflet tissue is held firmly in place by the frictional elements of the gripper (red arrow). *Source*: From Ref. 9.

In summary, the gross and microscopic examination of Mitra-Clips® explanted at different time intervals provides insights into the pathologic changes that may occur serially over time up to five years. The first phase of platelet/fibrin deposition is enhanced in the case of the MitraClip® by the presence of the woven polyester fabric, which surrounds the gripper arms, legs, and the threaded stud (Fig. 23.1). Fibrin deposition and inflammation enable formation of granulation tissue, and eventually collagen-rich fibrous tissue. The degree of encapsulation seen on gross and histologic examination depended on the duration of the implant, while taking into consideration physiologic healing variability and the artifactual loss of tissue during surgical explant.

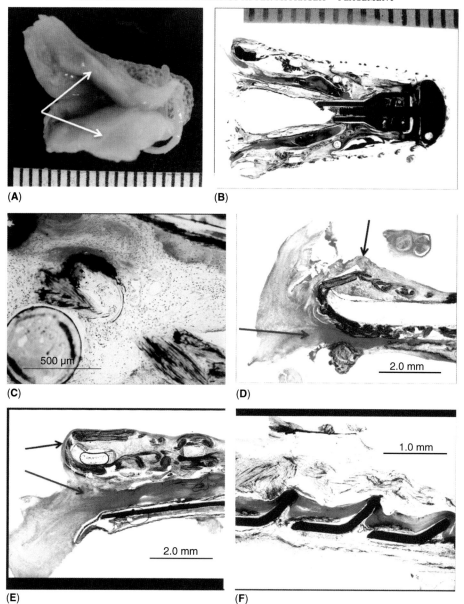

Figure 23.4 Subacute explant group (31–90 days). (A) Gross image demonstrating native mitral leaflet within the device (arrows) and (B) photomicrograph of the histologic section of a MitraClip® device explanted after 44 days. High magnification of the histologic section reveals (C), early organizing granulation tissue around the inner device components; (D, E) native leaflet between the arm and gripper components of the device (red arrows) with organized fibrous tissue outgrowth covering the outer arm surfaces (black arrows); (F) native mitral leaflet tissue inserted between the arm and gripper elements of the device held firmly in place by the frictional elements of the gripper. *Source*: From Ref. 9.

TISSUE BRIDGE

Over time, the tissue ingrowth increased between the arms of the device, resulting in the formation of a tissue bridge as was previously described in the porcine model (10). Interestingly, a similar tissue bridge was reported at autopsy by Privatera et al. in a 64-year-old male (11). In that case, a double orifice separated by a thick smooth surfaced tissue bridge connecting the anterior and posterior leaflets had formed four years after a successful Alfieri stitch repair.

It has been postulated that the MitraClip's® fibrous capsule and tissue bridge offload hemodynamic forces on the device over time. The tissue bridge coapting the two gripper arms and fibrous "transition zones" of organized dense collagen is continuous with the native leaflets thus providing structural

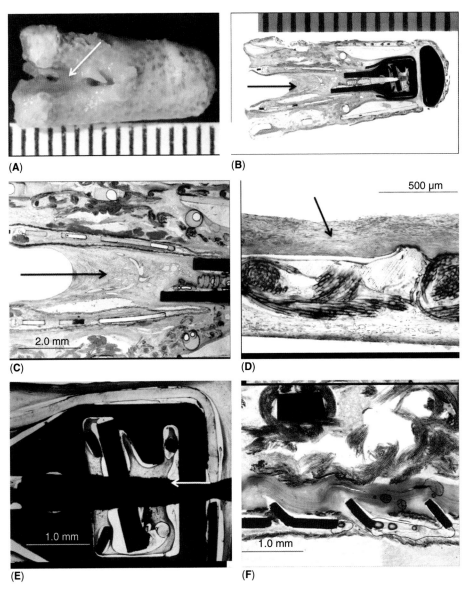

Figure 23.5 Chronic explant group (91–300 day). (A) Gross image demonstrating fibrous tissue bridging the area between the device arms (atrial tissue bridge, arrow), and (B) photomicrograph of the histologic section of a MitraClip® device explanted after 283 days demonstrating the tissue bridge (arrows). High magnification of the histologic section (C–F) reveals the tissue bridge between the device arms (C); organized fibrous capsule covering the outer arm surface (arrow) (D); fibrous tissue filling the areas within the internal device components (arrow) (E); and native mitral leaflet tissue inserted between the arm and gripper elements of the device held firmly in place by the frictional elements of the gripper arm. *Source:* From Ref. 9.

support to the double orifice. Over time, type III collagen is replaced by type I which cross links thereby stabilizing the transition zone in response to stress (12). This mature collagen does not appear to impede the ability to surgically dissect and repair the native leaflet tissue (13). Furthermore, since healing around the MitraClip® is limited to the device itself (fibrous capsule and tissue bridge) albeit with variable extension onto the mitral

scallop and adjacent chordae, we believe that treatment failures (persistence or return of MR) are not related to device healing per se but are more likely attributed to patient characteristics; for example, complex patient anatomy such as coexisting mitral annular dilatation and/or variability in chordal insertions, severity of degenerative disease, disease progression in DMR, or failure to address the primary disease in FMR.

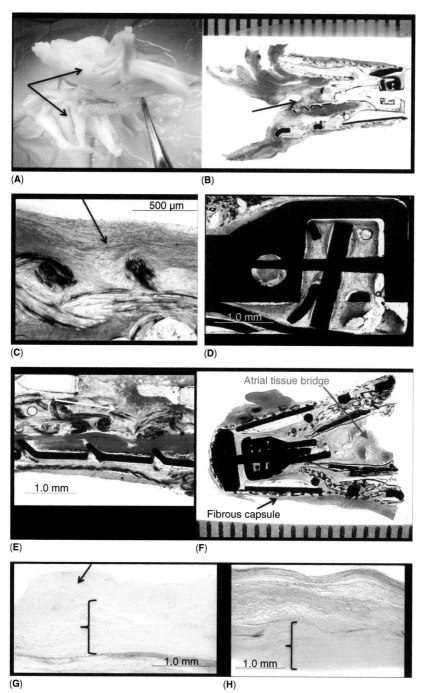

Figure 23.6 Long-term explant group (>300 days). (A) Gross image demonstrating native mitral leaflet tissue secured within the device arms (arrows) and (B) photomicrograph of the histologic section of a MitraClip® device explanted after 359 days demonstrating the fibrous outgrowth from the native leaflet bridging the area between the arms (atrial tissue bridge, arrow). High magnification of the histologic section (C–F) reveals organized fibrous capsule covering the outer arm surface (arrow) (C); fibrous tissue growth within the internal device components (arrow) (D); native leaflet tissue inserted between the arm and gripper elements of the device held firmly in place and secured in place by the frictional elements of the gripper (E); the difference between the atrial tissue bridge and ventricular fibrous capsule is delineated (F). (G–F) High magnification of the histologic section of native mitral leaflet demonstrates the expansion of the spongiosal layer from myxomatous tissue (arrow) ({) (G) and there is marked thickening of the ventricular surface with collagen ({) (H). *Source*: From Ref. 9.

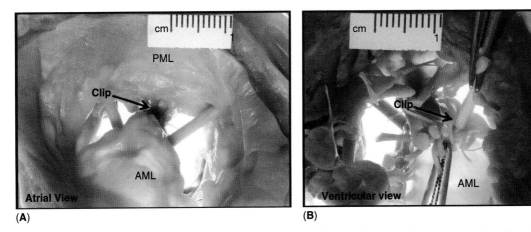

(A)   **(B)**

Figure 23.7 Autopsy case, gross images. (A, B) Mitral valve with surrounding myocardial tissue showing atrial and ventricular views of the clipped leaflets. The atrial view shows close apposition of mid-leaflet points leaving patent flow channels on either side of the clip (arrow). The valve orifices on either side of the clip are being propped open to illustrate double orifice.

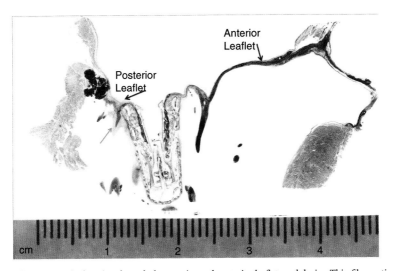

Figure 23.8 Autopsy case. Whole mount sagittal section through the anterior and posterior leaflets and device. Thin fibrous tissue coverage is shown here between device arms mitral leaflets. There was focal incorporation of chordal structure adjacent to the device (red arrow). Note calcification in posterior mitral annulus (black nodules).

NATIVE LEAFLET TISSUE

Thirty-five patients had sufficient leaflet tissue retained in at least one arm of the MitraClip® device to allow histopathologic review. There was no inflammatory reaction or obvious degradation of the leaflet tissue, with the exception of mild atrophy noted in rare leaflets. Fibrous tissue "transition zones" were clearly demarcated in the sections of two long-term devices. These transition zones originated from the native leaflet tissue and formed a fibrous capsule over the MitraClip®. The transition zones were composed of intact, organized collagen that became continuous with the native leaflet.

Five devices were submitted with native valve tissue remote from the device. All histologic sections of the native leaflets showed myxomatous expansion of the spongiosa with fibro-elastic thickening on both the atrial and ventricular surfaces (Fig. 23.6G and 23.6H).

FMR VERSUS DMR

Interestingly, there were no significant differences in healing between the FMR and DMR groups with the exception of fibrous capsule thickness and tissue bridge areas in the long-term group (>300 days) which showed greater tissue growth in

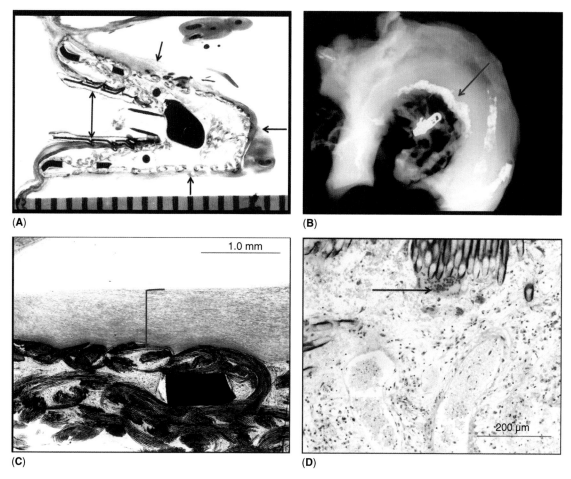

Figure 23.9 Autopsy case. (A) Photomicrograph of the histologic section of the MitraClip® demonstrating complete fibrous tissue incorporation of the outer surface and between the arms. (B) Radiograph (superior view). Clip is in the center of the leaflets. The posterior leaflet annulus shows heavy calcification (red arrow). (C) Well-organized smooth muscle cell and collagen-rich tissue growth covering the outer arm. (D) Granulation tissue filling the inner areas of the device composed of a loose collagen matrix with angiogenesis, chronic inflammation, and giant cell reaction to the fabric (black arrow).

FMR compared with DMR (Table 23.3). The reasons for greater tissue growth in the FMR group are not completely understood and deserve further study. Previous pathologic studies analyzing prosthetic heart valve explants have highlighted chronic inflammation, turbulent blood flow, valve orifice area, endocarditis, and surgical technique as contributors to neointimal growth (14).

GENERAL HEALING MECHANISMS

The pathologic changes observed following placement of the MitraClip® device are comparable to those observed around the sewing ring of a bioprosthetic heart valves or annuloplasty rings at the prosthesis-tissue interface (Fig. 23.10). In bioprosthetic heart valves, host tissue growth typically forms at the interfaces of the native tissues with the Dacron polyester covering the prosthetic sewing ring (15). Luk et al. recently characterized the pathologic response of 39 annuloplasty rings removed at the time of reoperation (16). A host tissue response (pannus) was found on the synthetic material on the surface of the ring and was identified as early as 29 days post implantation. Further it was demonstrated that up to one year, pannus growth was essentially limited to the sewing ring. Pannus growth, which extended onto the leaflet tissue itself occurred one year after repair suggesting that over time an inflammatory reaction is initiated with pannus growth at the site of the ring followed by growth onto the leaflet tissue.

Tissue healing follows a characteristic sequence of events in virtually all types of cardiac prosthetic devices following implantation. Early after deployment, there is platelet-fibrin deposition and acute inflammation. This is followed by chronic

Table 23.3 Histological Healing Response to the MitraClip®
Stratified by Etiology of Mitral Regurgitation

Implant Duration (Days)	Fibrous Capsule Thickness (mm)			Tissue Bridge (mm²)		
	DMR	FMR	P value	DMR	FMR	P value
31–90	0.13 ± 0.06	0.38 ± 0.47	0.35	4.0 ± 1.1	6.8 ± 4.9	0.82
91–300	0.26 ± 0.24	NAª	NAª	5.8 ± 4.0	NAª	NAª
> 300	0.31 ± 0.17	0.74 ± 0.29	0.043	5.2 ± 1.9	11.9 ± 0.1	0.037

ªNo specimens were available for measurements because of surgical disruption.*Abbreviations*: DMR, degenerative mitral regurgitation; FMR, functional mitral regurgitation.
Source: From Ref. (9).

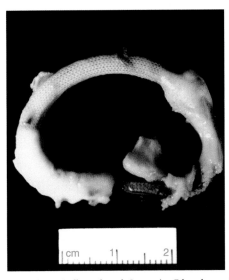

Figure 23.10 (**A**) Surgically explanted Carpentier–Edwards annuloplasty ring at 9 months. Note variable pannus formation around Dacron sewing ring. Identical tissue formation is seen forming around the polyester cover of MitraClips® at similar time-points.

inflammation, granulation tissue with smooth muscle cell/fibroblast infiltration, and proteoglycan-collagen (17,18). In addition, it has been proposed that the sewing ring induces a chronic inflammatory response to the foreign material characterized by a persistent macrophage reaction with recruitment of cells such as fibroblasts and smooth muscle cells causing a gradual thickening of the fibro muscular tissue over the cloth surface (16) (Fig. 23.11).

CLINICAL AND PATHOLOGIC PERSPECTIVES
Some investigators have reported failure of annuloplasty rings leading to clinical symptoms of mitral stenosis due to excessive

pannus formation originating from the annuloplasty ring (19,20). Over time, given the increased tissue growth around the MitraClip® device and formation of a tissue bridge between the two leaflets, the development of mitral stenosis might be of concern. Hermann et al. followed 18 patients after MitraClip® implantation and found no evidence of clinically significant mitral stenosis either immediately after device deployment or at 12 months follow-up (21). Clinical and pathologic data were collected from 50 patients studied by our laboratory for up to a maximum time-point of 5.1 years following MitraClip® implantation; no case of mitral stenosis due to device implantation has been documented thus far.

Additionally, it is well known that 20–30% of aortic bioprosthetic valves become dysfunctional in 10 years, through progressive structural deterioration. This rate is even higher in the mitral position (22). The reasons for accelerated failure are not completely understood but may relate to the higher closing pressures in the mitral position. The major mechanism underlying structural valve deterioration is calcification; calcific deposits may develop in the leaflets and/or neointimal tissue growth. In light of the risk of calcific failure for implanted valvular devices, it is important to note that none of the MitraClips® examined in our study showed gross or histologic evidence of calcification.

Another condition that can cause valves to fail is infective endocarditis. It has been reported to occur in 3–6% of patients receiving prosthetic valves, its incidence being lower in the mitral position as compared with the aortic position and is associated with greater than 30–80% mortality (23). Although it has been reported that MV repair has a decreased risk of infective endocarditis compared with MV replacement, the risk for patients with MV repair is still of concern (24). Notably, none of the explanted MitraClips® analyzed in our study demonstrated vegetative growths or histologic evidence of infective endocarditis.

CONCLUSION
The MitraClip® is an innovative percutaneous technology used to treat MR, which for decades has been treated through either surgical repair or replacement. There was long-term encapsulation of the device with formation of a tissue bridge increasing the stability of the device and mechanical integrity was maintained for up to five years. Clinically, in the vast majority of patients there was an observed reduction in MR. The recurrence of MR however, early or late after implantation deserves further study. The long-term durability of this percutaneous approach for the treatment of MR has not been established and requires additional study. Continued left ventricular remodeling and papillary muscle displacement in FMR add to the pathologic burden over time and severe degenerative disease remains a challenge. Future studies and longer-term follow-up will establish which disease etiologies and valve morphologies are likely to benefit the most, which is dependent on both clinical and morphologic factors, in particular the unique pathophysiologic anatomy of individual patients.

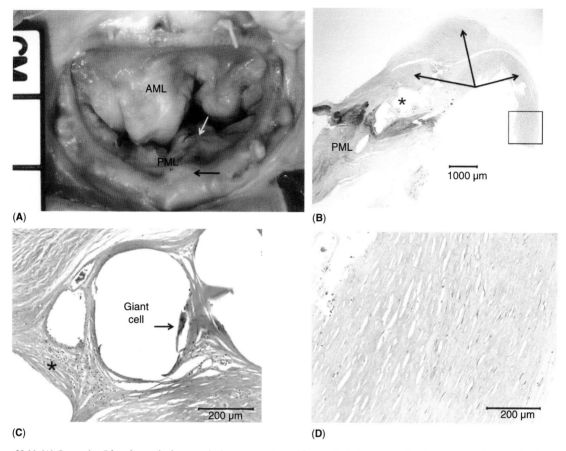

Figure 23.11 (A) Carpentier–Edwards annuloplasty repair ring seen at autopsy. The annuloplasty ring was placed seven years prior to death. Note marked thickening of both anterior mitral leaflet and posterior mitral leaflet (PML). Note row of blue valvuloplasty sutures (yellow arrow) in the PML. Fibrous pannus coats the ring with focal extension onto leaflets. Histologic section was taken from the ring adjacent to the PML (black arrow). (B) Low power Movat stained section shows fibrous tissue growth (black arrows) which had formed around the ring. The black asterisk denotes suture spaces. Note extension of fibrous tissue growth onto the PML. (C). Focal mild chronic inflammation (asterisk) and giant cell (H&E 20x). (D) Higher magnification of boxed inset in B highlights mature dense collagen-rich tissue growth (Movat 40x). Gross and histologic findings in the repaired mitral valve are comparable to those observed in long-term MitraClips®.

REFERENCES

1. Nkomo VT, Gardin JM, Skelton TN, et al. Burden of valvular heart diseases: a population-based study. Lancet 2006; 368: 1005–11.
2. Enriquez-Sarano M, Akins CW, Vahanian A. Mitral regurgitation. Lancet 2009; 373: 1382–94.
3. Perloff JK, Roberts WC. The mitral apparatus. functional anatomy of mitral regurgitation. Circulation 1972; 46: 227–39.
4. Duren DR, Becker AE, Dunning AJ. Long-term follow-up of idiopathic mitral valve prolapse in 300 patients: a prospective study. J Am Coll Cardiol 1988; 11: 42–7.
5. Bonow RO, Carabello BA, Kanu C, et al. Acc/aha 2006 guidelines for the management of patients with valvular heart disease: a report of the american college of cardiology/american heart association task force on practice guidelines (writing committee to revise the 1998 guidelines for the management of patients with valvular heart disease): developed in collaboration with the society of cardiovascular anesthesiologists: endorsed by the society for cardiovascular angiography and interventions and the society of thoracic surgeons. Circulation 2006; 114: e84–231.
6. Perlowski A, St Goar F, Glower DG, et al. Percutanenous therapies for mitral regurgitation. Curr Probl Cardiol 2012; 37: 42–68.
7. Alfieri O, Maisano F, De Bonis M, et al. The double-orifice technique in mitral valve repair: a simple solution for complex problems. J Thorac Cardiovasc Surg 2001; 122: 674–81.
8. Gillinov AM, Cosgrove DM, Lytle BW, et al. Reoperation for failure of mitral valve repair. J Thorac Cardiovasc Surg 1997; 113: 467–73; discussion 73–5.
9. Ladich E, Michaels MB, Jones RM, et al. Pathological healing response of explanted MitraClip® devices. Circulation 2011; 123: 1418–27.
10. Luk A, Butany J, Ahn E, et al. Mitral repair with the evalve MitraClip® device: histopathologic findings in the porcine model. Cardiovasc Pathol 2009; 18: 279–85.

11. Privitera S, Butany J, Cusimano RJ, et al. Images in cardiovascular medicine. alfieri mitral valve repair: clinical outcome and pathology. Circulation 2002; 106: e173–4.

12. Verma S, Mesana TG. Mitral-valve repair for mitral-valve prolapse. N Engl J Med 2009; 361: 2261–9.

13. Rogers JH, Yeo KK, Carroll JD, et al. Late surgical mitral valve repair after percutaneous repair with the MitraClip® system. J Card Surg 2009; 24: 677–81.

14. Vitale N, Renzulli A, Agozzino L, et al. Obstruction of mechanical mitral prostheses: analysis of pathologic findings. Ann Thorac Surg 1997; 63: 1101–6.

15. Siddiqui RF, Abraham JR, Butany J. Bioprosthetic heart valves: modes of failure. Histopathology 2009; 55: 135–44.

16. Luk A, Jegatheeswaran A, David TE, et al. Redo mitral valve surgery: morphological features. Cardiovasc Pathol 2008; 17: 309–17.

17. Virmani R, Farb A. Pathology of in-stent restenosis. Curr Opin Lipidol 1999; 10: 499–506.

18. Butany J, Collins MJ, Nair V, et al. Morphological findings in explanted toronto stentless porcine valves. Cardiovasc Pathol 2006; 15: 41–8.

19. Bisoi AK, Rajesh MR, Talwar S, et al. Mitral stenosis after duran ring annuloplasty for non-rheumatic mitral regurgitation a foreign body response? Heart Lung Circ 2006; 15: 189–90.

20. Ibrahim MF, David TE. Mitral stenosis after mitral valve repair for non-rheumatic mitral regurgitation. Ann Thorac Surg 2002; 73: 34–6.

21. Herrmann HC, Rohatgi S, Wasserman HS, et al. Mitral valve hemodynamic effects of percutaneous edge-to-edge repair with the MitraClip® device for mitral regurgitation. Catheter Cardiovasc Interv 2006; 68: 821–8.

22. Jamieson WR, Munro AI, Miyagishima RT, et al. Carpentier-edwards standard porcine bioprosthesis: clinical performance to seventeen years. Ann Thorac Surg 1995; 60: 999–1006; discussion 7.

23. Vongpatanasin W, Hillis LD, Lange RA. Prosthetic heart valves. N Engl J Med 1996; 335: 407–16.

24. Lawrie GM. Mitral valve repair vs replacement. current recommendations and long-term results. Cardiol Clin 1998; 16: 437–48.

24 Future directions in percutaneous mitral therapy
Ted Feldman and Frederick St. Goar

This book has described the development and utilization of percutaneous leaflet repair for mitral regurgitation (MR) using the MitraClip®. Several other approaches to percutaneous mitral repair are in various stages of development. In fact, at the time of this writing, one of these devices, Carillon from the Cardiac Dimensions, has already received CE approval for use in Europe.

As the field of percutaneous therapy for mitral repair advances, the greatest level of interest is in the development of devices for annuloplasty. Annuloplasty is used in virtually every surgical mitral valve repair (1,2). Leaflet repair including surgical edge-to-edge repair is most often practiced in conjunction with annuloplasty using implantation of a ring on the atrial side of the mitral annulus, to diminish the annular circumference, facilitate leaflet coaptation, and in some cases restore the geometry of the saddle shape of the mitral valve (3,4).

In addition to methods for percutaneous annuloplasty, several other surgical therapies are being adapted as catheter-based therapies. These other approaches include replacement of ruptured chordae tendineae (5) and left ventricular (LV) reshaping (6,7).

As therapy for MR develops in the future, the greatest challenge is restoration of LV geometry, as LV dysfunction is the root cause of functional MR. Historically, annuloplasty has been used to treat these patients, but with limited success. Annuloplasty may reduce the degree functional MR, but does not address the fundamental problem of LV chamber dilatation or deformity. A percutaneous approach to LV geometric restoration will thus be highly attractive.

We will review the current status of catheter-based approaches to indirect and direct annuloplasty, chordal replacement, and LV geometric remodeling.

INDIRECT ANNULOPLASTY
Annuloplasty approaches have included indirect and direct methods. For indirect annuloplasty, the coronary sinus has been employed. The coronary sinus encircles almost two-thirds of the mitral annulus, including the posterior mitral leaflet on the atrial side of the annulus. It is thus possible to implant a device in the coronary sinus that applies constraining forces to the mitral annulus with resultant diminution of the mitral annular circumference (8,9). Early animal studies have demonstrated that coronary sinus devices can reduce annular circumference in models of MR using pacing-mediated heart failure models (10,11). Several methods for coronary sinus annuloplasty have developed. All of them place a device that applies tension on the mitral annulus via the coronary sinus. This approach is especially appealing because of the simplicity of access to the coronary sinus.

The CARILLON mitral contour system (Cardiac Dimensions, Kirkland, Washington, USA) has the largest experience in humans (12). This device is a nitinol wire form that has been engineered to have distal and proximal anchors connected by a bridge element (Fig. 24.1). After jugular puncture, a 9-French guiding catheter is placed into the coronary sinus. The distal anchor is released first, and using the guide catheter, tension is pulled from the jugular to place a constricting force on the coronary sinus. The guide catheter is then withdrawn further to expose and release the proximal or coronary sinus ostium anchor. This anchor maintains the constricting force placed on the bridge by the guide catheter pullback. The first generation of this device did not anchor adequately. Re-engineering was easily accomplished and several patients were treated. The early findings with this device demonstrated its ability to reduce MR significantly, with improved LV volumes and dimensions. Clinical measures such as the six-minute walk test and New York Heart Association functional class were improved as well.

Several patients treated with the second-generation device experienced fracture of the wire form at one of the anchor points. Fractures were noticed on follow-up radiographs. Importantly, this did not result in clinical events. Interestingly, the fractures did not affect the efficacy of MR reduction. Further engineering improvements have resulted in a more robust device. In fact, bench testing was able to reproduce the wire fracture in the second-generation device, and the third generation of the Carillon does not fracture with this bench model. This latest-generation device has now received CE approval for use in Europe. A 50-patient trial has recently been reported (12).

Several other coronary sinus implant devices have come and gone. A system that employed two self-expanding stents, one in the anterior interventricular vein and one in the coronary sinus os, connected by a bridge element, was plagued by wire fracture (13). The occurrence of nitinol wire fracture in both this device and the Carillon illustrates the complex forces that a coronary sinus device is subjected to. While there is a long history of use of pacing leads in the coronary sinus without wire fracture complications, the rigid devices needed to place a constricting force on the mitral annulus appear to suffer from complex torsional forces. This has been one of the unanticipated challenges of working in the coronary sinus to accomplish annuloplasty. Another limitation is the ability to access and deliver the device into the coronary sinus, which has been largely overcome as experience with this approach has accumulated.

Another challenge with coronary sinus annuloplasty results from the fact that the coronary sinus crosses over the circumflex coronary artery in more than half of patients.

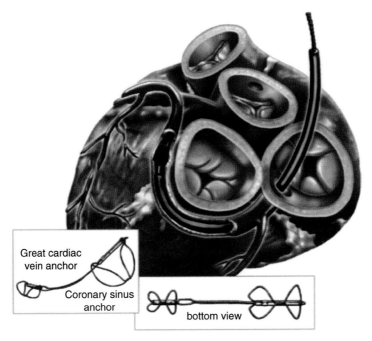

Figure 24.1 Coronary sinus annuloplasty: the cardiac dimensions carillon device. The guide catheter is introduced through the jugular venous access. The device is delivered in the distal coronary sinus, and then the guide catheter is pulled back to release the device in the coronary sinus ostium. The insets show the wire form, made of nitinol wire. Figure illustration by Craig Skaggs. Source: Courtesy of Feldman T, Cilingiroglu M. Percutaneous leaflet repair and annuloplasty for mitral regurgitation. J Am Coll Cardiol 2011; 57: 529–37.

Experience with the Carillon device has shown that this limits therapy in about 15–20% of patients. Coronary angiography during device implantation is necessary to assess the potential for coronary constriction at the time of device implantation.

Despite the indirect nature of coronary sinus annuloplasty, it is highly attractive because of the simplicity of the approach. Simple venous access is all that is required, so that the caliber of the device is less concerning than for transarterial approaches. A transvenous implant approach makes the procedure applicable to a potentially large population of patients with a wide level of physician operator experience.

DIRECT ANNULOPLASTY

Direct annuloplasty approaches involve implantation of a device directly into the mitral annulus. This might overcome some of the important limitations of the indirect coronary sinus approach, in particular circumflex coronary artery compression. Direct annuloplasty more closely mimics surgical annuloplasty ring implantation.

The anatomic approach to direct annuloplasty is clearly more challenging than the indirect coronary sinus approach. Direct annuloplasty is accomplished using retrograde transarterial access (14). A guide catheter is placed retrograde across the aortic valve and manipulated within the left ventricle to reach the space between the posterior mitral leaflet and the LV wall, adjacent to

the mitral annulus. There are two device approaches under development that utilize this direct transaortic-left ventricular route. Although these devices use the same route for access to the mitral annulus, each of them is unique.

The Mitralign® system (Mitralign, Inc., Tewksbury, Massachusetts, USA) places the guide catheter in the middle scallop of the posterior mitral leaflet via retrograde access (Fig. 24.2). Radiofrequency wires are utilized to go through the mitral annulus and deliver the wires to the left atrial side of the annulus. A pair of pledgets are passed over the wires as anchors and connected with a drawstring. Two pairs of pledgets are placed, one medial and one lateral. Tension on the drawstring brings the pledgets of each pair closer together to effect shortening of the mitral circumference. This system employs two pairs of pledgets on either side of the mitral annulus adjacent to the middle scallop. The mitral annulus circumference can be shortened between 1 and 3 cm with this method. This system has been utilized in preclinical and early human experiences. Evaluation of clinical outcomes achievable with this system will require additional experience.

The second direct annuloplasty system is the Accucinch® device (Guided Delivery Systems, Santa Clara, California, USA) (Fig. 24.3). Access to the annulus is achieved in a similar manner as with Mitralign. A specially designed delivery catheter is passed under the posterior leaflet, along the annulus. Through a series of evenly spaced openings in the deliver

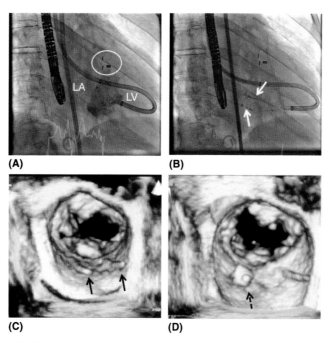

Figure 24.2 Direct annuloplasty. The Mitralign System. (**A**) A guide catheter has been passed retrograde from the aorta into the left ventricle. The catheter has a preformed curve that places the distal tip between the papillary muscles and under the midpart of the posterior mitral annulus. (**B**) A "bident" has been passed through the guide catheter and two wires placed through the mitral annulus from the left ventricular (LV) side to the left atrial (LA) side, as shown by the arrows. (**C**) A three-dimensional echocardiographic image from the "surgeon's view", or from the left atrial side looking down at the mitral valve, shows the two wires through the annulus in the LA cavity, shown by the black arrows. (**D**) The arrow points at a pledget that has been used to anchor one of the two wires. After a second pledget is placed on the second LA wire the pledgets can be drawn together to reduce the circumference of the mitral annulus. A second pair of pledgets can be used to further diminish the mitral annular circumference.

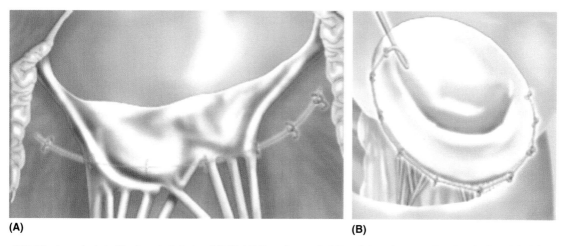

Figure 24.3 Direct annuloplasty. The Accucinch device of Guided Delivery Systems is delivered through retrograde catheterization of the left ventricle. (Left) Anchors are placed in the posterior mitral annulus and (Right) connected with a "drawstring" to cinch the annular circumference. Figure illustration by Craig Skaggs. Source: Courtesy of Feldman T, Cilingiroglu M. Percutaneous leaflet repair and annuloplasty for mitral regurgitation. J Am Coll Cardiol 2011; 57: 529–37.

catheter, as many as 12 nitinol anchors can be placed in the annulus. These anchors are connected with a cord or tether. Tension on the tether draws the anchors together with reduction of the mitral circumference, after which an anchor fixes the tension on the tether. This device has been implanted surgically and demonstrated feasibility in early human experience. A percutaneous method has been employed in a small number of patients as well.

Direct annuloplasty has the advantage of alleviating the potential for coronary artery compression. The guide catheters for these systems are larger than for coronary angioplasty and stenting, and thus have the risk for arterial injury and bleeding compared with a transvenous coronary sinus approach. The indirect coronary sinus approach places forces above the true annulus, on the atrial side of the annulus, while the direct devices do not have this issue and more closely mimic the surgical approach.

Yet another approach to direct annuloplasty utilizes an energy source to shrink the collagen in the mitral annuls. There are two companies with devices in this category. Quantum Cor has a ring electrode that is placed on the left atrial side of the annulus to deliver radiofrequency energy to the annulus (15). Preclinical and cadaver heart studies have shown that the annular circumference can be decreased significantly, without apparent damage to adjacent tissue, without recoil or loss of effect over a period of several months. A second energy-based technology, ReCor Medical, used a balloon centered in the mitral annulus to deliver energy and this technology is no longer developed.

LEFT VENTRICULAR REMODELING WITH ANNULAR COMPRESSION

For most patients with functional MR, the primary problem is abnormal LV function. Patients with ischemic functional MR have dilatation of the chamber associated with low ejection fraction and distortion of the chamber geometry. Papillary muscle disorientation contributes significantly to MR. Tethering of the chordae displaces the leaflets. Thus, therapies directed only at correcting the leaflet coaptation abnormality, such as annuloplasty, have no impact on the LV component of the MR. The results of surgical annuloplasty have been at best mixed in this population of patients with functional ischemic MR. Some attempts at LV remodeling therapies such as "stocking cap" devices to constrain the left ventricle have not yet been successful.

A novel therapy for surgical LV remodeling was developed and tested in a randomized trial. The Coapsys system (Myocor, Inc., Maple Grove, Minnesota, USA) is a ventricular reshaping device that simultaneously compresses the mitral annulus and subvalvular apparatus to decrease functional MR. The change in LV geometry decreases LV wall stress and creates favorable ventricular remodeling (6,7).

The Coapsys system consists of extracardiac epicardial pads connected by a flexible transventricular chord that pass through the LV chamber. The posterior pad compresses both the mitral annulus and papillary muscle levels. The device was placed intraoperatively during a coronary artery bypass graft surgery via a close heart, off pump, beating-heart approach. The invasiveness of this approach compared with conventional surgery was significantly less, since the left atrium did not have to be opened as it is for annuloplasty. An initial feasibility study, RESTOR-MV (Randomized Evaluation of Surgical Treatment for Off-pump Repair of the Mitral Valve) was a prospective, randomized, multicenter trial. The Coapsys system was compared with standard-of-care control in patients with functional MR undergoing coronary artery bypass graft surgery. The patients were randomized one to one. Ultimately, 235 patients were assessed for eligibility and 165 were randomized.

An intention-to-treat analysis of all patients randomized showed a survival advantage for Coapsys treatment (6). The mean follow-up interval was 28.3 months. There was a two-year survival rate of 87% for the Coapsys device compared with 77% for control patients treated with conventional annuloplasty and bypass (P = 0.038). At two years, 18 deaths had occurred in the control arm and 10 in the treatment arm. As-treated analysis confirmed the advantage in overall survival at two years for the Coapsys group, 89% versus 76% in the control group (P = 0.02). Control and Coapsys both produced decreases in LV end-diastolic dimension and MR at two years (p < 0.001); Coapsys provided a greater decrease in LV end-diastolic dimension (p = 0.021). Control had lower MR grades during follow-up (p = 0.01), but despite this Coapsys showed a survival advantage as noted above. Complication-free survival (including death, stroke, myocardial infarction, and valve reoperation) was significantly greater with Coapsys at two years (85% vs. 71%) p = 0.019).

There was a significantly greater decrease in LV chamber dimensions in the Coapsys group. Coapsys patients started with an average resting transventricular chordal length of 8.6 cm, which was shortened to 6.4 cm with the transventricular chord. The percentage of patients with New York Heart Association functional class improvement of I or more grades also showed an advantage for the Coapsys group.

This study is remarkable in that Coapsys is the first mechanical therapy for MR that resulted in immediate successful and favorable LV remodeling, and more importantly was associated with a survival advantage. On the basis of intention-to-treat analyses, the RESTOR-MV trial found that patients with FMR who required revascularization and were treated with ventricular reshaping rather than the standard surgical approach had hazard ratios of less than one-half for both mortality and major adverse outcomes. This trial validates the concept of the ventricular reshaping strategy in this subset of patients with heart failure.

A percutaneous method to perform this procedure was developed and two patients were treated (7). To accomplish this via catheter therapy, access to the pericardium is necessary. A dry pericardial tap was performed using a unique needle and 0.018-inch wire system. The wire was delivered across the anterior surface of the right ventricle and after a series of dilators were passed, a large subxiphoid pericardial introducer sheath was placed. A catheter was placed both on the anterior left ventricular surface at the junction of the right and left ventricles, and the posterior surface of the left ventricle adjacent to the circumflex, usually between the first and second obtuse marginal branches. Intracardiac echocardiographic catheters were used for "sighting" to line up the locations on the anterior and posterior myocardial surfaces. A nitinol wire was passed through one sighting catheter and a snare through the other to grab the wire and pull it all the way through the LV chamber. This established a wire system to place pads on the anterior and posterior surfaces with a tether traversing the left ventricular chamber between them. Ultimately, the pads were tensioned to diminish the LV chamber size and compress the mitral orifice. Tension could be increased on the pads until MR was too diminished or disappeared. Coronary arteriography was used during the placement of the pad to be sure that coronary impingement was not created.

Unfortunately, the company lost funding due to the financial crisis in 2008 and there has been no further development. Hopefully, some version of this approach will be brought back into investigation.

Ultimately, a therapy like Coapsys that reduces MR and also reshapes the left ventricle may provide the best solution for functional ischemic MR, since early work with this approach has been the only therapy to associate reduced MR with LV geometric remodeling with a resultant mortality improvement.

PERCUTANEOUS CHORDAL REPLACEMENT

Some research is being done to accomplish replacement of the chordae tendineae (5). Surgical transapical beating-heart implantation of neo-chordae using a novel device remains experimental with most of the work still in the preclinical phase. The NeoChord device is used to grasp the mitral leaflets and implant polytetrafluoroethylene sutures. This can be accomplished in the animal model without tearing of leaflets. This will hopefully be developed into a percutaneous procedure, but there are many hurdles, including the development of catheter-based apical access and repair systems.

PERCUTANEOUS MITRAL VALVE REPLACEMENT

Several approaches to percutaneous mitral valve replacement therapy are being developed. The challenges to accomplish this procedure successfully are very different from those for percutaneous aortic valve replacement.

In the situation of aortic stenosis, the calcific deposits in the native leaflets provide anchoring for the stent valve system. This is not the case for a mitral annulus and MR and some method to anchor the valve is necessary. Among those being investigated is the use of ridges or cuffs on either side of the annulus to help with fixation, or the modular use of an annuloplasty like ring to serve as the anchor for the stent valve system.

Percutaneous mitral valve replacement is highly attractive because it is clearly going to be completely effective for reducing MR. The great limitation of this approach is the

same problem faced with many surgical therapies for MR in patients with LV dysfunction and the therapy does not address in any way the problem of LV dysfunction and chamber distortion.

IMPROVEMENT OF THE MITRACLIP®

As described in an earlier chapter the effective clinical applicability of the MitraClip® goes well beyond what the inventors of this technology originally imagined. The edge-to-edge repair was originally described by Alfieri and his colleagues in the surgical community as only applicable in patients suffering from degenerative mitral insufficiency. It was thus assumed these would be the patients in whom the MitraClip® would be most effective. The data from the EVEREST trials support this application in selected patients, but expanded clinical experience with the MitraClip® has demonstrated that it can also be effectively utilized in patient's suffering from functional MR, a population who presently are not well served by either medical therapy or surgical intervention. The MitraClip® thus appears to be an effective therapy for both degenerative and functional mitral pathologies.

At present the extent of pathology for which the MitraClip® is being considered as a therapeutic alternative is limited. The anatomic inclusion criteria for the EVEREST and REALISM trials were narrow. As previously described, pathology was limited to the A2–P2 leaflet location. In the degenerative MR population, the flail gap was required to be less than 10 mm and the flail width less than 15 mm. In the functional population, leaflet apposition had to be measured at greater than 2 mm and the point of apposition could not be greater than 11 mm below the mitral annulus. This led to a large proportion of the patients presented for consideration for enrollment in the U.S. trials by informed echocardiographers to be turned down based on anatomic exclusion criteria. While our European colleagues have demonstrated that the MitraClip® can be effectively utilized in a patient population with a broader range of pathologies there are some potential design improvements which could broaden its range of effective. The two improvements that have been proposed are redesigning the gripper deployment system and lengthening the clip arms. As described in chapter 7, the present gripper design requires that leaflet tissue be stabilized simultaneously and the grippers are then dropped down together on the stabilized tissue. During the course of grasping it is not uncommon to capture only one of the leaflets frequently requiring multiple grasp attempts to eventually catch both leaflets. Because the gripper design has the ability to deploy one gripper at a time and thus grasp leaflets independently, the problem of missing one or the other leaflet should become less common. It will also facilitate pulling together leaflets which initially have limited tissue apposition, that is, situations with an oversized annulus or tethered leaflets. The iteration of independent gripper deployment will likely further demonstrate that the MitraClip® performs not simply an edge-to-edge repair but, as our surgical colleagues have taught us, a true cinching annuloplasty.

In a nondiseased mitral valve, the normal length of leaflet tissue apposition during systolic closure is 6–8 mm, which is the present length of the grasping portion of the MitraClip® arms (8 mm). In the patient population suffering from degenerative mitral pathology, with flail leaflets and/or leaflet tissue redundancy an increased length of leaflet to leaflet apposition is frequently required to reestablish functional coaptation. The MitraClip® in its present length is thus limited in its ability to deal with these pathologies. A next-generation design with longer grasping arms will certainly facilitate effective use in a broader range of pathologies.

CONCLUSION

In summary, the heterogeneous valve pathologies leading to MR and the inherent complexity of the mitral valve apparatus strongly supports the need for developing a variety of catheter-based therapeutic options. The addition of annuloplasty systems, methods for LV reshaping, and percutaneous mitral replacement technologies, as well as improvements in the technology and technique of the present MitraClip®, will lead to a dramatic increase in beneficial therapeutic options for patients suffering from MR.

REFERENCES

 1. Wu AH, Aaronson KD, Bolling SF, et al. Impact of mitral valve annuloplasty on mortality risk in patients with mitral regurgitation and left ventricular systolic dysfunction. J Am Coll Cardiol 2005; 45: 381–7.
 2. Mihaljevic T, Lam BK, Rajeswaran J, et al. Impact of mitral valve annuloplasty combined with revascularization in patients with functional ischemic mitral regurgitation. J Am Coll Cardiol 2007; 49: 2191–201.
 3. Alfieri O, Maisano F, De Bonis M, et al. The double-orifice technique in mitral valve repair: a simple solution for complex problems. J Thorac Cardiovasc Surg 2001; 122: 674–81.
 4. Maisano F, Viganò G, Blasio A, et al. Surgical isolated edge-to-edge mitral valve repair without annuloplasty: clinical proof of the principle for an endovascular approach. EuroIntervention 2006; 2: 181–6.
 5. Seeburger J, Leontjev S, Neumuth M, et al. Trans-apical beating-heart implantation of neo-chordae to mitral valve leaflets: results of an acute animal study. Eur J Cardiothorac Surg 2012; 41: 173–6.
 6. Grossi E, Woo Y, Schwartz C, et al. Comparison of coapsys annuloplasty and internal reduction mitral annuloplasty in the randomized treatment of functional ischemic mitral regurgitation: impact on the left ventricle. J Thorac Cardiovasc Surg 2006; 131: 1095–8.
 7. Pedersen WR, Block PC, Feldman TE. The icoapsys repair system for the percutaneous treatment of functional mitral insufficiency. EuroIntervention 2006; 1(Suppl A): A44–8.
 8. Choure A, Garcia M, Hesse B, et al. In vivo analysis of the anatomical relationship of coronary sinus to mitral annulus and left circumflex coronary artery using cardiac multidetector computed tomography: implications for percutaneous coronary sinus mitral annuloplasty. J Am Coll Cardiol 2006; 48: 1938–45.
 9. Tops L, Van de Veire N, Schuijf J, et al. Noninvasive evaluation of coronary sinus anatomy and its relation to the mitral valve annulus: implications for percutaneous mitral annuloplasty. Circulation 2007; 115: 1426–32.
10. Byrne MJ, Kaye DM, Mathis M, et al. Percutaneous mitral annular reduction provides continued benefit in an ovine model of dilated cardiomyopathy. Circulation 2004; 110: 3088–92.
11. Maniu CV, Patel JB, Reuter DG, et al. Acute and chronic reduction of functional mitral regurgitation in experimental heart failure by percutaneous mitral annuloplasty. J Am Coll Cardiol 2004; 44: 1652–61.
12. Schofer J, Siminiak T, Haude M, et al. Percutaneous mitral annuloplasty for functional mitral regurgitation: results of the amadeus trial. Circulation 2009; 120: 326–33.
13. Webb JG, Harnek J, Munt BI, et al. Percutaneous transvenous mitral annuloplasty; initial human experience with device implantation in the coronary sinus. Circulation 2006; 113: 851–5.
14. Nagy ZL, Peterffy A. Mitral annuloplasty with a suture technique. Eur J Cardiothorac Surg 2000; 18: 739–41.
15. Heuser RR, Witzel T, Dickens D, Takeda PA. Percutaneous treatment for mitral regurgitation: the quantumcor system. J Interv Cardiol 2008; 21: 178–82.

Index